Modern Microtia Reconstruction

John F. Reinisch, MD • Youssef Tahiri, MD
Editors

Modern Microtia Reconstruction

Art, Science, and New Clinical Techniques

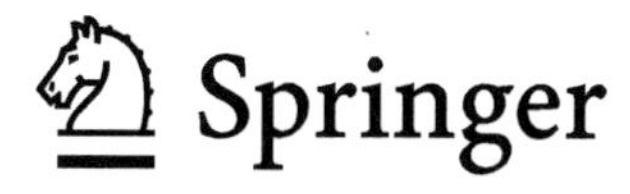

Editors
John F. Reinisch, MD, FACS
Keck School of Medicine
University of Souther California
Los Angeles, CA
USA

Craniofacial and Pediatric
Plastic Surgery
Cedars Sinai Medical Center
Los Angeles, CA
USA

Youssef Tahiri, MD, MSc, FRCSC,
FACS, FAAP
Plastic and Reconstructive Surgery
Cedars-Sinai Medical Center
Los Angeles, CA
USA

Additional material to this book can be downloaded from https://link.springer.com/book/10.1007/978-3-030-16387-7

ISBN 978-3-030-16389-1 ISBN 978-3-030-16387-7 (eBook)
https://doi.org/10.1007/978-3-030-16387-7

© Springer Nature Switzerland AG 2019
This work is subject to copyright. All rights are reserved by the Publisher, whether the whole or part of the material is concerned, specifically the rights of translation, reprinting, reuse of illustrations, recitation, broadcasting, reproduction on microfilms or in any other physical way, and transmission or information storage and retrieval, electronic adaptation, computer software, or by similar or dissimilar methodology now known or hereafter developed.
The use of general descriptive names, registered names, trademarks, service marks, etc. in this publication does not imply, even in the absence of a specific statement, that such names are exempt from the relevant protective laws and regulations and therefore free for general use.
The publisher, the authors, and the editors are safe to assume that the advice and information in this book are believed to be true and accurate at the date of publication. Neither the publisher nor the authors or the editors give a warranty, expressed or implied, with respect to the material contained herein or for any errors or omissions that may have been made. The publisher remains neutral with regard to jurisdictional claims in published maps and institutional affiliations.

This Springer imprint is published by the registered company Springer Nature Switzerland AG
The registered company address is: Gewerbestrasse 11, 6330 Cham, Switzerland

To our microtia patients, who taught us the art of ear reconstruction.

John and Youssef

First Preface: Ear Reconstruction in the Twenty-First Century

Personal History

In 1950, a month after my sixth birthday, my father died at age 42. He was an obstetrician whose early death occurred in the exact middle of the twentieth century. Surgical practice has changed markedly in the last 70 years. I often wonder what my father would think if he could see today's operating suite.

Indirectly, his death gave me a connection to ear reconstruction. Growing up in a fatherless home with two younger sisters, my mother felt that I needed male influence in my life and enrolled me in a boy's boarding school in the eighth grade. The education I obtained was superior to that in my local high school and facilitated my early acceptance to Dartmouth College in Hanover, New Hampshire.

Before my graduation from high school, I saw a dilapidated 1931 Model A Ford in a classmate's garage. I bought the car for $150. That car became my obsession. I spent the next two summers meticulously restoring the Ford to its original condition (Fig. 1). I drove the Model A the 100 miles from my home to Hanover at the beginning of my sophomore year.

As I was polishing my car outside my dormitory, an older man on a bicycle, possibly a college professor, stopped to admire my car (Fig. 2). He wore a tweed jacket and had a thin briefcase in the front basket. He told me that he owned a similar Ford when he was younger. Over the next year, we would wave and smile in passing, acknowledging our car bonding experience.

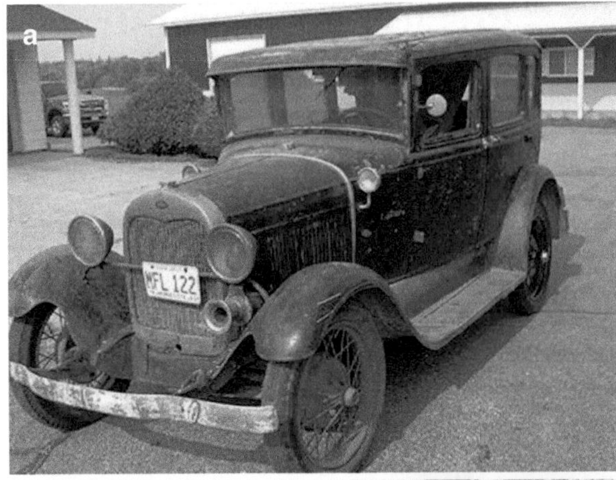

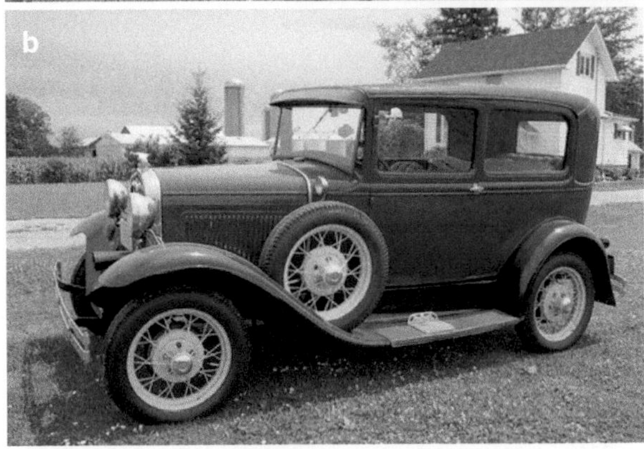

Fig. 1 Model A Ford before (**a**) and after (**b**) restoration

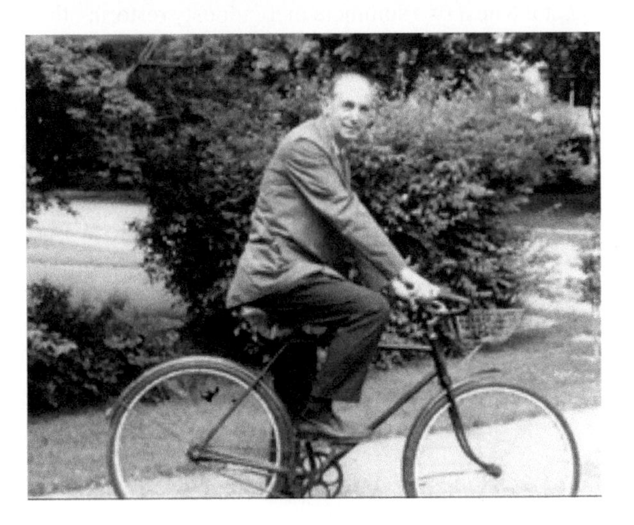

Fig. 2 Older man on a bicycle admiring the restored car

I was a premed student and worked one night a week at the local hospital as a blood draw technician. One night, I was paged to the emergency room where a patient needed to have labs drawn. I was surprised to see the "college professor" repairing a facial laceration on a patient in the next bay. I watched the repair and learned that the man who had stopped his bike to admire my car was a plastic surgeon named Dr. Radford Tanzer. He was the first plastic surgeon I had ever met. Years later, when I decided to do a plastic surgery residency, I learned that Radford Tanzer was considered the father of ear reconstruction.

Ear Reconstruction in the Nineteenth and Twentieth Centuries

In the 1950s, Dr. Tanzer operated on two boys with microtia using their own costal cartilage as the framework. In 1958, he presented the two completed cases at the ASPS meeting in Chicago and received a standing ovation. His seminal paper was published in the *Plastic and Reconstructive Surgery (PRS)* journal in January 1959.

Prior to Tanzer's paper, there was no reliable method for total ear reconstruction. A variety of materials for structural support (bone, ivory, silver wire, dental rubber, steel, and maternal costal and cadaver ear and costal cartilage) have been used. Schmieden (1908) was the first to use costal cartilage placed under remote chest or arm skin prior to waltzing the skin and cartilage to the head. In the nineteenth and early twentieth centuries, well-known surgeons (Dieffenback, Zeis, Fritze and Reich, Konig, Lexer, Beck, Davis, Gilles) discouraged ear reconstruction because of the poor results. Reconstruction was done by waltzing flaps from the arm, chest, supraclavicular region, and neck. Gilles, Esser and Esser, and Aufricht implanted carved cartilage in the mastoid area and are the early pioneers of ear reconstruction.

Tanzer's results were significantly better than prior attempts. His method of ear reconstruction became the worldwide paradigm for ear reconstruction. His basic method, modified by subsequent surgeons, is the gold standard that every reconstructive surgeon has been taught for the past 60 years.

When Tanzer's paper was published in 1959, the available implant materials and the social attitudes were different than they are now in the twenty-first century. The best available material for an ear was costal cartilage. Parents accepted a physician's recommendation with little question. Surgical options for ear reconstruction were limited. Although Tanzer advocated early ear reconstruction "in the preschool period" to address the "psychic trauma of a conspicuous deformity," subsequent surgeons have delayed intervention to obtain more cartilage for increased projection and to minimize secondary chest wall deformity. Biomaterials such as silicone, porous polyethylene, and cultured cartilage were not available. Patient's attitudes and knowledge were also very different. Today's ready access to medical information, greater awareness of childhood bullying, and parental expectation of shared decision-making with their surgeon would come decades after Tanzer's publication.

Ear Reconstruction in the Twenty-First Century

When one considers the revolutionary changes that have occurred in all surgical specialties, it is striking that thc most common method of ear reconstruction today is still very similar to the method described by Tanzer almost 60 years ago. Although today's rib cartilage reconstruction is safer and more efficient (fewer stages), the basic method of cartilage harvest, framework assembly with stainless steel wire, placement of the framework under the mastoid skin, and suction of the skin over the cartilage frame with a catheter has not changed significantly from Tanzer's original description.

Interestingly, the automobile that connected me to Dr. Tanzer holds an interesting evolutionary parallel. The majority of today's cars are basically refined versions of the automobile that Dr. Tanzer drove in the mid-1950s. Although today's models are certainly safer and more efficient, they are still based on the internal combustion engine that uses gasoline, pistons, and an exhaust. Today's automobile has evolved for over a century, yet it is still based on the technology used in the 1931 Model A Ford that prompted a chance meeting between Radford Tanzer and me in 1964.

In the twenty-first century, the automobile industry is undergoing a revolution, with the introduction of electric and fuel cell vehicles. Ear reconstruction is also undergoing a revolutionary change, with the increasing popularity of the porous polyethylene implant procedure (PPIP). This method is completely different from the traditional cartilage technique of reconstruction. The PPIP is not a simple substitution of a plastic implant for the autologous cartilage framework beneath the mastoid skin. The PPIP uses an alternative soft tissue coverage, which, together with the alloplastic implant, provides a markedly improved reconstructive experience for the patient. The implant permits early reconstruction without the discomfort or the potential chest deformity of a cartilage harvest. The large covering fascia permits sufficient projection of the ear framework to obviate the need for a second surgery. Together, the alloplastic framework and covering soft tissue allows ear reconstruction to be done as a single, outpatient surgery before a child begins school. Additionally, an aural atresia repair can be performed before or at the same time so that a true "total ear reconstruction" can be done in a single stage during the early critical period of brain development.

Transition to Newer Technology

While surgeons have been slow to adopt this newer PPIP method of ear reconstruction, parents easily see its advantages and increasingly seek this technique for their children.

Porous polyethylene ear reconstruction is analogous to this century's electric vehicles. Automobile manufacturers, recognizing the public's interest, are introducing more electric vehicles as they anticipate a gradual transition away from cars based on internal combustion technology. Companies that are slow to provide this alternative will lose market share.

Many surgeons, especially those who have invested years learning the rib cartilage technique, are resistant to change and still prefer last century's method of reconstruction. Some surgeons, attempting to improve projection of their cartilage framework, now use a postauricular or scalp fascia flap to cover wedges of cartilage or porous polyethylene. Using a combination of the old and the new, these surgeries have improved projection and, in my transportation metaphor, are analogous to today's hybrid cars. By incorporating traditional and newer technologies, hybrid cars are more efficient but are also heavier and more expensive. As battery technology improves and charging stations become more abundant, the transitional hybrid cars will disappear.

Both internal combustion and electric vehicles provide equally safe and reliable transportation. Similarly, in experienced hands, one can obtain excellent ear reconstructions outcomes with both the traditional cartilage method and the more recent porous polyethylene method of ear reconstruction.

Changing Social Attitudes

The transition away from vehicles based on last century's technology is a response to society's increasing interest in renewable, less polluting energy. In a similar sense, parent's attraction to alloplastic reconstruction is also related to changing societal attitudes. In the twenty-first century, society looks at deformity more holistically. The psychological impact, the loss of function, and the cosmetic appearance are considered together. Rather than focusing solely on the external deformity, we have become more aware of the presence and deleterious effects of teasing.

We also have becoming more cognizant of auditory processing, the early influence of hearing on brain maturation, and the lost opportunity when hearing restoration occurs after the critical periods of auditory development. PPE ear reconstruction appeals to parents because it allows for the early treatment of both the outer cosmetic deformity and functional conductive hearing loss better than the traditional cartilage method.

Future of Ear Reconstruction

While it is impossible to accurately foresee what ear reconstruction may be like further into the twenty-first century, it is clear that the material of the ear framework will change in the future. Neither hyaline rib cartilage nor PPE frameworks are adequate substitutes for the more supple fibrous cartilage structures found in the normal ear. While the rigidity of both rib and PPE can resist the early contractile forces of the covering soft tissue, they do not mimic the flexible structure of a

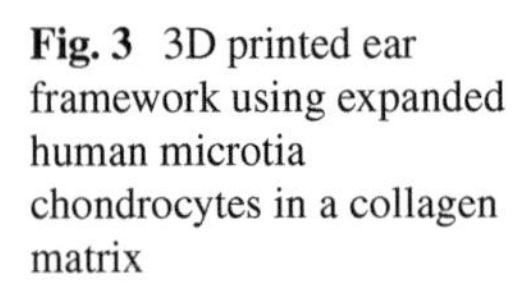

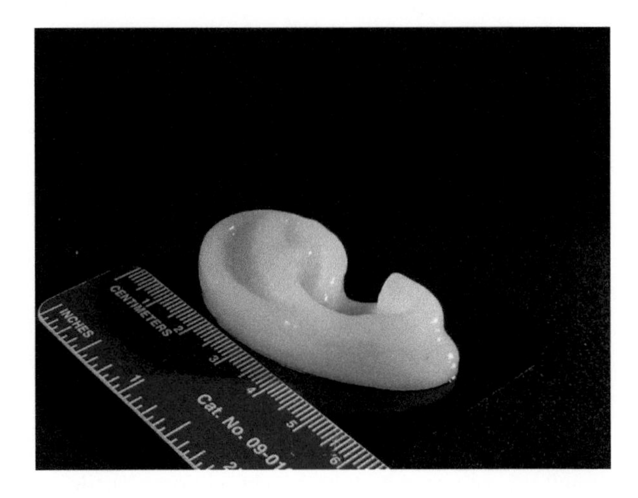

Fig. 3 3D printed ear framework using expanded human microtia chondrocytes in a collagen matrix

natural ear. Rib cartilage tends to calcify over time and often loses substance and shape. PPE may be better than costal cartilage at retaining its shape over time, but it is at greater risk of implant fracture and exposure.

Tissue engineering, the blending of biology and engineering, became a reality at the end of the last century. Because of its relatively simple structure and low metabolic requirements, cartilage was one of the first tissues studied. The use of ink-jet layering of biologic material has captured the imagination of scientists and very likely will produce a biologically active ear scaffold for ear reconstruction in the coming years. Harvested humane chondrocytes, which have been expanded and printed with collagen ink, have been shown to become normal-appearing fibrous cartilage when implanted in an immunologically altered animal model (Fig. 3).

In the next decade or two, an engineered framework, either from autologous chondrocytes or stem cells, will be developed that can maintain its shape and its flexibility over time. It will offer a significantly better option to the currently used ear frameworks.

Los Angeles, CA, USA John F. Reinisch, MD, FACS

Second Preface: Benefits of Connecting the Dots and Staying Hungry and Foolish

This preface is inspired by a commencement speech that Steve Jobs delivered in 2005 at Stanford University. In it, he spoke of "connecting the dots" and recommended that the graduates "stay hungry, stay foolish." I will address both of those points and how they inspired me as I reflect on my life and career.

Connecting the Dots

During his speech, Jobs stated, "You can't connect the dots looking forward; you can only connect them looking backwards." He explained how he was adopted, went to college 17 years later, dropped out because it was expensive and he did not see how it would benefit him, sat in on a calligraphy class, started Apple, designed the first Apple computer using the typography and spacing knowledge he gained in the calligraphy class, and ended up getting fired from Apple. He explained that he was devastated after getting fired from Apple and that "The only thing that kept [him] going was that he loved what he did." He explained that ultimately, "Getting fired from Apple was the best thing that could have ever happened to [him]. The heaviness of being successful was replaced by the lightness of being a beginner again, less sure about everything. It freed [him] to enter one of the most creative periods of [his] life." Following this, he started Next and Pixar, which became the most successful animation studio in the world. After Apple purchased Next, Jobs returned to work for Apple.

Jobs' speech resonates with me because, like Jobs, as I reflect on my life, it is evident how each event in my life has successively lead to the next. As a young boy growing up in Casablanca, Morocco, I worked extremely hard in school to become fluent in Mathematics and Science. My dedication to school enabled me to move to Montreal, Canada, where I attended a competitive high school and college programs. I ultimately was accepted into McGill University School of Medicine. My continued dedication to my studies allowed me to gain acceptance into McGill

University's Plastic Surgery Residency Program during which I also earned a Master of Experimental Surgery Degree.

After this, I completed a craniofacial fellowship at the University of Pennsylvania. As with Jobs when he founded Pixar, my time at the University of Pennsylvania was both creative and productive because I was surrounded by incredible mentors. During that year, in 2014, I presented on "*A Comparative Analysis of Complications Associated with Intracranial Procedures in 746 Patients with Nonsyndromic Single Suture Craniosynostosis*" at the American Association of Plastic Surgeons Meeting, in Miami. Immediately following my presentation, Dr. John F. Reinisch presented on "*Porous Polyethylene Ear Reconstruction for Microtia.*" After our respective presentations, I introduced myself to Dr. Reinisch and expressed an interest in visiting him in Los Angeles to observe his technique. He agreed to host me.

At the end of my fellowship, I hesitated between returning to Montreal and accepting a position at McGill University, where my friends and family were located, and accepting a position at Indiana University's Riley Hospital for Children. The immediate demand for my services coupled with the fact that I would inherit both Dr. Robert J. Havlik and Dr. Roberto Flores' practices, both of whom had accepted positions at alternate universities, leads me to accept the position at Indiana University. During my first year in practice, I traveled to Los Angeles to observe Dr. Reinisch perform a porous polyethylene ear reconstruction (Fig. 1). After returning to Indianapolis, I began performing porous polyethylene ear reconstructions.

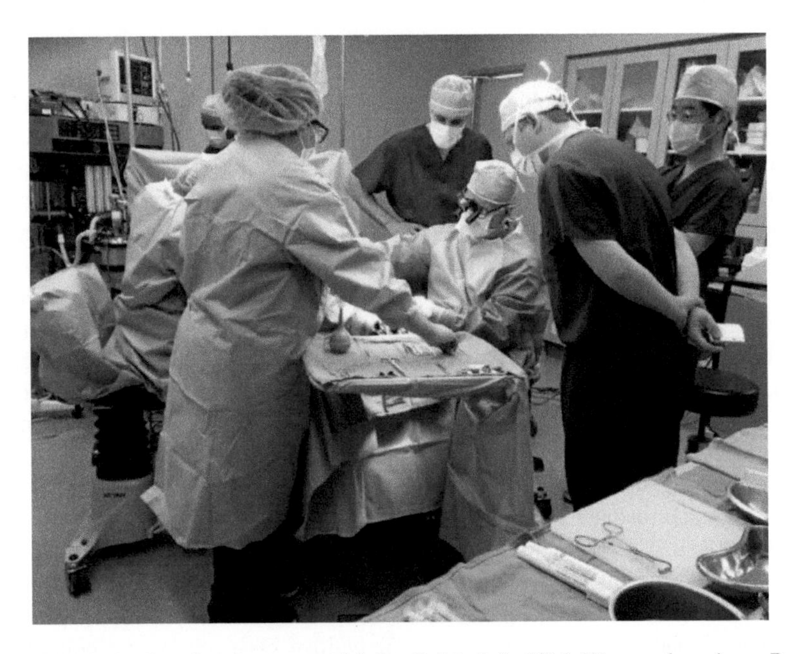

Fig. 1 This is the first time I came to visit Dr. Reinisch in 2014. We are observing a Porous Polyethylene Ear reconstruction. Dr. Reinisch is operating. I am right behind him, on his right side. My fellow at that time, Dr. Travis Greathouse, is on his left. Dr. Reinisch had a third observer (in the back) from South Korea

I maintained contact with Dr. Reinisch and enjoyed lunch with him and his wife Nancy in 2015 after I presented on "*Mandibular Distraction Osteogenesis in the Very Small with Robin Sequence: Is It Safe?*" at the American Association of Plastic Surgeons Meeting, in Scottsdale, Arizona. Shortly thereafter, I received a phone call from Dr. Reinisch asking me if I was interested in joining his practice. After visiting Los Angeles a few more times and joining Dr. Reinisch in China for a patient conference, I decided to join his practice.

As I reflect on the events that have occurred throughout my life, it is evident how each event paved the way for the next. As a young child in Casablanca, I could not have connected the dots looking forward. However, as an ear reconstruction specialist and craniofacial surgeon living in Los Angeles, I can connect the dots looking backward.

Stay Hungry, Stay Foolish

In his speech, Jobs told the graduates "Stay hungry, stay foolish." He stated, "Have the courage to follow your heart and intuition, they somehow already know what you truly want to become."

During medical school and residency, I knew I was passionate about pediatric plastic and craniofacial surgery. Specifically, I had fallen in love with craniofacial surgery. I was drawn to cranial distraction, craniosynostosis surgery, mandibular distraction, and cleft lip and palate. My interest in craniofacial surgery continued to increase during my first few years of practice as I obtained great functional and cosmetic outcomes.

However, I followed my heart and intuition when I joined Dr. Reinisch's practice. I knew that I would no longer spend the majority of my time and energy performing the craniofacial surgeries that I had grown to love but would instead spend my time and energy perfecting the art of ear reconstruction. My hunger to perfect the surgery drove me to observe and assist Dr. Reinisch in performing many ear reconstructions. I also began performing many ear reconstructions on my own. The more I performed these, the better my technique and results became, and the more I loved the surgery. Currently, Currently I performed approximately 100 ear reconstruction per year. During each surgery, I extensively analyze the various surgical steps that directly affect cosmetic details to ensure the best outcomes for my patients.

Dr. Reinisch and I wrote this book to share our passion for ear reconstruction with you and to provide you with the most comprehensive and up-to-date information about modern microtia surgery. We hope you enjoy this book!

Los Angeles, CA, USA Youssef Tahiri, MD, MSc, FRCSC, FACS, FAAP

Contents

Contributors

Scott Bartlett, MD Division of Plastic and Reconstructive Surgery, University of Pennsylvania and The Children's Hospital of Philadelphia, Philadelphia, PA, USA

Randall A. Bly, MD Pediatric Otolaryngology, Seattle Children's Hospital, Department of Otolaryngology-Head and Neck Surgery, University of Washington School of Medicine, Seattle, WA, USA

Neil Bulstrode, BSc(Hons), MBBS, MD, FRCS(Plast) Department of Plastic and Reconstructive Surgery, Great Ormond Street Hospital, London, UK

Patricia Cecchi, MD Bambino Gesu Hospital, Plastic Surgery Unit, Rome, Italy

Michael W. Chu, MD Indiana University, Department of Surgery, Indianapolis, IN, USA

Sabrina Cugno, MD, MSc, FRCSC, FACS, FAAP Department of Plastic and Reconstructive Surgery, Montreal Children's Hospital, Shriners Hospital for Children, CHU Sainte-Justine, Montreal, QC, Canada

Christopher A. Derderian, MD Department of Plastic Surgery, University of Texas Southwestern Medical Center, Dallas, TX, USA

Daniel J. Gould, MD, PhD University of Southern California, Plastic and Reconstructive Surgery, Los Angeles, CA, USA

Darina Krastinova, MD Clinique Chateaux de la Maye, Paris, France

Daniel Mazzaferro, MD, MBA Division of Plastic and Reconstructive Surgery, University of Pennsylvania and The Children's Hospital of Philadelphia, Philadelphia, PA, USA

Craig Miller, MD Department of Otolaryngology – Head and Neck Surgery, University of Washington School of Medicine, Seattle, WA, USA

Ananth S. Murthy, MD, FACS Pediatric Plastic and Reconstructive Surgery, Akron Children's Hospital, Akron, OH, USA

Sanjay Naran, MD Division of Pediatric Plastic Surgery, Advocate Children's Hospital, Chicago, IL, USA

Section of Plastic and Reconstructive Surgery, University of Chicago Medicine & Biological Sciences, Chicago, IL, USA

Department of Plastic Surgery, University of Pittsburgh School of Medicine, Pittsburgh, PA, USA

Richard J. Novak, MD Adjunct Clinical Professor of Anesthesiology, Perioperative and Pain Medicine, Stanford University, Stanford, CA, USA

Caitlin L. Pray, PA-C Plastic and Reconstructive Surgery, Cedars-Sinai Medical Center, Los Angeles, CA, USA

John F. Reinisch, MD, FACS Keck School of Medicine, University of Souther California, Los Angeles, CA, USA

Craniofacial and Pediatric Plastic Surgery, Cedars Sinai Medical Center, Los Angeles, CA, USA

Joseph B. Roberson Jr., MD California Ear Institute, Global Hearing – International Center for Atresia and Microtia Repair, East Palo Alto, CA, USA

Kathleen C. Y. Sie, MD, FACS Pediatric Otolaryngology, Childhood Communication Center, Seattle Childrens Hospital, Department of Otolaryngology – Head and Neck Surgery, University of Washington School of Medicine, Seattle, WA, USA

Youssef Tahiri, MD, MSc, FRCSC, FACS, FAAP Plastic and Reconstructive Surgery, Cedars-Sinai Medical Center, Los Angeles, CA, USA

Jesse A. Taylor, MD, FACS Children's Hospital of Philadelphia, Division of Plastic Surgery, University of Pennsylvania, Philadelphia, PA, USA

Sunil S. Tholpady, MS, MD, PhD Riley Hospital for Children, Department of Surgery, Indianapolis, IN, USA

Indiana University, Department of Surgery, Indianapolis, IN, USA

Claire van Hövell tot Westerflier, MSc, MD University Medical Center Utrecht, Department of Pediatric Plastic Surgery, Utrecht University, Utrecht, The Netherlands

Ari M. Wes, BA Children's Hospital of Philadelphia, Division of Plastic Surgery, University of Pennsylvania, Philadelphia, PA, USA

Chapter 1
Anatomy and Anthropometry of the Ear

Ari M. Wes and Jesse A. Taylor

Auricular Skeleton and Cutaneous Covering

Auricular topography is in part defined by the complex underlying cartilaginous skeleton (Fig. 1.1a, b). This skeleton is characterized by multiple named concavities and convexities, which are somewhat unique in people, whether or not ear pathology is present [1]. A feature that infrequently varies between people is the antihelix, which runs parallel to the helical rim and divides into the superior and inferior crus superiorly.

Centered around the external auditory canal, the auricle exists to funnel sound waves towards the auditory canal. The external ear also assists in locating a sound's origins, and functions to amplify sounds with frequencies around 3 kHz, a figure within the frequency range of human speech [2].

Both anterior and posterior aspects of the ear's cartilaginous framework are covered in the perichondrium. Though relatively adherent across the external ear's entirety, the perichondrium is particularly adherent to the helical border and cartilaginous folds of the auricle. The perichondrium can be dissected away from the underlying cartilage relatively easily, as is done during auricular cartilage harvest.

As big a contributor to ear shape is the cutaneous covering. Anteriorly, the cartilaginous framework of the external ear is covered by extremely thin, hairless, and sensitive skin. Between these layers of cartilage and skin reside only the aforementioned perichondrium and a thin subcutaneous fat layer. It is in this subcutaneous fat layer that an array of vessels and nerves are distributed. This fact remains important when considering flap creation and harvesting techniques. The proximity between cartilage and skin in this location is closer than in any other anatomical region [3].

A. M. Wes · J. A. Taylor (✉)
Children's Hospital of Philadelphia, Division of Plastic Surgery, University of Pennsylvania, Philadelphia, PA, USA
e-mail: Taylorj5@email.chop.edu

© Springer Nature Switzerland AG 2019

J. F. Reinisch, Y. Tahiri (eds.), *Modern Microtia Reconstruction*,
https://doi.org/10.1007/978-3-030-16387-7_1

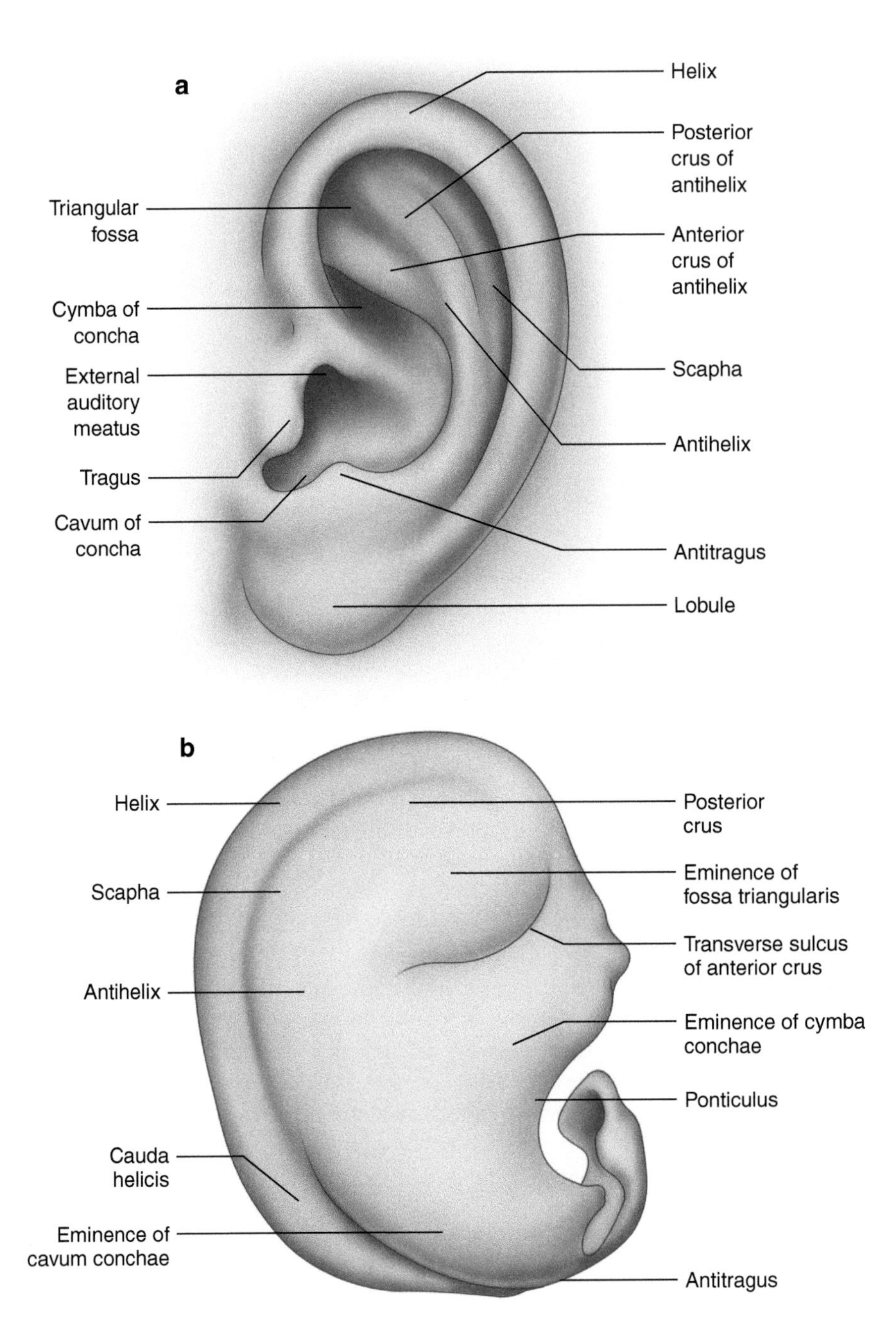

Fig. 1.1 Lateral view with skin (**a**) and medial view without skin (**b**) of the auricle

Posteriorly, the cartilaginous skeleton is covered by skin that is largely distinct from the auricle's anterior surface. Specifically, this skin is thick, very smooth, and relatively mobile with respect to the underlying cartilage. These characteristics help to explain the region's popularity as a donor site for skin grafts to the face [4]. Deep to this skin is the superficial, or areolar fat layer, which contains vessels running perpendicular to the plane of overlying skin. This layer makes up the first of two fatty layers on the ear's posterior aspect, the deeper of which is the lamellar layer. It is this layer that helps to explain the overlying skin's ability to glide with respect to auricular cartilage. A fascial layer containing a complex neurovascular network lies sandwiched between the two aforementioned fat layers [3].

The third and last unique type of skin found in the ear is that of the lobule. With both anterior and posterior aspects largely resembling one another, the lobule is covered in skin that is both thin and soft. No cartilage is present in the lobule; instead, the bulk of this region is composed of fatty tissue containing vasculature that helps to supply the lower portion of the auricle [5].

Ligaments and Muscles

Auricular muscles can be classified as either extrinsic or intrinsic. As the name suggests, extrinsic muscles of the ear originate at a location other than the auricle itself. Intrinsic muscles, on the other hand, both originate from and insert on the auricle.

There are three extrinsic auricular muscles: the anterior, posterior, and superior muscles. The primary role of these muscles is to stabilize the ear against the temporal region, though they also impact the ear's position and angle of projection. The anterior muscle is the smallest of the extrinsic muscles, originating from the zygomatic arch and inserting into the spina auricularis. Its function, while extremely limited, is to pull the auricle anteriorly. The posterior muscle originates from the mastoid and inserts into the concha's posterior surface. The third and largest of the extrinsic muscles is the superior muscle. This muscle originates from the galea aponeurotica and inserts into the posterior, or cranial, surface of the triangular fossa (Fig. 1.2a, b). To underscore the role of these muscles in ear stabilization, one can look to reports of ear hypermobility in the case of external auricular muscle agenesis [6].

The intrinsic auricular muscles, of which there are six, determine the auricle's cartilaginous topography. This group includes the major helical, minor helical, tragal, and antitragal muscles on the auricle's anterior surface. Posteriorly, one finds the auricular oblique and transverse muscles (Fig. 1.2a, b) [7].

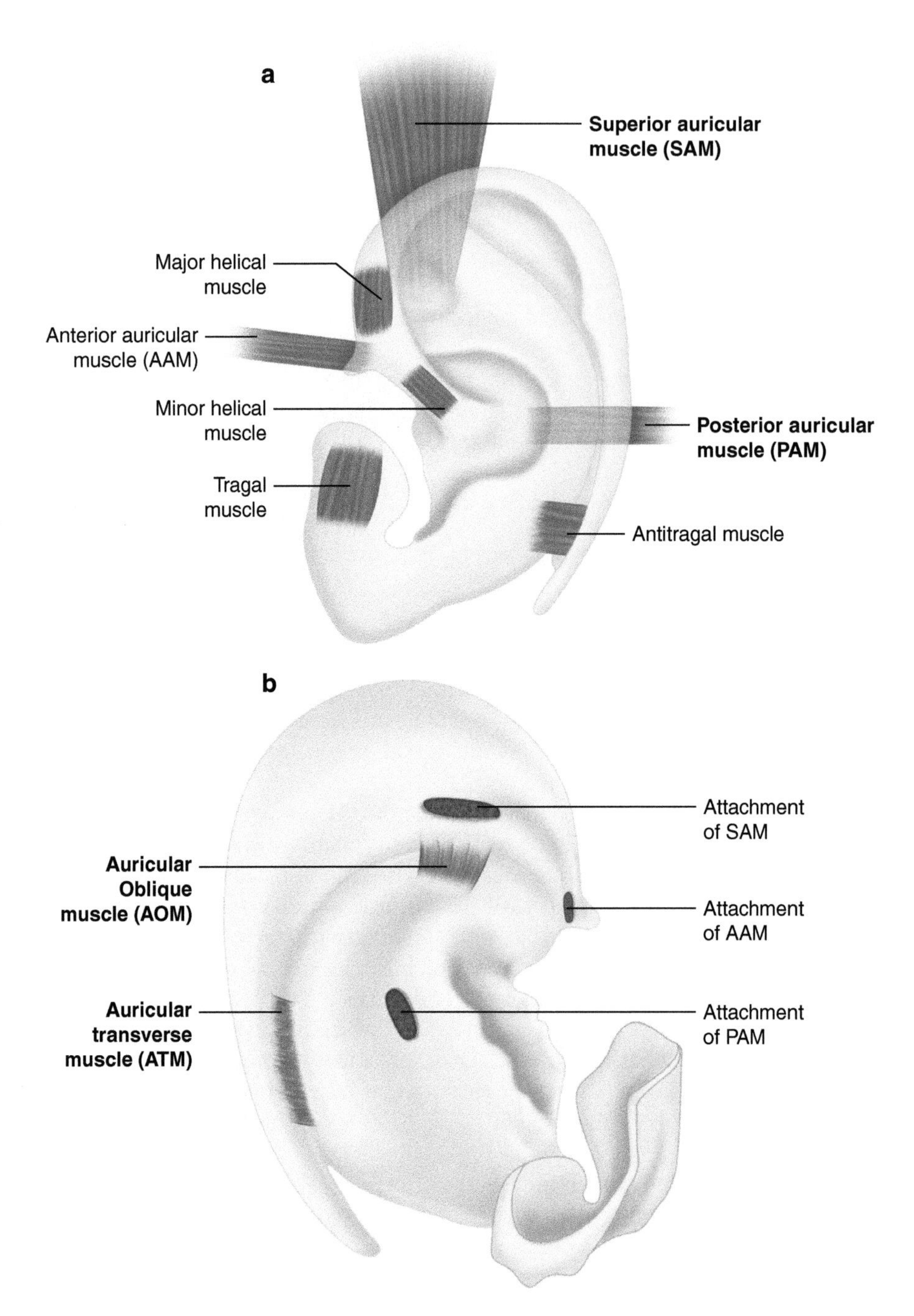

Fig. 1.2 Schematic of intrinsic and extrinsic muscles of the auricle: (**a**) lateral view; (**b**) medial view

Blood Supply

Arterial

The auricle's arterial supply comes from two branches of the external carotid artery: the superficial temporal artery (STA) and the posterior auricular artery (PAA). More specifically, the STA gives rise to three additional branches, the superior-, middle-, and inferior-anterior auricular arteries. The superior and inferior branches provide arterial flow to the helical rim, ultimately meeting and forming the helical rim arcade. The middle-anterior auricular branch supplies the tragus, the helical root, and the superior portion of the external auditory meatus (Fig. 1.3a) [8].

The PAA, also a branch of the external carotid artery, ascends superficially to course in the subcutaneous fat layer at the level of the mastoid. From here, the artery continues to course superiorly along the posterior aspect of the auricle, giving off a variable number of radially directed branches that ultimately connect with the helical rim arcade (Fig. 1.3b). Importantly, the PAA also gives off perforating vessels that penetrate the auricular cartilage to emerge on the anterior surface. Though somewhat variable in number across the population, these perforators consistently emerge near the helical root and near the antitragus in the auricle's concha. A thorough understanding of this vasculature is critical in that it allows a surgeon to creatively and reliably construct local flaps for the reconstruction of congenital or traumatic defects.

Venous

The auricle's venous system largely follows the course of the aforementioned arterial system. On the anterior surface of the auricle, venous blood drains through the anterior auricular veins, and subsequently, the superficial temporal vein. The superficial temporal vein ultimately contributes to the posterior facial vein. Posteriorly, the venous system returns blood to the posterior auricular vein that, together with the posterior branch of the posterior facial vein, makes the external jugular vein.

Lymphatic

Coursing in the auricle's subcutaneous fat, the lymphatic vessels in the region coalesce into four groups of collecting branches. The anterior branch represents the convergence of lymph vessels from most of the auricle's lateral surface; it courses along the cruz of the helix and drains into the pre-auricular lymph nodes. The superior branches are made up of lymph vessels that arise in the superior helix and course along the posterior aspect of the auricle to the infra-auricular lymph node. Arising from the scaphoid fossa, the middle branches course over the helical rim, to

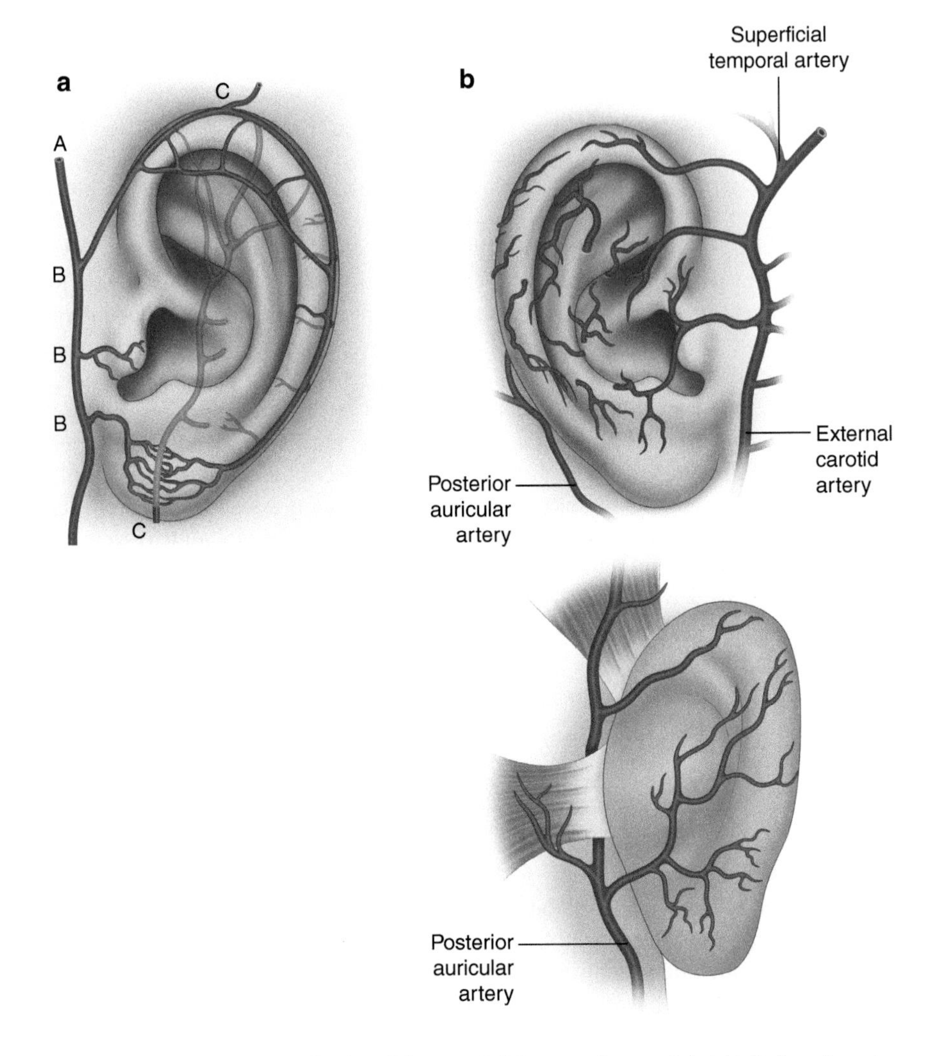

Fig. 1.3 (**a**) Schematic of distribution of the superficial temporal artery (label A), its three branches (label B), the posterior auricular artery (label C), and resulting arcades. (**b**) Vascularity of the ear: Lateral view (top) and medial view (bottom)

the auricle's posterior aspect, then drain into the infra-auricular lymph node. Finally, the inferior branches arise from the lobule and course down to drain into the infra-auricular lymph node [9].

Innervation

A thorough understanding of the locations and relationships between innervating nerves and the various regions of the auricle remains critical for surgeons.

Sensory

Four nerves carry sensory information from the external ear: the great auricular nerve (GAN), the auricular branch of the vagus nerve (ABVN), the auriculotemporal nerve (ATN), and the lesser occipital nerve (LON) (Figs. 1.4 and 1.5).

The GAN arises from the cervical plexus (C2 and C3), courses beneath the posterior border of the sternocleidomastoid muscle, then travels superficially until just deep to the platysma. At the parotid gland, the GAN divides into anterior and posterior branches. Disagreement exists with respect to the individual contributions of each of these branches, but together the branches of the GAN provide sensation to the lobule and lower half of the auricle both laterally and medially [10].

The ABVN, after a deep and circuitous route from the jugular ganglion, rises superficially between the mastoid process and the tympanic portion of the temporal bone. This nerve provides sensation to the cymba concha and antihelix laterally, and to the middle and (less often) lower thirds of the auricle medially (Figs. 1.4 and 1.5).

The mandibular branch of the trigeminal nerve gives way to the ATN, which courses alongside the superficial temporal artery, and provides sensory innervation primarily to the spine and crus of the helix.

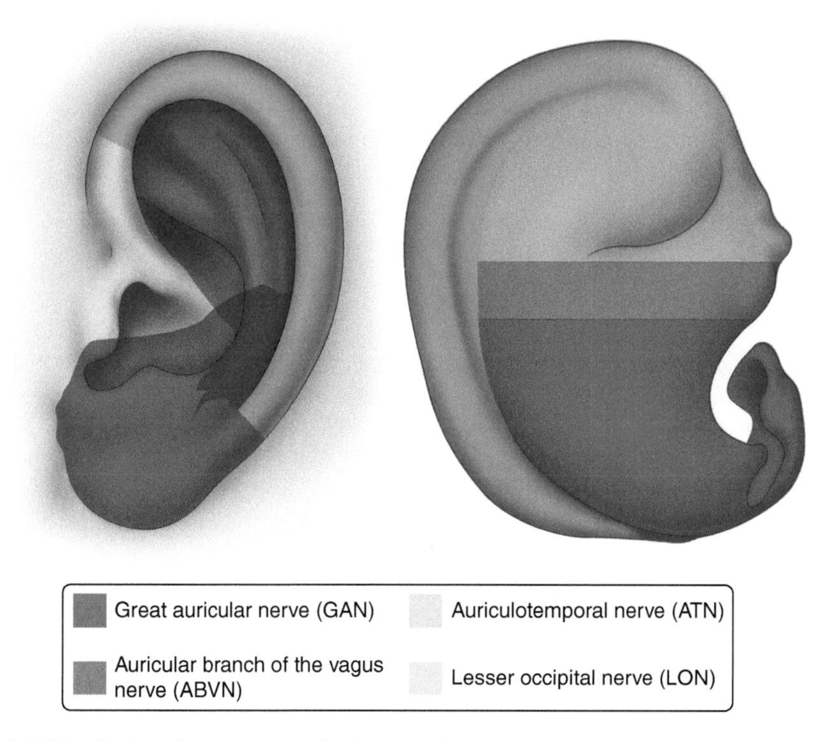

Fig. 1.4 Distribution of sensory nerves in the external ear

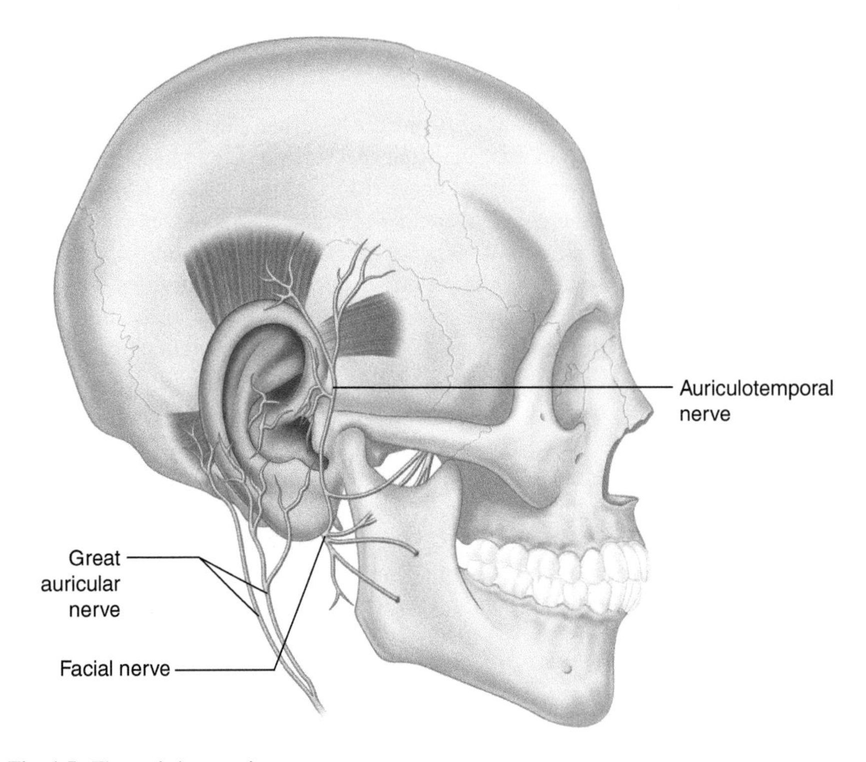

Fig. 1.5 The ear's innervation

Finally, the LON provides sensation to the upper third of the medial auricle, and its course mirrors that of the GAN.

Motor

Motor innervation of the auricle, while of less relative importance due to the minimal role of auricular musculature, is less convoluted than the ear's sensory innervation. Two nerves, both of which arise from the facial nerve, are responsible for all motor innervation of the ear: the posterior auricular nerve (PAN) and the temporal branch of the facial nerve (TBFN).

The PAN ascends just anterior to the mastoid process and innervates the posterior auricular muscle as well as the intrinsic muscles on the auricle's medial surface. The TBFN on the other hand, travels laterally over the zygomatic arch, where it innervates the anterior and superior auricular muscles. Intrinsic muscles on the auricle's lateral surface are also innervated by branches of the facial nerve [10].

Embryology and Development

The branchial arches are an embryological successor of the pharyngeal arches, and play a central role in auricular development. Specifically, it is the interface between the first and second branchial arches that is of particular interest for our purposes. In the sixth week of development, six small mounds, called the hillocks of His, form on the dorsal surfaces of the first and second branchial arches; these mounds will go on to form the external ear. At approximately week 8 of gestation, the groove between the first and second branchial arches (termed the "first branchial groove") invaginates, creating the external auditory meatus. It is this invagination that allows for the simultaneous migration and fusion of the six hillocks of His, forming the early cartilaginous precursor to the auricle. Evidence suggests that the first hillock originates from the first branchial arch, and gives rise to the tragus, while the origins of the remaining hillocks remain debated [5, 11]. At 12 weeks of gestation, the auricle's peculiar topographical characteristics begin to develop, and at 18 weeks the auricle detaches from the head. By 22 weeks, the auricle resembles that of an adult, and development is complete (Fig. 1.6a–c) [5, 12].

Anthropometry

A thorough understanding of the sizes and proportions of the "normal" external ear is critical for a reconstructive surgeon. With respect to size, the normal adult ear measures approximately 5.5–6.5 cm in height, with a width of 50–60% of that. Along a line connecting the brow and the columella, approximately one ear length separates the lateral orbital rim and the root of the helix.

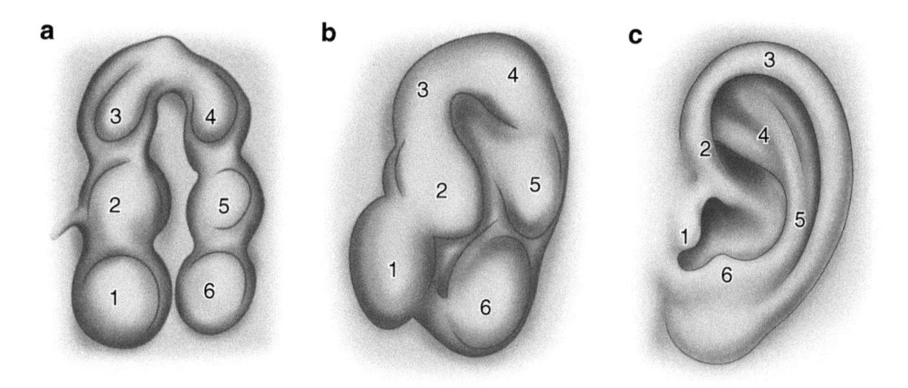

Fig. 1.6 Embryological development of the auricle. Migration of the six hillocks can be seen from (**a**) the early fetus, through (**b**) the primitive ear, and finally (**c**) the fully developed ear

Box 1.1 Anthropometric characteristics of the normal auricle

Height is approximately 5.5–6.5 cm.
Width is 3–4.5 cm, or 50–60% of auricular height.
The root of the helix lies approximately one ear length lateral to the lateral orbital rim.
Projection from the plane of the mastoid process is approximately 20° in females and 25° in males.
The auricle's long axis is rotated 20° posteriorly from a perfect vertical.

The auricle has been noted to grow more rapidly in width than in length, with 90% of adult-ear-width being reached in the first year of life, and 75% of adult-ear-length in the same time period [13].

Ear projection, as measured by the angle between mastoid and concha, is approximately 20° in females, and 25° in males. Furthermore, on frontal view, the helix should project 2–5 mm more laterally than the antihelix. With respect to ear rotation, the long axis of the auricle is normally rotated posteriorly, approximately 20° from vertical [14]. See Box 1.1.

Conclusion

The auricle is a complex organ, and its appearance remains important to the patients of reconstructive and aesthetic surgeons alike. Importantly, the intricacy and distinctiveness of the ear's topography poses a particular challenge to the reconstructive surgeon treating a patient with microtia. In this chapter, we discussed the auricular skin, cartilage, vasculature, innervation, embryological development, and shape. A deep understanding of this anatomy is a crucial component of the reconstructive surgeon's arsenal, but represents only the first step in understanding microtia repair.

References

1. Baker S. Local flaps in facial reconstruction. 3rd ed. Philadelphia: WB Saunders; 2014.
2. Middlebrooks JC, Green DM. Sound localization by human listeners. Annu Rev Psychol. 1991;42:135–59.
3. Avelar JM. Ear reconstruction. Berlin/Heidelberg: Springer-Verlag; 2013.
4. Fujino T, Harashina T, Nakajima T. Free skin flap from the retroauricular region to the nose. Plast Reconstr Surg. 1976;57:338–41.
5. Siegert R, Weerda H, Remmert S. Embryology and surgical anatomy of the auricle. Facial Plast Surg. 1994;10:232–43.

6. Hoogbergen MM, Schuurman AH, Rijnders W, Kon M. Auricular hypermobility due to agenesis of the extrinsic muscles. Plast Reconstr Surg. 1996;98:869–71.
7. Yotsuyanagi T, Yamauchi M, Yamashita K, Sugai A, Gonda A, Kitada A, et al. Abnormality of auricular muscles in congenital auricular deformities. Plast Reconstr Surg. 2015;136:78e–88e.
8. Zilinsky I, Erdmann D, Weissman O, Hammer N, Sora MC, Schenck TL, et al. Reevaluation of the arterial blood supply of the auricle. J Anat. 2017;230:315–24.
9. Pan W-RR, le Roux CM, Levy SM, Briggs CA. Lymphatic drainage of the external ear. Head Neck. 2011;33:60–4.
10. Peuker ET, Filler TJ. The nerve supply of the human auricle. Clin Anat. 2002;15:35–7.
11. Sauter R, Villavicencio E, Schwager K. Doubling of the pinna, a rare branchial arch developmental disorder. Laryngorhinootologie. 2006;85:657–60.
12. Anthwal N, Thompson H. The development of the mammalian outer and middle ear. J Anat. 2016;228:217–32.
13. Pawar SS, Koch CA, Murakami C. Treatment of prominent ears and otoplasty: a contemporary review. JAMA Facial Plast Surg. 2015;17:449–54.
14. Janis JE, Rohrich RJ, Gutowski KA. Otoplasty. Plast Reconstr Surg. 2005;115(4):60e–72e.

Chapter 2
Classification and Prevalence of Microtia

Daniel J. Gould, Caitlin L. Pray, Youssef Tahiri, and John F. Reinisch

Introduction

The anatomy of the external ear is complex. The external ear develops from several branchial arches and can present with multiple developmental anomalies at birth. In this chapter, we discuss the classification and prevalence of microtia.

Microtia

Microtia exists as a broad phenotypic spectrum with little consensus on terminology. Figure 2.1 shows the types of microtia that one may see. Some clinicians refer to all points on the spectrum as "microtia," while others delineate "microtia" (underdeveloped ear) from "anotia" (absent ear) [1–4]. Throughout this textbook, we will refer to the spectrum as "microtia" with anotia simply being one end of the spectrum.

Microtia not only has a wide range of phenotypic expressions as seen in Fig. 2.1, but can also be associated with various craniofacial abnormalities. These defects include mandibular hypoplasia, facial nerve weakness or paralysis, soft tissue hypoplasia, palatal dysfunction, and macrostomia. These associated findings almost always occur on the same side as the microtia. Microtia may also be seen be seen as part of various syndromes such as Treacher-Collins and Goldenhar Syndromes [1, 5–9].

D. J. Gould (✉)
University of Southern California, Plastic and Reconstructive Surgery, Los Angeles, CA, USA

C. L. Pray · Y. Tahiri · J. F. Reinisch
Plastic and Reconstructive Surgery, Cedars-Sinai Medical Center, Los Angeles, CA, USA

© Springer Nature Switzerland AG 2019
J. F. Reinisch, Y. Tahiri (eds.), *Modern Microtia Reconstruction*,
https://doi.org/10.1007/978-3-030-16387-7_2

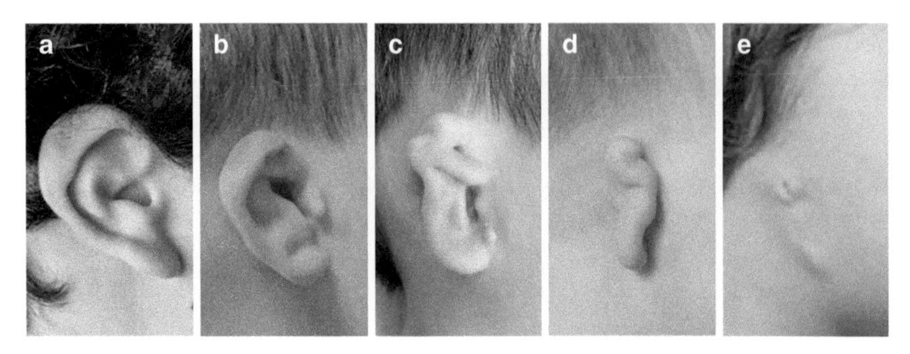

Fig. 2.1 The spectrum of microtia presentation from small to absent ear. (**a**) Marx grade 1 or Nagata atypical type microtia. (**b**) Marx grade 2 or Nagata concha type microtia (**c**) Marx grade 2 or Nagata small concha type microtia (**d**) Marx grade 3 or Nagata's lobule type microtia (**e**) Marx grade 3, Rogers grade 4, or Nagata anotia

In the great majority of cases, microtia is also associated with an ipsilateral conductive hearing loss secondary to either aural atresia (absent ear canal) or aural stenosis (narrowed ear canal). The ipsilateral cochlea is typically normal, as it is unrelated embryologically to the development of the outer ear and canal.

Anotia, which is relatively uncommon, is often seen with more severe forms of microsomia, including severe nerve involvement, as well as conductive and sensorineural hearing loss [8].

Prevalence

The prevalence of microtia varies depending on the population studied. Reported rates vary widely between 0.8 and 12 per 10,000 patients in the literature [2–5, 10–14]. Because many of these studies included live birth, stillbirth, and elective terminations of pregnancy, these population studies may not reflect the prevalence among viable pregnancies. Several of these studies also specified rates of anotia, which fell between 0.2 and 0.5 per 10,000. Recently, a large study identified the global prevalence rates for microtia-anotia to be 2.06 (CI: 2.02–2.10), with microtia 1.55 (CI: 1.50–1.60), and anotia 0.36 (CI: 0.34–0.38) [14]. Microtia is more common in males with an estimated increase in risk of approximately 20–40% compared with females [2, 15–18]. Ninety-three percent of microtia occurs in a unilateral fashion [2, 11, 12], with most experiencing hearing loss only in the affected ear [17]. Some evidence supports a higher rate of right-sided disease [2, 12, 17].

Microtia tends to be more severe and is more commonly bilateral in syndromic patients. Patients with more severe forms and bilateral microtia tend to exhibit Mendelian patterns of inheritance [19]. This contrasts with sporadic cases, where epigenetic and environmental influences are believed to be involved [20].

It is worth noting that because microtia has a range of presentation, very mild forms are likely underreported in some studies, and thus prevalence rates actually may be higher. This may account for some of the disparity in reported prevalence rates [3, 4, 13, 16]. For the same reason, mild or "isolated" cases of microtia may not be followed by university craniofacial clinics. This may explain why published series of microtia patients from these centers tend to have a higher incidence of associated anomalies as these teams have been selectively referred more severely affected patients.

A discussion on the prevalence of microtia must include consideration of ethnicity, as significantly higher rates have been identified in Asian and Hispanic populations compared with Caucasian and African populations [3, 4, 13, 14, 18]. Additionally, some studies have suggested higher prevalence rates among Chilean, Native American, and Ecuadorian populations, which may be due to environmental and genetic factors [15, 21–23]. See Table 2.1. Importantly, Table 2.1 describes prospective population based studies of stillbirth and live birth, and though it includes China, it leaves out other studies which have shown rates as high as 2.71 in China Beijing (1.2 million population study = n) and 3.11 in mainland China (3.9 Million = n) [14].

Anotia involves absence of the ear in its entirety. Anotia is thought to represent the most severe form of microtia, though this has not been shown mechanistically [1]. Using a Der Simonian–Laird random effects model, Van Nunen and colleagues reported a rate of 7% of anotia among microtia patients [24]. Anotia is rare in Caucasians and Africans, compared to higher rates in Hispanic and Asian children [2].

Classification

Due to the variety of anatomic presentation of microtia, understanding existing classification systems can be difficult [16, 25, 26].

The Marx classification system was published in 1926 and was the first classification system developed for microtia. It describes auricle grades 1, 2, and 3 [27]. Marx Grade 1 is a small auricle with all identifiable landmarks; Marx Grade 2 is an abnormal auricle without some identifiable landmarks; Marx Grade 3 is very small auricular tag or anotia [27].

Rogers added Grade 4 to the Marx system in 1974 to separately classify anotia. Rogers believed that anotia represented a much more severe deformity, and thus it should have a discrete category [27]. This remains a popular international grading system. However, though it does give some idea of severity, it does not expand description beyond the external ear.

Tanzer designed a classification, which grouped all congenital ear deformities by the surgical approach required for correction [28]. This included anotia as Type 1; a completely hypoplastic ear (microtia) with external canal atresia as Type 2a; a completely hypoplastic ear without aural atresia as Type 2b; hypoplasia of the middle third of the auricle as Type 3; hypoplasia of the superior third in the form of constriction (cup and lop ear) as Type 4a; hypoplasia of the superior third in the form of cryptotia as Type 4b; hypoplasia of the entire superior third as Type 4c; and prominent ear as Type 5.

Table 2.1 Prevalence of microtia in several studies from the literature

Study	Age of ascertainment	Prevalence of microtia/anotia (per 10.000)	Prevalence of anotia (per 10,000)	Prevalence of microtia (per 10, 000)	Types of microtia included (Marx)	References
Population based						
Central-East France	LB + SB	0.8	0.4	0.4	1–4	Harris et al. [2]
California	LB + SB	2.0	0.2	1.8	1–4	Harris et al. [2]
Sweden	LB + SB	2.4	0.2	2.1	1–4	Harris et al. [2]
California	LB + SB	2.2	Nr	Nr	Nr	Shaw et al. [4]
Hawaii	LB + SB + TP	3.8	0.3	3.5	2–4	Forrester and Merz [17]
Finland	LB + SB	4.3	0.2	4.1	1–4	Sumaria et al.[a]
Texas	LB + SB + TP	2.8	Nr	Nr	Nr	Husain et al.
Texas	LB + SB + TP	2.9	0.2	2.7	2–4	Canfield [13]
Hospital based						
Navajo	>21	9.7	Nr	Nr	Nr	Jaffe
New Mexico	Any age	1.3	Nr	Nr	1–4	Aase and Tegtmeier[b]
Navajo	4–14	12.0	Nr	Nr	Nr	Nelson and Berry [22]
South America	LB	3.2	Nr	Nr	1–4	Castilla and Orioli [12]
Italy	LB + SB	1.5	0.3	1.2	1–4	Mastroiacovo et al. [11]
China	LB + SB	1.4	Nr	Nr	Nr	Zhu et al.
Chile	LB + SB	8.8	0.5	8.3	1–4	Nazer et al. [10]

There are varying population frequencies, and the variation between populations is thought to be due to complex genetic, environmental, and epigenetic factors

LB livebirth, *SB* stillborn, *TP* terminated pregnancy

[a]Suutarla et al. [5]

[b]Aase and Tegtmeier [23]

In 1988, Weerda modified Marx and Tanzer's definitions and expanded his classification to include all congenital abnormalities of the external ear, including macrotia [29].

In 1993, Nagata created the Nagata classification system, which focuses on reconstructive surgical algorithms and options [30]. His classification is broken into concha type, small concha type, lobule type, and anotia.

In 2009, Hunter et al. published an article in conjunction with the *American Journal of Medical Genetics* to more precisely standardize ear terminology [31].

This system modified the Weerda classification, but emphasized the importance of measuring the longitudinal length of the ear to define first, second, and third degrees of microtia based on standard deviations from the mean.

The above classification systems focus solely on the external ear structure. However, microtia can be associated with other craniofacial anomalies and syndromes. These patients, such as those with craniofacial microsomia and Treacher Collins syndrome are more frequently seen at regional or university craniofacial centers where more inclusive multisystem classifications are useful. An early multisystem classification system, developed by David, was called the SAT system. It included (S)keletal, (A)uricular, and soft (T)issue anomalies [32].

The OMENS classification created by Vento, La Brie, and Mulliken expanded the SAT system by splitting the Skeletal component into Orbital and Mandibular scores, and separated facial nerve function from the soft tissue component (see Table 2.2) [33]. The OMENS-Plus classification expanded OMENS to include extra-craniofacial features of the disease, such as heart, renal, or vertebral anomalies [34]. This classification has become a powerful tool in the assessment of craniofacial microsomia (CFM), as it helps identify and describe patients with associated or additional severe deformities [35–39]. The OMENS-Plus has also helped identify that the diagnostic criteria of Goldenhar syndrome remains unclear, and that subjectively, Goldenhar syndrome is over-diagnosed in patients who show more severe CFM features [38].

Table 2.2 OMENS classification for hemifacial microsomia. Data from Vento et al. [35] OMENS classification was originally developed to better classify hemifacial microsomia patients. It considers the orbit, mandible, ear, facial nerve, and soft tissue. It can differentiate those that will require mandible surgery and was an early attempt at standardizing severity

Orbit	Mandible	Ear	Facial nerve	Soft tissue
$O = 0$ normal orbital size	$M = 0$	$E = 0$ normal ear	$N = 0$ no facial nerve involvement	$S = 0$ no soft tissue or muscle involved
$O = 1$ abnormal orbital volume/shape	$M = 1$ mandible and glenoid small, short ramus	$E = 1$ ear with cupping, hypoplasia but all structures present	$N = 1$ temporal and zygomatic branches involved	$S = 1$ minimal soft tissue muscle involved
	$M = 2$ ramus short and abnormal shape subdivisions based on position of the condyle and TMJ		$N = 2$ buccal mandibular and cervical branches involved	$S = 2$moderate lack of soft tissue and muscle
	$M = 3$ absence of glenoid fossa, ramus, and TMJ		$N = 3$ all branches involved	$S = 3$ severe lack of soft tissue and or muscle
			$N = 5$ sensory involved	
			$N = 12$ hypoglossal involved	

Several authors have identified important correlations between disease severity and the organ systems represented by the OMENS-Plus classification system. For example, one retrospective study of 105 patients demonstrated a correlation among orbital, soft tissue, and mandibular deformities, as well as a correlation between facial nerve involvement and degree of ear deformity [40].

The OMENS classification focuses more on patients with craniofacial microsomia and less on those with microtia. For example, hearing function, an important aspect of microtia, is not part of the O.M.E.N.S. classification.

The HEAR MAPS system (Table 2.3) was developed by Reinisch, Roberson, and colleagues to better describe patients with microtia [40]. The system includes

Table 2.3 HEAR MAPS is a concise method of classifying ear and facial aspects in patients with microtia. It is the only system that includes hearing function

Hear bone/ear (PTA2 db HL)		
	Bone PTA2/Air PTA2	
Ear (microtia)		
	Grade 1	Normal
	Grade 2	Mild malformation
	Grade 3	Moderate malformation
	Grade 4	Anotia
Atresia Jahrsdoerfer CT Scale		
	Grade 1–10	
Remnant earlobe		
	Grade 1	Normal
	Grade 2	Mildly reduced
	Grade 3	Moderately reduced
	Grade 4	Severely reduced/ absent
Mandible		
	Grade 1	Normal
	Grade 2	Mildly reduced
	Grade 3	Moderately reduced
	Grade 4	Severely reduced/ absent
Asymmetry soft tissue		
	Grade 1	Normal
	Grade 2	Mildly reduced
	Grade 3	Moderately reduced
	Grade 4	Severely reduced/ absent
Paresis of facial nerve (House–Brackmann scale)		
	Grade 1–6	
Syndrome		
	Grade 1	None
	Grade 2	Yes

Adapted with permission of Elsevier from Roberson et al. [40]

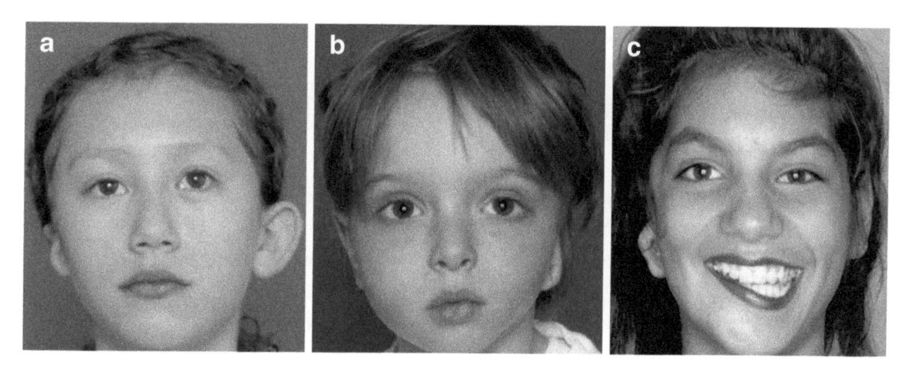

Fig. 2.2 HEAR MAPS. The HEAR MAPS classification system was developed for grading microtia and considers associated craniofacial abnormalities and syndromes. (**a**) This patient is classified as H1.6E9A1R1 M2A1P1S1. Her bone conduction is normal in the 10–20 dB range with an air conduction in the 60–70 dB range. She has grade 3 microtia with a Jahrsdoerfer atresia score of 9 by CT scan. She has no other associated craniofacial anomalies and no evidence of a syndrome. (**b**) This patient is classified as H1.6E3A3R1 M2A3P1S1. He has Grade 3 microtia with a Jahrsdoerfer atresia score of 3 by CT scan. His ear lobe is a similar size to his right ear. His mandible is shifted slightly with significant soft tissue hypoplasia. He has no facial nerve deficit and no evidence of a syndrome. (**c**) This patient is classified as H1.6E3A4R1 M1A1P4MS1, She has a Jahrsdoerfer atresia score of 4 and a marginal mandibular palsy

bone and air conduction hearing levels. It also grades the severity of the ear remnant, the atresia score as determined by CT scan, the size of the lobular remnant, mandibular deviation, the degree of cheek soft tissue hypoplasia, and facial nerve weakness. It also recognizes the presence or absence of an associated syndrome. The letters of HEAR defines the microtic ear while the MAPS portion of the classification refers to the face. The letters of HEAR represent Hearing, Ear grade, Atresia score, and Remnant lobe. MAPS refers to the face with the letters representing Mandible, Asymmetry of soft tissue, Paralysis, and Syndrome. This system provides the most concise and comprehensive phenotypic description of individuals with microtia (Fig. 2.2).

Constricted Ear

The term "constricted ear" was coined by Tanzer to better categorize a group of congenital ear deformities [41]. Tanzer noted the subtle findings of hooding of the helix and flattening of the antihelix and included lop ear and cup ear within the grading system for constricted ear. It can be debated whether some constricted ears are true grade 1 microtia versus a separate category of ear deformity.

Tanzer's original description included three groups and two subgroups (Table 2.4). Group 1 constricted ear is lidding only of the helix or lop ear. Group 2 involves the helix and the scapha. This form of constriction involves hooding and gives a "cup" appearance (cup ear), and is subdivided into two subgroups. Group 2A is fairly moderate and does not require extra skin to expand the helix.

Table 2.4 Tanzer's classification of the constricted ear demonstrates the different severities of constriction

Group	Description
Group 1	Involvement of helix only
Group 2	Involvement of helix and scapha
2A	No supplemental skin needed at the margin of the auricle
2B	Supplemental skin required at margin of auricle
Group 3	Extreme cupping deformity: often associated with incomplete migration, forward tilt, stenosis of external auditory canal, and deafness

Adapted with permission of Wolters Kluwer Health from Tanzer [28, 41]

There is failure of folding of the superior antihelical crus, which along with helical hooding, causes a purse string effect of skin over the auricle. Group2B is more severe with a flattened anti-helix, severe hooding, and reduced ear height. Importantly, in this form of cup ear, the constriction limits reconstruction. The skin in the upper ear is not sufficient for the reconstruction of the superior auricle with repositioned cartilage framework: such repair typically requires supplemental flap and skin graft. Group 3 represents a tubular ear, where the deformity is due to the attachment of the anterior helix close to the lobule. These ears are low-set with abnormal hairlines and superior anterior rotation of the auricle toward the orbit. This deformity is usually accompanied by a stenotic canal and hearing impairment.

Conclusion

Microtia presents with spectrum of ear morphology. A number of classification systems have been developed to guide diagnosis and treatment of microtia. In order to properly evaluate and treat each patient, one must appropriately differentiate the subtype of the external ear deformity and identify associated craniofacial issues. The goal of treatment should be the restoration of both facial symmetry and hearing function. With efficient planning and awareness of the patients' concerns, one should strive for the maximum benefit with the least number of interventions.

References

1. Stevenson RE, Hall JG. Human malformations and related anomalies. Oxford: Oxford University Press; 2005.
2. Harris J, Källén B, Robert E. The epidemiology of anotia and microtia. J Med Genet. 1996;33:809–13.
3. Forrester MB, Merz RD. Descriptive epidemiology of anotia and microtia, Hawaii, 1986–2002. Congenit Anom. 2005;45:119–24.

4. Shaw GM, Carmichael SL, Kaidarova Z, Harris JA. Epidemiologic characteristics of anotia and microtia in California, 1989-1997. Birth Defects Res A Clin Mol Teratol. 2004;70:472–5.
5. Suutarla S, Rautio J, Ritvanen A, Ala-Mello S, Jero J, Klockars T. Microtia in Finland: comparison of characteristics in different populations. Int J Pediatr Otorhinolaryngol. 2007;71:1211–7.
6. Ishimoto S, Ito K, Karino S, Takegoshi H, Kaga K, Yamasoba T. Hearing levels in patients with microtia: correlation with temporal bone malformation. Laryngoscope. 2007;117:461–5.
7. Calzolari F, Garani G, Sensi A, Martini A. Clinical and radiological evaluation in children with microtia. Br J Audiol. 1999;33:303–12.
8. Bassila MK, Goldberg R. The association of facial palsy and/or sensorineural hearing loss in patients with hemifacial microsomia. Cleft Palate J. 1989;26:287–91.
9. Tekes A, Ishman SL, Baugher KM, Brown DJ, Lin SY, Tunkel DE, et al. Does microtia predict severity of temporal bone CT abnormalities in children with persistent conductive hearing loss. J Neuroradiol J de neuroradiologie. 2013;40:192–7.
10. Nazer J, Lay-Son G, Cifuentes L. Prevalence of microtia and anotia at the maternity of the University of Chile Clinical Hospital. Rev Med Chil. 2006;134:1295–301.
11. Mastroiacovo P, Corchia C, Botto LD, Lanni R, Zampino G, Fusco D. Epidemiology and genetics of microtia-anotia: a registry based study on over one million births. J Med Genet. 1995;32:453–7.
12. Castilla EE, Orioli IM. Prevalence rates of microtia in South America. Int J Epidemiol. 1986;15:364–8.
13. Canfield MA, Langlois PH, Nguyen LM, Scheuerle AE. Epidemiologic features and clinical subgroups of anotia/microtia in Texas. Birth Defects Res A Clin Mol Teratol. 2009;85:905–13.
14. Luquetti DV, Leoncini E, Mastroiacovo P. Microtia-anotia: a global review of prevalence rates. Birth Defects Res A Clin Mol Teratol. 2011;91:813–22.
15. Luquetti DV, Saltzman BS, Lopez-Camelo J, Dutra MG, Castilla EE. Risk factors and demographics for Microtia in South America: a case-control analysis. Birth Defects Res A Clin Mol Teratol. 2013;97:736–43.
16. Luquetti DV, Heike CL, Hing AV, Cunningham ML, Cox TC. Microtia: epidemiology and genetics. Am J Med Genet A. 2012;158A:124–39.
17. Forrester MB, Merz RD. Descriptive epidemiology of anotia and microtia, Hawaii, 1986-2002. Congenit Anom (Kyoto). 2005;45:119–24.
18. Deng K, Dai L, Yi L, Deng C, Li X, Zhu J. Epidemiologic characteristics and time trend in the prevalence of anotia and microtia in China. Birth Defects Res A Clin Mol Teratol. 2016;106:88–94.
19. Hunter AGW, Yotsuyanagi T. The external ear: more attention to detail may aid syndrome diagnosis and contribute answers to embryological questions. Am J Med Genet Part A. 2005;135(3):237–50.
20. Llano-Rivas I, et al. Microtia: a clinical and genetic study at the National Institute of Pediatrics in Mexico City. Arch Med Res. 1999;30(2):120–4.
21. Yang J, Carmichael SL, Kaidarova Z, Shaw GM. Risks of selected congenital malformations among offspring of mixed race-ethnicity. Birth Defects Res A Clin Mol Teratol. 2004;70:820–4.
22. Nelson SM, Berry RI. Ear disease and hearing loss among Navajo children–a mass survey. Laryngoscope. 1984;94:316–23.
23. Aase JM, Tegtmeier RE. Microtia in New Mexico: evidence for multifactorial causation. Birth Defects Orig Artic Ser. 1977;13:113–6.
24. Van Nunen DPF, Kolodzynski MN, van den Boogaard M-JH, Kon M, Breugem CC. Microtia 537 in the Netherlands: clinical characteristics and associated anomalies. Int J Pediatr 538 Otorhinolaryngol. 2014;78:954–9.
25. Luquetti DV, Saltzman BS, Vivaldi D, Pimenta LA, Hing AV, Cassell CH, et al. Evaluation of ICD-9-CM codes for craniofacial microsomia. Birth Defects Res A Clin Mol Teratol. 2012;94:990–5.
26. Luquetti DV, Saltzman BS, Heike CL, Sie KC, Birgfeld CB, Evans KN, et al. Phenotypic sub-grouping in microtia using a statistical and a clinical approach. Am J Med Genet A. 2015;167:688–94.

27. Rogers B. Anatomy, embryology, and classification of auricular deformities. In: Tanzer R, Edgerton M, editors. Symposium on reconstruction of the auricle, vol. 10. St. Louis: CV Mosby; 1974. p. 3–11.
28. Tanzer RC. Microtia. Clin Plast Surg. 1978;5(3):317–36.
29. Weerda H. Classification of congenital deformities of the auricle. Facial Plastic Surg. 1988;5:385–8.
30. Nagata S. A new method of total reconstruction of the auricle for microtia. Plast Reconstr Surg. 1993;92:187–201.
31. Hunter AG. The elements of morphology: ear–an initial approach for the incisura. Am J Med Genet A. 2010;152a:401–3.
32. David DJ, Mahatumarat C, Cooter RD. Hemifacial microsomia: a multisystem classification. Plast Reconstr Surg. 1987;80:525.
33. Vento M, LaBrie R, Mulliken J. The O.M.E.N.S. classification of hemifacial microsomia. Cleft Palat Craniofac. J. 1991;28:68.
34. Horgan JE, Padwa BL, LaBrie RA, Mulliken JB. OMENS-plus: analysis of craniofacial and extracraniofacial anomalies in hemifacial microsomia. Cleft Palate Craniofac J. 1995;32:405–12.
35. Vento AR, LaBrie RA, Mulliken JB. The O.M.E.N.S. Classification of hemifacial microsomia. Cleft Palate Craniofac J. 1991;28:68–76; discussion 77.
36. Gougoutas AJ, Singh DJ, Low DW, Bartlett SP. Hemifacial microsomia: clinical features and pictographic representations of the OMENS classification system. Plast Reconstr Surg. 2007;120:112e–20e.
37. Tuin J, Tahiri Y, Paliga JT, Taylor JA, Bartlett SP. Distinguishing Goldenhar syndrome from Craniofacial Microsomia. J Craniofac Surg. 2015;26:1887–92.
38. Tuin AJ, Tahiri Y, Paine KM, Paliga JT, Taylor JA, Bartlett SP. Clarifying the relationships among the different features of the OMENS+ classification in craniofacial microsomia. Plast Reconstr Surg. 2015;135:149e–56e.
39. Poon CC, Meara JG, Heggie AA. Hemifacial microsomia: use of the OMENS-Plus classification at the Royal Children's Hospital of Melbourne. Plast Reconstr Surg. 2003;111:1011–8.
40. Roberson JB Jr, Goldsztein H, Balaker A, Schendel SA, Reinisch JF. HEAR MAPS a classification for congenital microtia/atresia based on the evaluation of 742 patients. Int J Pediatr Otorhinolaryngol. 2013;77:1551–4.
41. Tanzer RC. The constricted (cup and lop) ear. Plast Reconstr Surg. 1975;55:406–15.

Chapter 3
Microtia

Christopher A. Derderian

Introduction

Microtia can be used to describe a wide spectrum of malformations of the external ear, ranging from minor irregularities in the contour and size of the ear to a complete absence of the ear, known as anotia. Tanzer described the most commonly observed form of microtia – the Marx grade III or Nagata "lobular type" – as "the full-blown or complete form of microtia, comprising about 50% of significant ear deformities, represented by a lobule lying usually in a vertical position, capped by a nubbin containing a small mass of rolled up, elastic cartilage, bearing a vague resemblance to the auricle" [1]. The vast majority of patients with microtia also have conductive hearing loss making this a complex problem that affects both function and psychosocial well-being due to appearance. Microtia can occur in isolation, as part of a genetic syndrome, or in association with other anomalies such as those observed in craniofacial microsomia. This chapter will address relevant embryology, epidemiology, genetics, grading systems, and anatomic variants of microtia that may impact the clinical workup and surgical treatment of affected patients.

Embryology

The pharyngeal arches are composed of mesenchymal cells of mesodermal and neural crest origin. Wilhelm His introduced the traditional model of external ear development in which the ear is derived from three anterior hillocks on the first branchial

---

C. A. Derderian (✉)
Department of Plastic Surgery, University of Texas Southwestern Medical Center, Dallas, TX, USA
e-mail: Christopher.derderian@utsouthwestern.edu

© Springer Nature Switzerland AG 2019

J. F. Reinisch, Y. Tahiri (eds.), *Modern Microtia Reconstruction*,
https://doi.org/10.1007/978-3-030-16387-7_3

arch and three posterior hillocks on the second branchial arch [2–4]. These hillocks appear between fifth and sixth weeks of development as seen in Fig. 3.1a–d [2–5]. Streeter described the hillocks as "foci of more active proliferation of the condensed mesenchymal primordium" that outpace the proliferation of the surrounding mesenchyme until their rates of proliferation equalize at about week 7 of development (Figs. 3.1a–d and 3.2a–l) [4, 5]. The hillocks on first branchial arch are smaller, appear later, and disappear first compared to those of the second arch. His believed that the hillocks correlated to specific structures of the ears, but the importance of the hillocks to specific structures is now downplayed [5–7]. In the traditional model, the anterior hillocks contribute to the root of the helix, the anterior helical rim, the tragus, and the intertragic notch. The mesynchyme from the first pharyngeal arch also forms the malleus and incus of the ossicular chain [3]. The posterior hillocks from the second pharyngeal arch form the remaining posterior portion of the auricle, including the concha, antihelix, the inferior crus, triangular fossa, superior crus, helix, antitragus, and lobule. The mesenchyme of the second arch contributes to the stapes of the ossicular chain [3]. The proximity of the origins of the mandibular prominence of the first arch and the auricular hillocks is appreciable in Fig. 3.1a–d. Figure 3.2a–l demonstrates the development of the ear from the rising of the auricular hillocks to the fully developed form. The ear begins development in the anterior neck and migrates dorsal and cephalad to reach the adult position by about 20 weeks gestation.

Recently, several new concepts of ear development have been presented that amend the simple hillock model of His. In 2005, Porter and Tan presented a new model of how the posterior structures of the auricle form [5]. In their model, the anterior hillocks still contribute to the root of the helix, tragus, and antitragus. The contribution of the posterior hillocks is reduced to the concha, the body of the antihelix, the triangular fossa, and the inferior crus. The helix, scapha, and superior crus are derived from the "free ear fold" as delineated by the arrow and red dotted line in Fig. 3.1d. The free ear fold develops separately from tissue immediately caudal to the second pharyngeal arch hillocks [5–7].

Additional insight into development of the ear has come from transgenic animal models. The first branchial cleft between the first and second branchial arches has long been thought to develop into the external auditory canal, and that fusion of the cleft with the first branchial pouch (endoderm) forms the tympanic membrane. Cox and colleagues recently reviewed the effects of genetic mutations of *Hoxa2* on branchial arch derivatives in mouse models and presented evidence that the external auditory canal may be derived from an invagination within the first branchial arch that is separate from the first branchial cleft [7, 8]. These mouse models also suggest that the first branchial arch contributions to the ear may be more limited than previously thought, perhaps only contributing to the tragus [7]. The rapidly expanding number of animal models will continue to provide a deeper understanding of the genes important in the normal and abnormal development of the ear.

The common tissue origins of the external ear, the external auditory canal (meatus), and the middle ear structures from the first and second branchial arches

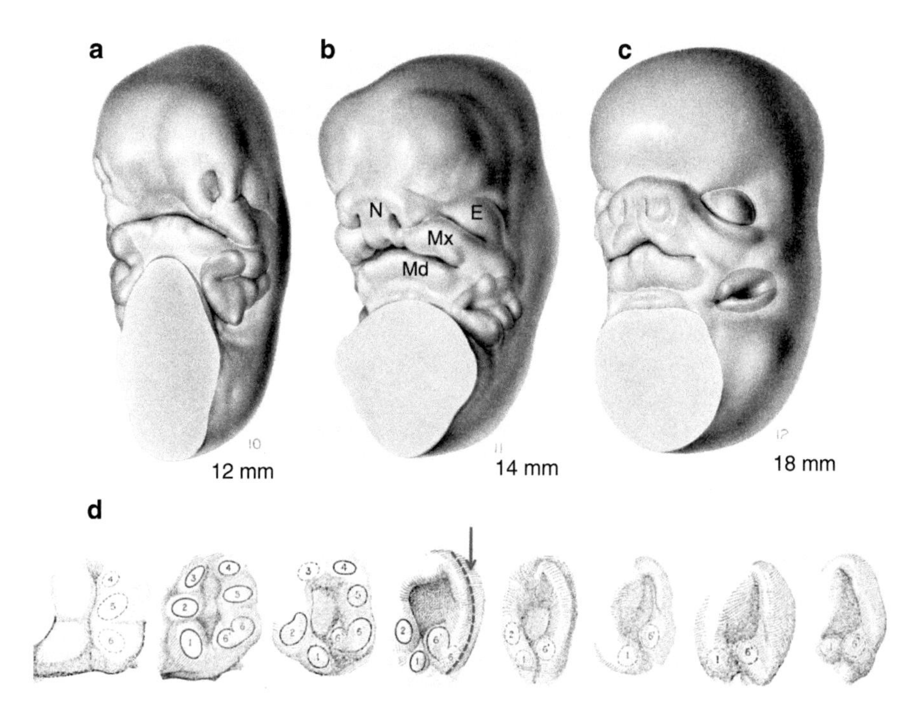

Fig. 3.1 These images are from Streeter's *Development of the Auricle in the Human Embryo*. The crown-rump length of the embryo is in the bottom left corner of (**a–c**). In A, the shaded anterior and posterior hillocks of His are seen arising from the first and second branchial arches. The separate mandibular and maxillary prominences are visible with the maxillary prominence fused to the medial and lateral nasal processes consistent with the sixth week of development. (**b**) Rapid proliferation of the tissues within the auricular hillocks. The proximity of the origins of the mandibular prominence of the first arch and auricular hillocks is appreciable. (**c**) Confluence of the auricular hillocks that are no longer appreciable. (**d**) Drawings from Streeter demonstrating the appearance of the individual, numbered hillocks and the sequence of their eventual confluence in the early phases of development of the external ear. The red arrow and dotted line in the fourth image demonstrate the approximate location and phase of development that the "free ear fold" appears as described by Porter and Tan. (Used with permission of the Carnegie Institute of Washington from Streeter [4])

including the ossicular chain likely explains the 80–90% incidence of congenital aural atresia and >90% incidence of conductive hearing loss in the setting of microtia (Fig. 3.3) [2, 9, 10]. The severity of the deformity of the external ear and middle ear are generally proportionate to one another [11]. The common tissue origins of the ear and the skeletal, muscular, and neural components of the face from the first and second branchial arches explains the high coincidence microtia with macrostomia, facial clefts, facial palsy, and facial asymmetry as seen in craniofacial microsomia (CFM) and the oculo-auricular-vertebral spectrum (OAVS). Approximately 65% of patients with CFM have microtia [12]. Our understanding of the function of genes

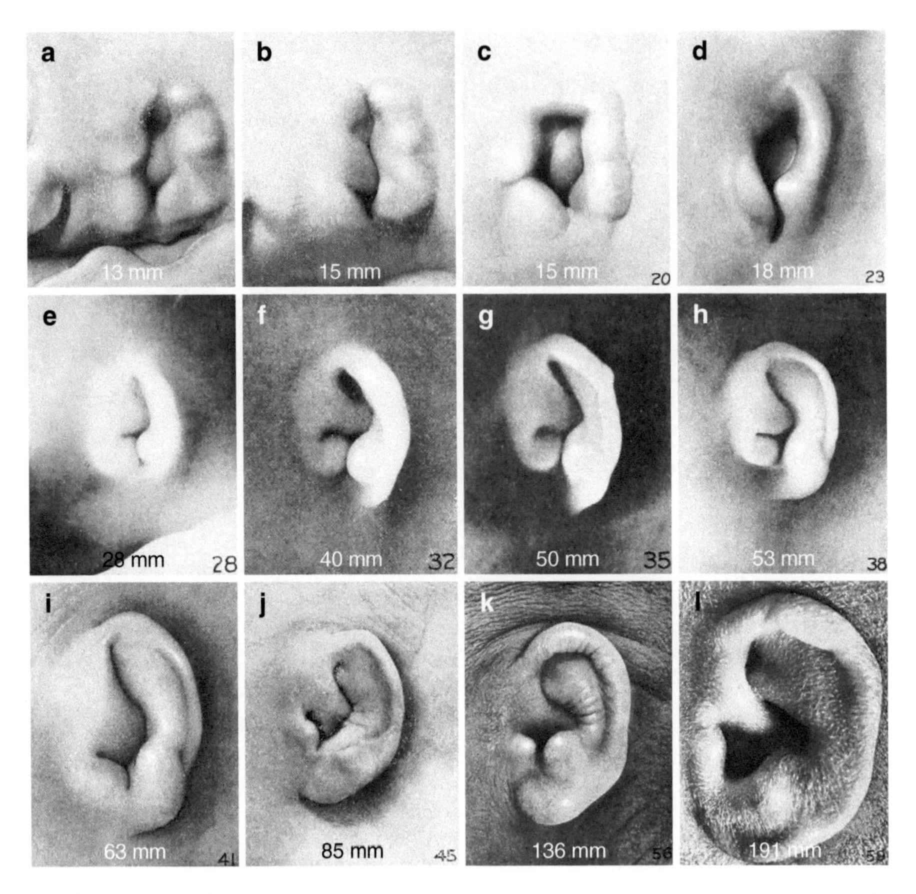

Fig. 3.2 (**a–d**) are drawings from Plates 2 and 3 of Streeter's *Development of the Auricle in the Human Embryo*. The crown-rump length is in the bottom center of the photo. Note the proliferation and confluence of the auricular hillocks in drawings (**a-d**). (**e–l**) are magnified photographs from Plates 4–6 Plate of Streeter's *Development of the Auricle in the Human Embryo*. (Used with permission of the Carnegie Institute of Washington from Streeter [4])

involved in cell migration, proliferation, patterning, and tissue identity within the structures derived from the first and second branchial arches is growing rapidly. It is important to note that patients with microtia may have malformations of distant structures developing synchronously with the ear including the heart, kidney, and/or eye [5].

The cochlea and semicircular canals of the inner ear develop from the otic placode, which is an ectodermal thickening not associated with the branchial arches, that invaginates to form the otic vesicle (Fig. 3.3) [3]. The distant tissue origin of the inner ear structures explains why the inner ear structures are usually normal in the setting of microtia.

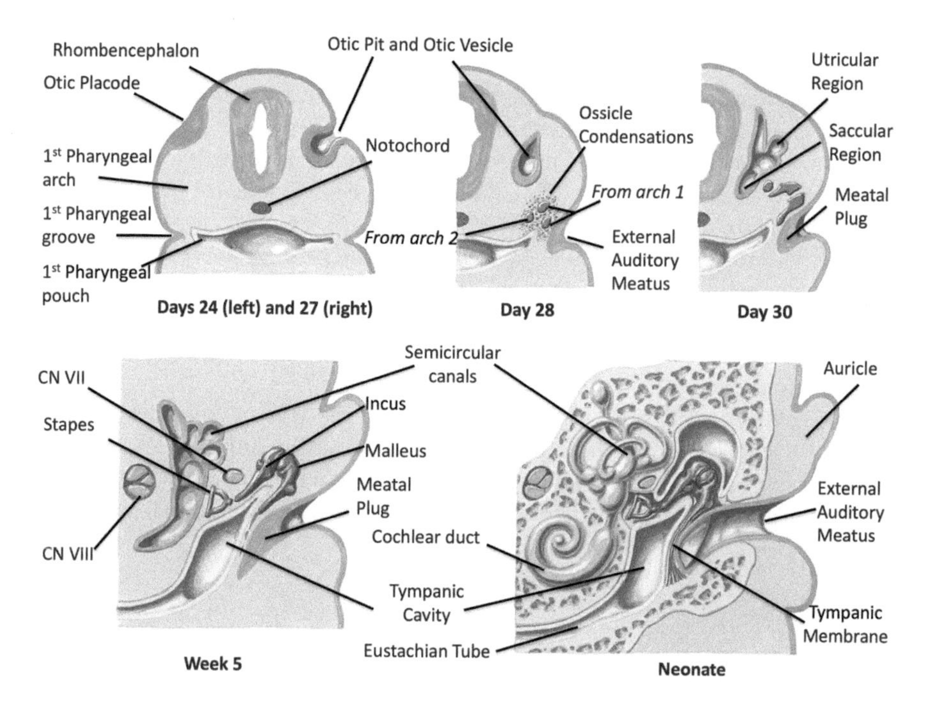

Fig. 3.3 This Netter illustration presents the cross-sectional development of the inner, middle, and outer ear elements. Note the distant ectodermal origin of the otic placode, pit, and vesicle with regard to the pharyngeal arches. The external ear and the ossicles are derived from first and second pharyngeal arch mesenchyme. The first pharyngeal cleft/groove eventually becomes the external acoustic meatus, and the first pharyngeal pouch eventually becomes the tympanic cavity. (Netter Illustration. Used with permission of Elsevier, Inc. All rights reserved. www.netterimages.com)

Incidence/Prevalence

The epidemiology of microtia and anotia may be described separately in the literature, but anotia will be included as part of the spectrum of microtia in this chapter. Microtia has a wide range of incidence depending on the population studied. Population studies from Western Europe, Asia, and the USA have shown rates of microtia ranging from 0.83 to 4.34 per 10,000 births [13–18]. The wide range in incidence may be due to several factors. Variations in inclusion and exclusion criteria between studies likely impacts this number to some degree, but there are also clearly populations at distinctly higher and lower risks for microtia. In general, Caucasians and Blacks have a lower risk for microtia than Hispanics and Asians. US population studies in Texas, California, and Hawaii demonstrated the incidence of microtia were 2.86, 2.5, and 3.79 cases per 10,000 births, respectively [13–16, 18]. Compared to Caucasians, African Americans have an equivalent or reduced relative risk of microtia. Compared to Caucasians, Asians and Pacific Islanders have a relative risk of 1.8–3.2, whereas Hispanics have a relative risk of 2.2–6.7 [13, 18]. Non-population-based studies have shown that Native Americans (particularly Navajo), Chileans, and Ecuadorians have even higher rates of microtia [19–24].

Microtia is more common in males who comprise 54–73% of all cases, depending on the study [14, 15, 17, 21, 25–27]. The majority of cases are unilateral (75–93%), with a right-sided propensity (60%) [14, 15, 17, 21, 25–27]. About 15–20% of all cases are bilateral, and those with bilateral microtia are more likely to have other anomalies present, such as in OAVS, or a genetic syndrome [13, 15, 17, 18]. As many as 85% and as few as 25% of the cases of microtia reported in the literature have been classified as "isolated" cases, perhaps due to the scrutiny with which other anomalies were identified and included [14, 15, 17, 21, 25–27].

Conductive hearing loss is present on the affected side in more than 90% of patients with microtia. In those patients with unilateral microtia, the majority of patients have normal hearing in the unaffected ear; however, a high index of suspicion for hearing loss is critical because 10% of patients have sensorineural hearing loss.

Risk Factors

Many risks factors have been identified for microtia. Maternal diabetes type I, maternal anemia, acute maternal illness in the first trimester, and maternal exposure to high altitude (above 2000 meters/6500 feet) have been identified as carrying a significant increased risk for microtia [6, 12, 15, 20, 26, 28, 29]. Other associated risks factors include high maternal or paternal age, multiple births, nonspecific maternal use of medication, and low birth weight. Racial and ethnic groups at increased risk include Native Americans (particularly Navajo), Hispanics, Ecuadorians, Chileans, Asians, Filipinos, and Pacific Islanders [13–19, 21, 22, 24].

Teratogens associated with microtia include retinoic acid, thalidomide, mycophenolate mofetil, and alcohol consumption [30–33]. Folic acid supplementation has been shown to reduce the risk of microtia [12, 34].

Pathogenesis

Vascular disruption or reduced blood flow leading to ischemia and poor growth or tissue necrosis has long been hypothesized as a possible cause of microtia. The strong association of microtia with anomalies of other derivatives of the first and second branchial arches, as observed in CFM and OAVS, and that these typically occur unilaterally supports such a global disruption theory. Much of the early scientific support for this hypothesis came from studies by Poswillo who showed that monkeys exposed to thalidomide and mice exposed to triazine exhibited hematomas at the junction of the pharyngeal and hyoid arteries [33, 35]. The animals demonstrated unilateral ear and mandible defects on the same side as the vascular disruption. Later, Otani and colleagues demonstrated that a transgenic mouse model of microtia with features of hemifacial microsomia exhibited rupture of the vasculature at the dorsal aspect of the second branchial arch [36–38]. No human correlate to this mutation has been found. Recently, Johnston and Bronsky examined Poswillo's experiments and concluded that the time frame in which the hematomas developed in Poswillo's animal models was too late in relation to drug delivery to be the cause of the observed deformities [12, 39, 40]. An expanding body of evidence for genetic causes of microtia and/or CFM and OAVS unrelated to vascular disruption has further weakened the vascular disruption theory.

Accumulating evidence now supports disturbances in the regulation of neural crest cell (NCC) proliferation and/or migration as a key causative factor for microtia. The causative mutation in Treacher Collins syndrome *TCOF1* causes abnormal ribosome function that decreases NCC proliferation and migration into the first and second pharyngeal arches [6, 12, 39, 41]. Abnormal development secondary to maternal diabetes or maternal retinoid exposure has been associated with abnormal NCC migration and differentiation in the pharyngeal arches [12]. As stated earlier, *Hoxa2* is expressed by NCC in the second pharyngeal arch and appears to play a critical role in defining the second pharyngeal arch identity. When expressed by first branchial arch NCC, *Hoxa2* causes the first pharyngeal arch to form second pharyngeal arch structures [7]. Conversely, *Hoxa2* knockout mice develop microtia [12, 42]. Therefore, it seems more likely that genetic influences on NCC migration, proliferation, and tissue identity play a more important role in the pathogenesis of microtia than vascular disruption.

Genetics of Microtia

The evidence of genetic causes of microtia comes from both human studies and animal models with known genetic mutations and microtia. The incidence of familial cases of microtia ranges from 3% to 34% [6, 12, 39, 43]. Artunduaga and colleagues published a study of twins demonstrating a higher concordance of microtia in monozygotic twins (38.5%) versus dizygotic twins (4.5%), strengthening the evidence for a genetic predisposition [44]. Several reports of familial cases with autosomal recessive or dominant modes of inheritance with variable expression and incomplete penetrance have been summarized [6, 12, 39].

Approximately 40% of patients with microtia have associated anomalies or a known syndrome [6, 12, 13, 18, 43]. Facial clefts, facial asymmetry, renal abnormalities, cardiac defects, microphthalmia, polydactyly, and vertebral anomalies are the most common abnormal findings found in patients with microtia [2, 6, 39, 43, 45]. Many of these associated anomalies fit within or overlap with the diagno-

Table 3.1 Common microtia syndromes

Syndrome	Frequency of Microtia	Genes Identified
Auriculo-condylar	100	*PLCB4, GNAI3*
Branchio-oto	80–90	*SIX1, EYA1*
Branchio-oto-renal	30–60	*SIX5, EYA1*
CHARGE	80–100	*CHD7*
Craniofacial microsomia	65%	*GSC*
Kabuki	80–85	*MLL2, KDM6a*
Mandibulofacial dysostosis	100	*HOXD*
Mandibulofacial dysostosis with microcephaly	98	*EFTUD2*
Meier-Gorlin (ear-patella-short stature)	100	*ORC1, ORC4, ORC6, CDT1, CDC6*
Microtia, hearing impairment, and cleft palate	100	*HOXA2*
Nager	80	*SF3B4*
Oculo-auricular	100	*HMX1*
Townes-Brocks	88	*SALL1*
Treacher Collins	60–80	*TCOF1*

Data from:
Alasti and Van Camp [43]
Bartel-Friedrich [6]
Gendron et al. [39]
Luquetti et al. [12]

sis oculo-auriculo-vertebral spectrum (OAVS) that has ear dysplasia including microtia as a major feature. There are several syndromes associated with microtia, but we will discuss only the more commonly associated sydromes in the following text. Table 3.1 summarizes the syndromes, mutations, and frequency of microtia.

OAVS

Oculo-auriculo-vertebral spectrum (OAVS) is a heterogeneous disorder that primarily affects structures derived from the first and second branchial arches [39, 45]. Characteristic features of OAVS overlap with other named syndromes and constellations of findings associated with microtia including craniofacial microsomia (CFM), first and second pharyngeal arch anomalies, and Goldenhar syndrome, which represents the severe end of the oculo-auriculo-vertebral spectrum [45].

Patients with OAVS have asymmetric ear deformities including preauricular pits and tags with variable dysplasia of the ear ranging from normal or mild abnormalities to microtia with the majority of patients experiencing some degree of hearing loss [6, 12, 45, 46]. Facial asymmetry is variably present due to hypoplasia of the jaws and/or hypoplasia of the overlying soft tissues. Facial palsy may also be present [6, 12, 45, 46]. It is important to note that patients with microtia and congenital aural atresia and facial nerve weakness have a 60% incidence of sensorineural hearing loss as compared to those who do not have facial nerve dysfunction (7%) [47].

Macrostomia is the most frequently occurring orofacial cleft in OAVS, but cleft lip and palate may also be present [45]. Epibulbar dermoids are the most common occular finding [45]. Coloboma and microphthalmia can occur but are less frequently present. Vertebral anomalies are also a common finding. The majority of patients with OAVS have one side affected. As in microtia, the right side is affected more commonly, and there is a male predilection [12, 25, 45]. When bilateral, most patients demonstrate asymmetry in severity [12, 25, 45, 46]. Some controversy exists as to whether all patients with microtia, including apparently "isolated microtia," should carry the diagnosis of OAVS that may cloud the reporting of the coincidence of microtia and OAVS. A case example of a patient with bilateral OAVS is shown in Fig. 3.4a–c. Note the significant asymmetry in the skeletal, soft tissue, and ear dysplasia in this 9-year-old female.

Most cases of OAVS are sporadic. Reports of familial transmission of AOVS following autosomal dominant and recessive patterns of inheritance, genetic linkage in familial transmission and overlapping features of OAVS with chromosomal aberrations have been reported [6, 45]. A strong allelic expression imbalance of the *BAPX1* gene has been identified in fibroblasts of patients with OAVS [39, 43, 48]. Human Goosecoid (GSC) is a transcription factor whose overlapping expression with BAPX1 during development appears to be important for ear development. In mouse models, disruption of the *Gsc* expression causes abnormal development of the mandible, the external auditory meatus, and the inner ear [39, 43].

Treacher Collins Syndrome

Treacher Collins syndrome (TCS) is an autosomal dominant condition with an estimated incidence of 1 in 50,000 live births [41]. The characteristic features of TCS include severe hypoplasia of the facial bones including characteristic hypoplasia or absence of the zygomata, down-slanting of the palpebral fissures, cleft palate, micrognathia, and microtia in 60–80% of patients. TCS demonstrates autosomal dominant inheritance with variable penetrance [41]. Mutations of the *TCOF1* gene cause the syndrome with 60% of cases occurring spontaneously and 40% of cases demonstrating familial inheritance [41, 43, 49]. *TCOF1* encodes the protein Treacle that is important in ribosome biogenesis. Mutations of *TCOF1* in mouse models results in abnormal proliferation and migration of cranial neural crest cells into the first and second branchial arches leading to severe hypoplasia of the ears, soft tissues of the face, and craniofacial skeleton [49].

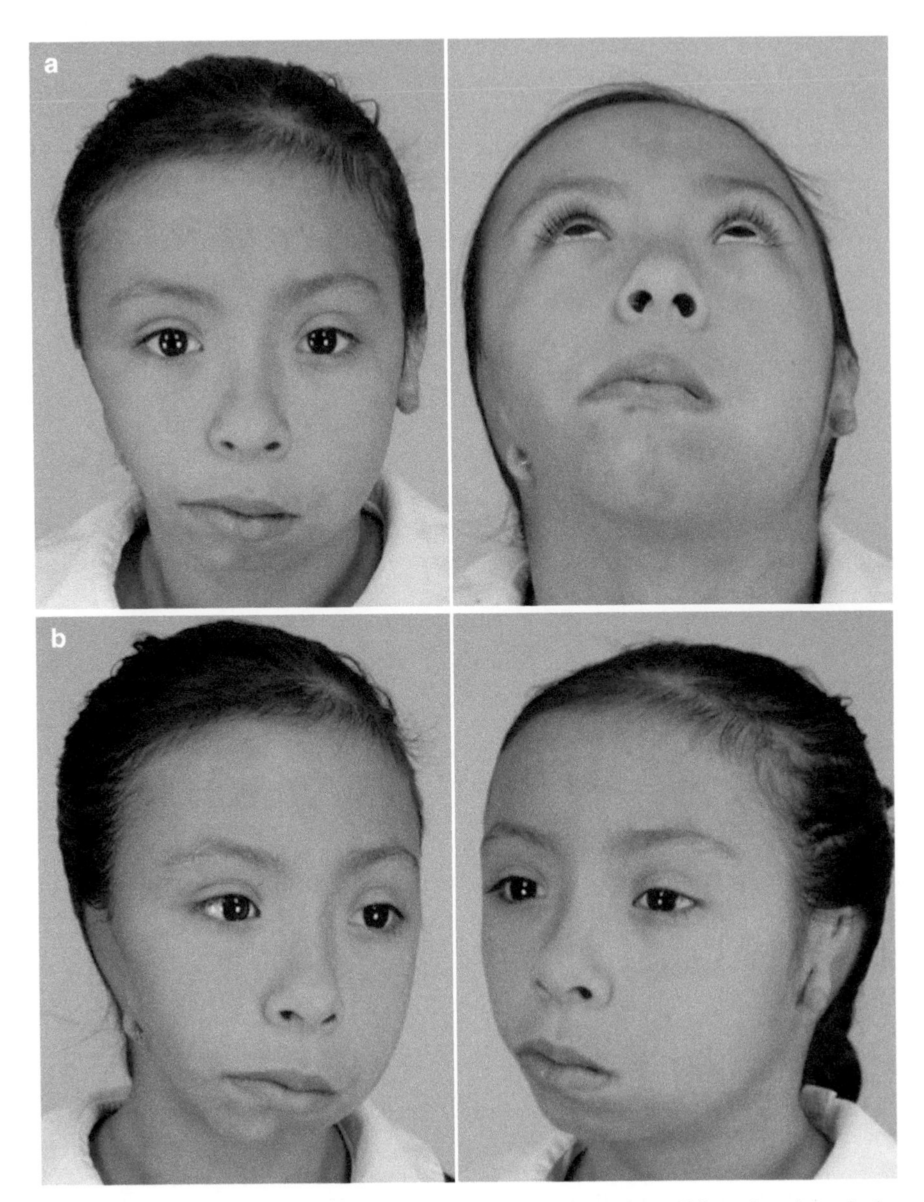

Fig. 3.4 (**a–c**) This 9-year old girl has bilateral microtia in the setting of bilateral oculo-auriculo-vetebral spectrum (OAVS). Note the significant asymmetry in the skeletal, soft tissue, and ear dysplasia in this 9-year-old female. Severe mandibular hypoplasia contributes to a depressed skeletal platform on the patient's right. Although the grade of microtia would be classified as similar in most systems, there is asymmetry in the size and position of the remnants and lobules. The hairline and lobule and remnant position are both lower on the patient's right side. The local soft tissues are more atrophic on the right, and the side burn is also ill defined on the right. In patients with this degree of skeletal and soft tissue dysplasia, there is often an aberrant course of the superficial temporal vessels with a low branch point

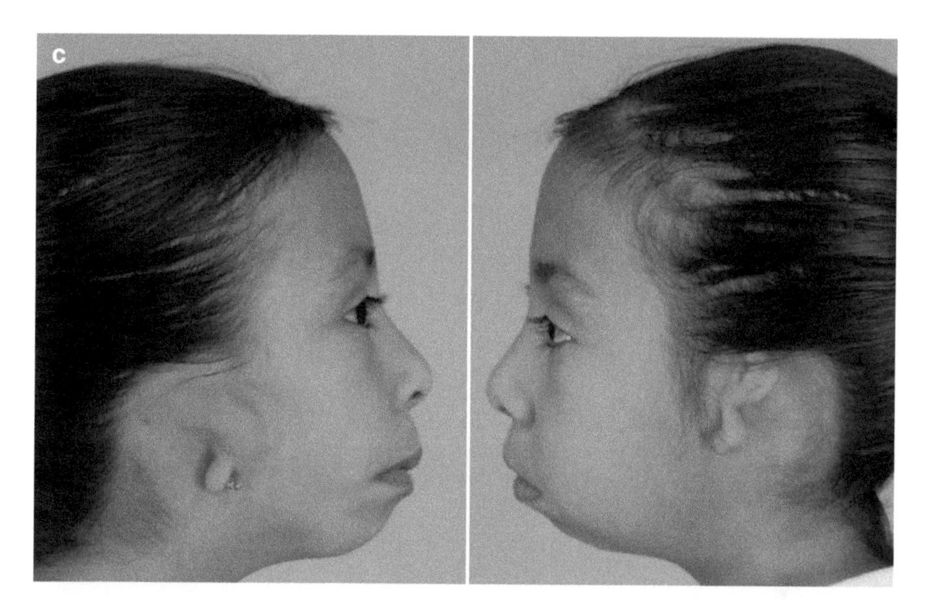

Fig. 3.4 (continued)

Classification Systems

Multiple classification systems for microtia have been proposed based upon recurrent patterns of malformation (Box 3.1). Simplified systems are the easiest to use, but they are the least specific with regard to the appearance of the ear. Marx introduced a simple system in 1926 that is still commonly used: grade I – small ear but normal features; grade II – microtia with some but not all normal structures; grade III – microtia with a small remnant and no recognizable features; and a later modification by Rogers added grade IV for anotia [50, 51]. Tanzer, Nagata, and Firmin created classification systems that correlated the microtic remnant classification with their surgical approaches to treatment [1, 52, 53]. Weerda presented a grading system of three degrees of severity of dysplasia of the ear including macrotia and abnormal morphology such as protruding ears and cryptotia [54]. Figure 3.5 demonstrates the full spectrum of microtia variants from anotia to nearly normal ears with minor irregularities.

Recent efforts in improving classification systems have been focused on more comprehensive and accurate description of the features of the ear that are present or absent and other relevant physical findings. A recent classification system by Roberson and Reinisch uses the acronym HEAR MAPS that combines grading of aural atresia, a modified Marx grading of microtia, and OMENS-type grading of

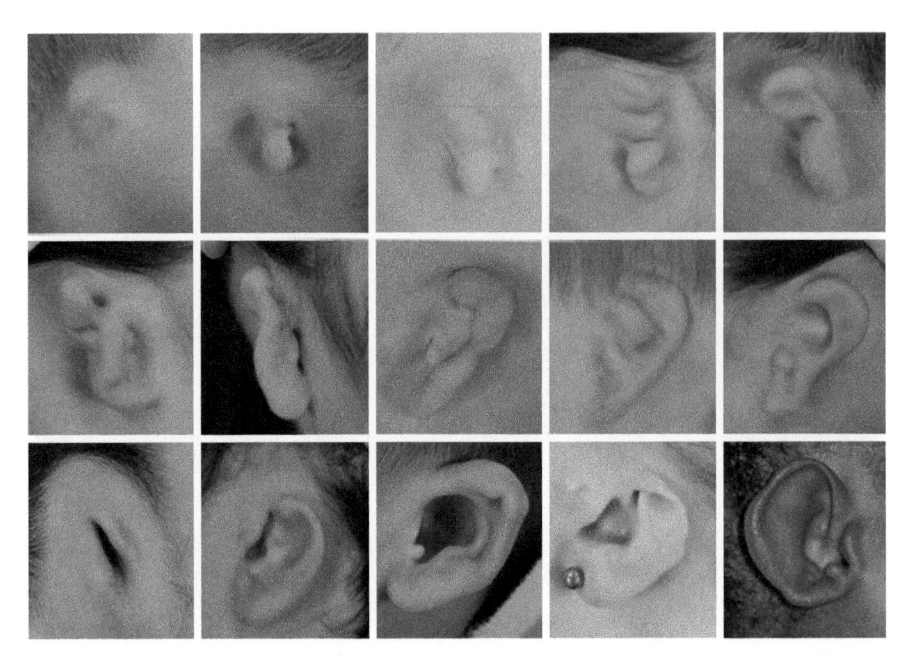

Fig. 3.5 The full spectrum of microtia is shown in this figure. The top left image demonstrates anotia (Marx grade IV), and the images change from left to right with variety of forms of Marx III/lobular type microtia with peanut-shaped nubbins of cartilage above vertically rotated lobules. The middle row demonstrates increasingly more "ear like" remnants with the lobule gradually assuming a more normal orientation, but no obviously recognizable features in the cartilaginous structures. The bottom row shows a wide range of microtia with recognizable features and some nearly normal appearing ears. (Copyright retained by Christopher A. Derderian, MD. Used with permission)

Box 3.1 Classification Systems for Microtia
Marx/Rogers (1, 2)

Grade I A smaller than normal auricle with all normal features of an ear
Grade II An abnormal auricle with some recognizable normal structures
Grade III An abnormal auricle with some no recognizable normal structures
Grade IV Anotia

Tanzer (3)

1. Anotia
2. Complete hypoplasia (microtia)
   (a) With atresia of the external auditory canal
   (b) Without atresia of the external auditory canal
3. Hypoplasia of the middle third of the auricle
4. Hypoplasia of the superior third of the auricle

(a) Constricted (cup and lop) ear
(b) Cryptoptia
(c) Hypoplasia of entire superior third

5. Prominent ear

Weerda (4)

I. **First-degree dysplasia**

Most structures of a normal auricle are recognizable (minor deformities)

A. Macrotia
B. Protruding ears (prominent ears)
C. Cryptotia
D. Absence of the upper helix
E. Small deformities: absence of tragus, satyr ear (pointed ear, "Devil's ear"), Darwin's tubercle, Stahl ear
F. Colobomata (transverse clefts)
G. Lobule deformities
H. Cup ear deformities

1. Type I: Cupped upper portion of the helix (lidding; mild lop/constricted ear)
2. Type II: Severe cup ear deformity

II. **Second-degree dysplasia**

Some structures of a normal auricle are recognizable
Synonym Marx grade II microtia

A. Cup ear deformity, type III – the severe cop ear is malformed in all dimensions
B. Mini ear

III. **Third-degree dysplasia**

None of the structures of a normal auricle are recognizable
Synonyms: peanut ear, Marx grade III microtia

A. Unilateral
B. Bilateral
C. Anotia

Nagata (5)

1. **Lobule type:** remnant ear and ear lobule without concha, acoustic meatus and tragus
2. **Concha type:** remnant ear, ear lobule, concha, acoustic meatus, tragus, and incisura intertragica

3. **Small concha type:** remnant ear and lobule and a small indentation representing the concha
4. **Anotia:** no ear or tissue with minute resemblance to an ear
5. **Atypical:** cases that do not fall into the above classifications

Hunter et al. (6)

Microtia first degree: presence of all the normal ear components and the median longitudinal length more than 2 SD below the mean

Microtia second degree: median longitudinal length of the ear more than 2 SD below the mean in the presence of some, but not all, parts of the normal ear

Microtia third degree: presence of some auricular structures, but none of these structures conform to recognized ear components

Anotia: complete absence of the ear

HEAR MAPS Roberson et al. (7)

Hear bone/air

Ear (microtia Marx grade)

Atresia Jahrsdoerder CT Scale (1–10)

Remnant earlobe

Grade 1 Normal
Grade 2 Mildly reduced
Grade 3 Moderately Reduced
Grade 4 Severely reduced/absent

Mandible

Grade 1 Normal
Grade 2 Mildly reduced
Grade 3 Moderately reduced
Grade 4 Severely reduced/absent

Asymmetry soft tissue

Grade 1 Normal
Grade 2 Mildly reduced
Grade 3 Moderately reduced
Grade 4 Severely reduced/absent

Paresis facial nerve

House-Brackmann scale (1–6)

Syndrome

Grade 1 None
Grade 2 Yes

Luquetti et al. (8)
Phenotypic assessment tool-Microtia (PAT-Microtia)

1. Marx H. Die Missbildungen des ohres. In: Handbuch der Spez Path Anatomie Histologie. Berlin: Springer; 1924. p.131.
2. Rogers B. Anatomy, embryology and classification of auricular defor-mites. In: Tanzer RC, Edgerton MT, editors. Symposium on reconstruction of the Auricle, vol 10. Saint Louis: C. V. Mosby Co.; 1974.
3. Tanzer RC. Microtia. Clin Plast Surg. 1978;5(3):317–36.
4. Weerda H. Classification of congenital deformities of the auricle. Facial Plast Surg. 1988;5(5):385–8.
5. Nagata S. Microtia: auricular reconstruction. In: Achauer BM, Eriksson E, Guyuron B, Coleman III JJ, Russell RC, Vander Kolk CA, editors. Plastic surgery: indications, operations and outcomes. vol 2. St. Louis, MO: Mosby; 2000.
6. Hunter A, Frias JL, Gillessen-Kaesbach G, Hughes H, Jones KL, Wilson L. Elements of morphology: standard terminology for the ear. Am J Med Genet A. 2009;149A(1):40–60.
7. Roberson JB, Jr., Goldsztein H, Balaker A, Schendel SA, Reinisch JF. HEAR MAPS a classification for congenital microtia/atresia based on the evaluation of 742 patients. Int J Pediatr Otorhinolaryngol. 2013;77(9):1551–4.
8. Luquetti DV, Saltzman BS, Sie KC, Birgfeld CB, Leroux BG, Evans KN, et al. Interrater reliability of a phenotypic assessment tool for the ear morphology in microtia. Am J Med Genet A. 2013;161A(6):1264–72.

features of craniofacial microsomia (CFM), and the presence or absence of syndromes [55, 56].

HEAR MAPS grades the atresia using the Jarhsdoerfer's 10-point scale, which deducts a point if the external ear is abnormal, but provides little information about the severity of the ear deformity or related craniofacial abnormalities [55]. Grading the severity of the skeletal and soft tissue abnormality is an important consideration that greatly impacts the outcomes of ear reconstruction, but these elements are omitted in most grading systems. In all patients, particularly those with facial asymmetry due to CFM or related syndromes, the position of the remnant ear, position of the hairline, amount and quality of local skin available for construct coverage, and adequacy of the underlying skeletal platform will all impact the quality of the reconstruction. However, most grading scales comment only on how normal the ear is. Figure 3.4a–c demonstrates how the patient with asymmetric position of remnants with the same Marx grading of III presents a much greater challenge on the right where the remnant is abnormally low when compared to the left that is in a much more favorable position, on a more stable skeletal platform, with a better hairline position and more local skin available.

In 2013, Luquetti and colleagues introduced a detailed, standardized phenotypic assessment tool (PAT-Microtia) [57]. This tool uses standardized terminology presented by Hunter and colleagues for normal and abnormal ear findings to more precisely characterize the anatomic changes and facilitate identification of patterns of microtia [58]. Using a more detailed assessment tool such as the PAT-Microtia can increase accuracy in detailing the appearance of the ear and associated findings with particular patterns that may be helpful in future clinical and genetic research efforts. The additional complexity of this type of tool may be more time consuming and may require a more experienced clinician for accurate diagnosis.

Hearing Issues

Congenital aural atresia (CAA) is present in 80–90% of the cases of microtia [2, 10, 30]. The severity of the deformity of the external and middle ear is generally proportionate to one another [11]. Eighty to 90% of these patients have conductive hearing loss only, but 10–15% of patients can have a sensorineural hearing loss (SNHL) also [2, 10, 30]. A notable exception to this statistic is when patients have CAA in the presence of facial nerve palsy, particularly in the setting of craniofacial microsomia, because of a much higher incidence of SNHL in this population [59, 60].

The majority of patients with microtia have unilateral disease and normal hearing in the contralateral ear that allows for normal speech and language development. When assessing newborns with unilateral microtia and CAA, it is important to know the hearing status of the non-microtic ear. If normal hearing is present on the newborn hearing screen, one can expect normal speech development. If there is any concern regarding the hearing status of the non-microtic ear in unilateral cases, or in bilateral microtia cases, diagnostic auditory brainstem response (ABR) testing should be performed. Any conditions affecting the normal ear such as recurrent otitis or effusions should be treated aggressively to protect hearing in the unaffected ear [2, 10, 30]. The management of aural atresia will be discussed in detail elsewhere in this book.

Summary

There is a wide spectrum of severity of microtia. Abnormal proliferation and migration of neural crest cells into the first and second branchial arches appears to be important in the pathogenesis of microtia. The common tissue origins of the external and middle ear structures from the first and second branchial arches result in the vast majority of patients with microtia also having congenital aural atresia and conductive hearing loss. Ten to 15% of patients with microtia also have sensorineural hearing loss. Patients with other constellations of anomalies – such as CFM, microtia, and facial nerve palsy – have an increased risk for sensorineural hearing loss.

Hispanics, Asians, Native Americans, and subpopulations of South America have an increased risk for microtia compared to Caucasians and Blacks. Isolated cases of microtia must be distinguished from syndromic cases and those that occur in the setting of other anomalies such as CFM and OAVS. Patients with bilateral microtia are more likely to have a syndrome, and/or other anomalies. In the setting of OAVS, bilateral microtia is often asymmetric. The skeletal and soft tissue dysplasia that can accompany microtia may significantly impact the potential reconstructive outcome, but the impact of the factors is not reflected in many grading systems.

References

1. Tanzer RC. Microtia. Clin Plast Surg. 1978;5(3):317–36.
2. Beahm EK, Walton RL. Auricular reconstruction for microtia: part I. Anatomy, embryology, and clinical evaluation. Plast Reconstr Surg. 2002;109(7):2473–82; quiz following 82.
3. Sadler TW. Langman's medical embryology. 13th ed. Philadelphia: Wolters Kluwer; 2015; xiii, 407 pages
4. Streeter GL. Development of the auricle in the human embryo. Carnegie Instn Wash Publ 277, Contrib Embryol. 1922;14:111–38.
5. Porter CJ, Tan ST. Congenital auricular anomalies: topographic anatomy, embryology, classification, and treatment strategies. Plast Reconstr Surg. 2005;115(6):1701–12.
6. Bartel-Friedrich S. Congenital auricular malformations: description of anomalies and syndromes. Facial Plast Surg. 2015;31(6):567–80.
7. Cox TC, Camci ED, Vora S, Luquetti DV, Turner EE. The genetics of auricular development and malformation: new findings in model systems driving future directions for microtia research. Eur J Med Genet. 2014;57(8):394–401.
8. Minoux M, Kratochwil CF, Ducret S, Amin S, Kitazawa T, Kurihara H, et al. Mouse Hoxa2 mutations provide a model for microtia and auricle duplication. Development. 2013;140(21):4386–97.
9. Dougherty W, Kesser BW. Management of conductive hearing loss in children. Otolaryngol Clin N Am. 2015;48(6):955–74.
10. Kelley PE, Scholes MA. Microtia and congenital aural atresia. Otolaryngol Clin N Am. 2007;40(1):61–80, vi.
11. Kountakis SE, Helidonis E, Jahrsdoerfer RA. Microtia grade as an indicator of middle ear development in aural atresia. Arch Otolaryngol Head Neck Surg. 1995;121(8):885–6.
12. Luquetti DV, Heike CL, Hing AV, Cunningham ML, Cox TC. Microtia: epidemiology and genetics. Am J Med Genet A. 2012;158A(1):124–39.
13. Canfield MA, Langlois PH, Nguyen LM, Scheuerle AE. Epidemiologic features and clinical subgroups of anotia/microtia in Texas. Birth Defects Res A Clin Mol Teratol. 2009;85(11):905–13.
14. Forrester MB, Merz RD. Descriptive epidemiology of anotia and microtia, Hawaii, 1986-2002. Congenit Anom (Kyoto). 2005;45(4):119–24.
15. Harris J, Kallen B, Robert E. The epidemiology of anotia and microtia. J Med Genet. 1996;33(10):809–13.
16. Husain T, Langlois PH, Sever LE, Gambello MJ. Descriptive epidemiologic features shared by birth defects thought to be related to vascular disruption in Texas, 1996-2002. Birth Defects Res A Clin Mol Teratol. 2008;82(6):435–40.
17. Mastroiacovo P, Corchia C, Botto LD, Lanni R, Zampino G, Fusco D. Epidemiology and genetics of microtia-anotia: a registry based study on over one million births. J Med Genet. 1995;32(6):453–7.

18. Shaw GM, Carmichael SL, Kaidarova Z, Harris JA. Epidemiologic characteristics of anotia and microtia in California, 1989-1997. Birth Defects Res A Clin Mol Teratol. 2004;70(7):472–5.
19. Aase JM, Tegtmeier RE. Microtia in New Mexico: evidence for multifactorial causation. Birth Defects Orig Artic Ser. 1977;13(3A):113–6.
20. Castilla EE, Lopez-Camelo JS, Campana H. Altitude as a risk factor for congenital anomalies. Am J Med Genet. 1999;86(1):9–14.
21. Castilla EE, Orioli IM. Prevalence rates of microtia in South America. Int J Epidemiol. 1986;15(3):364–8.
22. Jaffe BF. The incidence of ear diseases in the Navajo Indians. Laryngoscope. 1969;79(12):2126–34.
23. Nazer J, Lay-Son G, Cifuentes L. Prevalence of microtia and anotia at the maternity of the University of Chile Clinical Hospital. Rev Med Chil. 2006;134(10):1295–301.
24. Nelson SM, Berry RI. Ear disease and hearing loss among Navajo children--a mass survey. Laryngoscope. 1984;94(3):316–23.
25. Rollnick BR, Kaye CI, Nagatoshi K, Hauck W, Martin AO. Oculoauriculovertebral dysplasia and variants: phenotypic characteristics of 294 patients. Am J Med Genet. 1987;26(2):361–75.
26. Okajima H, Takeichi Y, Umeda K, Baba S. Clinical analysis of 592 patients with microtia. Acta Otolaryngol Suppl. 1996;525:18–24.
27. Suutarla S, Rautio J, Ritvanen A, Ala-Mello S, Jero J, Klockars T. Microtia in Finland: comparison of characteristics in different populations. Int J Pediatr Otorhinolaryngol. 2007;71(8):1211–7.
28. Luquetti DV, Cox TC, Lopez-Camelo J, Dutra Mda G, Cunningham ML, Castilla EE. Preferential associated anomalies in 818 cases of microtia in South America. Am J Med Genet A. 2013;161A(5):1051–7.
29. Luquetti DV, Saltzman BS, Lopez-Camelo J, Dutra Mda G, Castilla EE. Risk factors and demographics for microtia in South America: a case-control analysis. Birth Defects Res A Clin Mol Teratol. 2013;97(11):736–43.
30. Carey JC. Ear. In: Stevenson RE, Hall JG, editors. Human malformations and related anomalies. 2nd ed. Oxford/New York: Oxford University Press; 2006. p. 327–72.
31. Monga M. Vitamin A and its congeners. Semin Perinatol. 1997;21(2):135–42.
32. Perez-Aytes A, Ledo A, Boso V, Saenz P, Roma E, Poveda JL, et al. In utero exposure to mycophenolate mofetil: a characteristic phenotype? Am J Med Genet A. 2008;146A(1):1–7.
33. Poswillo D. The pathogenesis of the first and second branchial arch syndrome. Oral Surg Oral Med Oral Pathol. 1973;35(3):302–28.
34. Ma C, Carmichael SL, Scheuerle AE, Canfield MA, Shaw GM. National Birth Defects Prevention S. Association of microtia with maternal obesity and periconceptional folic acid use. Am J Med Genet A. 2010;152A(11):2756–61.
35. Poswillo D. Hemorrhage in development of the face. Birth Defects Orig Artic Ser. 1975;11(7):61–81.
36. Cousley R, Naora H, Yokoyama M, Kimura M, Otani H. Validity of the Hfm transgenic mouse as a model for hemifacial microsomia. Cleft Palate Craniofac J. 2002;39(1):81–92.
37. Naora H, Kimura M, Otani H, Yokoyama M, Koizumi T, Katsuki M, et al. Transgenic mouse model of hemifacial microsomia: cloning and characterization of insertional mutation region on chromosome 10. Genomics. 1994;23(3):515–9.
38. Otani H, Tanaka O, Naora H, Yokoyama M, Nomura T, Kimura M, et al. Microtia as an autosomal dominant mutation in a transgenic mouse line: a possible animal model of branchial arch anomalies. Anat Anz. 1991;172(1):1–9.
39. Gendron C, Schwentker A, van Aalst JA. Genetic advances in the understanding of microtia. J Pediatr Genet. 2016;5(4):189–97.
40. Johnston MC, Bronsky PT. Prenatal craniofacial development: new insights on normal and abnormal mechanisms. Crit Rev Oral Biol Med. 1995;6(1):25–79.
41. Trainor PA, Dixon J, Dixon MJ. Treacher Collins syndrome: etiology, pathogenesis and prevention. Eur J Hum Genet. 2009;17(3):275–83.
42. Gendron-Maguire M, Mallo M, Zhang M, Gridley T. Hoxa-2 mutant mice exhibit homeotic transformation of skeletal elements derived from cranial neural crest. Cell. 1993;75(7):1317–31.

43. Alasti F, Van Camp G. Genetics of microtia and associated syndromes. J Med Genet. 2009;46(6):361–9.
44. Artunduaga MA, Quintanilla-Dieck Mde L, Greenway S, Betensky R, Nicolau Y, Hamdan U, et al. A classic twin study of external ear malformations, including microtia. N Engl J Med. 2009;361(12):1216–8.
45. Beleza-Meireles A, Clayton-Smith J, Saraiva JM, Tassabehji M. Oculo-auriculo-vertebral spectrum: a review of the literature and genetic update. J Med Genet. 2014;51(10):635–45.
46. Cohen MM Jr, Rollnick BR, Kaye CI. Oculoauriculovertebral spectrum: an updated critique. Cleft Palate J. 1989;26(4):276–86.
47. Vrabec JT, Lin JW. Inner ear anomalies in congenital aural atresia. Otol Neurotol. 2010;31(9):1421–6.
48. Fischer S, Ludecke HJ, Wieczorek D, Bohringer S, Gillessen-Kaesbach G, Horsthemke B. Histone acetylation dependent allelic expression imbalance of BAPX1 in patients with the oculo-auriculo-vertebral spectrum. Hum Mol Genet. 2006;15(4):581–7.
49. Dixon J, Jones NC, Sandell LL, Jayasinghe SM, Crane J, Rey JP, et al. Tcof1/treacle is required for neural crest cell formation and proliferation deficiencies that cause craniofacial abnormalities. Proc Natl Acad Sci U S A. 2006;103(36):13403–8.
50. Rogers B. Anatomy, embryology and classification of auricular deformites. In: Tanzer RC, Edgerton MT, editors. Symposium on reconstruction of the Auricle, vol. 10. Saint Louis: C. V. Mosby Co.; 1974.
51. Marx H. Die Missbildungen des ohres. In: Handbuch der Spez path Anatomie Histologie. Berlin: Springer; 1924. p. 131.
52. Firmin F, Marchac A. A novel algorithm for autologous ear reconstruction. Semin Plast Surg. 2011;25(4):257–64.
53. Nagata S. Microtia: auricular reconstruction. In: Achauer BM, Eriksson E, Guyuron B, Coleman III JJ, Russell RC, Vander Kolk CA, editors. Plastic surgery: indications, operations and outcomes, vol. 2. St. Louis, MO: Mosby; 2000.
54. Weerda H. Classification of congenital deformities of the auricle. Facial Plast Surg. 1988;5(5):385–8.
55. Roberson JB Jr, Goldsztein H, Balaker A, Schendel SA, Reinisch JF. HEAR MAPS a classification for congenital microtia/atresia based on the evaluation of 742 patients. Int J Pediatr Otorhinolaryngol. 2013;77(9):1551–4.
56. Gougoutas AJ, Singh DJ, Low DW, Bartlett SP. Hemifacial microsomia: clinical features and pictographic representations of the OMENS classification system. Plast Reconstr Surg. 2007;120(7):112e–20e.
57. Luquetti DV, Saltzman BS, Sie KC, Birgfeld CB, Leroux BG, Evans KN, et al. Interrater reliability of a phenotypic assessment tool for the ear morphology in microtia. Am J Med Genet A. 2013;161A(6):1264–72.
58. Hunter A, Frias JL, Gillessen-Kaesbach G, Hughes H, Jones KL, Wilson L. Elements of morphology: standard terminology for the ear. Am J Med Genet A. 2009;149A(1):40–60.
59. Bassila MK, Goldberg R. The association of facial palsy and/or sensorineural hearing loss in patients with hemifacial microsomia. Cleft Palate J. 1989;26(4):287–91.
60. Carvalho GJ, Song CS, Vargervik K, Lalwani AK. Auditory and facial nerve dysfunction in patients with hemifacial microsomia. Arch Otolaryngol Head Neck Surg. 1999;125(2):209–12.

Chapter 4
Microtia-Associated Syndromes

Sunil S. Tholpady and Michael W. Chu

Abbreviations

OAVS	Oculo-auriculo-vertebral spectrum
OMIM	Online Mendelian Inheritance in Man
TCS	Treacher Collins syndrome

Introduction

External ear development occurs from derivations of the first (mandibular) and second (hyoid) pharyngeal arches, with the first pharyngeal cleft responsible for the external auditory meatus. At approximately 5 weeks of age, each arch develops three elevations that form into the six hillocks of His that create very specific auricular structures. From the mandibular arch, the three hillocks form the tragus, helix, and cymba concha, while the three hillocks from the hyoid arch form the concha, antihelix, and antitragus. The ear is attached to the skull by anterior and posterior extrinsic as well as intrinsic ligaments, external (auricularis anterior, superior, and posterior) and internal (helicis major and minor, tragicus, antitragicus, and the transverse and oblique) muscles, skin, and the external auditory canal cartilage. The ear lies in a horizontal posterior position relative to the mandible and only achieves its rotated and elevated position during mandibular and facial growth. The ear itself is composed of neural crest cells, which are a specialized cell type responsible for much of facial development and migrate a large distance to make their cognate structures [1–4].

S. S. Tholpady (✉)
Riley Hospital for Children, Department of Surgery, Indianapolis, IN, USA

Indiana University, Department of Surgery, Indianapolis, IN, USA

M. W. Chu
Indiana University, Department of Surgery, Indianapolis, IN, USA

© Springer Nature Switzerland AG 2019

J. F. Reinisch, Y. Tahiri (eds.), *Modern Microtia Reconstruction*,
https://doi.org/10.1007/978-3-030-16387-7_4

Several corollaries to abnormal external ear anatomy are derived from knowledge of the development of these structures. Problems specific to the first or second pharyngeal arches can affect one set of hillocks or the other (or both). Additionally, some chromosomal abnormalities lead to low set, rotated ears. This can then be seen as a growth and migration defect that can be generalized to the possibility of other neural crest or craniofacial developmental problems. Finally, neural crest problems in one location can lead to problems at other locations; the neural crest is responsible for multiple other cells types including cardiac tissue providing an explanation as to the association between external ear and cardiac defects [5].

The advent of large databases with an open-source, curated dataset makes the discussion of all ear anomalies beyond the scope of this chapter, which instead focuses on the most commonly encountered microtia-associated diseases. However, knowledge of these resources can help to identify new associations and diseases that are heretofore undescribed. A search of multiple websites yields greater than 100 syndromes that are associated with external ear anomalies.

Two major curated databases serve as repositories for rare disease information. The first is OMIM®, or the Online Mendelian Inheritance in Man® (Johns Hopkins University, Baltimore, MD, USA) (https://www.omim.org/). The database was created first in book format in the early 1960s by Victor McKusick and survived 12 editions as the Mendelian Inheritance in Man until 1998. The online version was created in 1985 and developed for the web by the NCBI (National Center for Biotechnology Information). As such it is freely available and contains all known Mendelian disorders.

As can be imagined, not all diseases have been indexed in OMIM due to their rarity or inability to be classified as a Mendelian disorder. Other databases exist that catalog rare diseases. One such database is Orphanet (INSERM, Paris, France) (https://www.orpha.net) which is established in France in 1997 with the purpose of gathering knowledge on rare diseases to improve the identification, diagnosis, care, and treatment of rare genetic diseases. In the intervening 20 years, it has grown to a consortium of 40 countries including most of Europe, Australia, and Canada. As OMIM assigns a unique identifier to each disease, so does Orphanet, which is cross referenced with OMIM.

This is not a complete listing of all resources available on the internet. Because multiple search terms that appear to be similar yield widely varying results, it is wise to search via multiple classification systems and in multiple databases. A search for external ear anomalies through an aggregator website (http://compbio.charite.de/hpoweb/) is demonstrated in Table 4.1, with over 140 OMIM and Orphanet instances of associated diseases. This would serve as the starting point for a complete list of all syndromes associated with external ear anomalies. Since the majority of these occur with such low frequency, it is likely that most would never be encountered by the practitioner evaluating the external ear.

Epidemiologic investigations demonstrate a worldwide birth prevalence of microtia/anotia to be between 1/3000 and 1/20000 [6, 7]. The knowledge of associations between an ear malformation and other organ systems helps to fully describe the challenges and difficulties that may face the patient and provide a larger

Table 4.1 Total data from data query from HPO:0008551 (microtia) from compbio.charite.de/hpoweb/showterm?id=HP:0008551. Disease IDs can be used to specifically search for disease by typing number into OMIM® (Johns Hopkins University, Baltimore, MD, USA) (https://www.omim.org/) or Orphanet (INSERM, Paris, France) (http://www.orpha.net/consor/cgi-bin/Disease_Search_Simple.php?lng=EN&diseaseGroup=Search+a+disease)

Disease ID	Disease name	Associated genes
OMIM:613805	Meier-Gorlin syndrome 5	CDC6 (990)
ORPHA:857	Townes-Brocks syndrome	SALL1 (6299)
OMIM:311900	Tarp syndrome	RBM10 (8241)
OMIM:141750	Alpha-thalassemia/mental retardation syndrome, chromosome 16-related	
ORPHA:2438	Hand-foot-genital syndrome	HOXA13 (3209)
ORPHA:2036	Scalp-ear-nipple syndrome	KCTD1 (284252)
ORPHA:2305	Isotretinoin syndrome	
ORPHA:163976	X-linked intellectual disability, van Esch type	
OMIM:614643	Muscular dystrophy-dystroglycanopathy (congenital with brain and eye anomalies), type a, 7	ISPD (729920)
OMIM:606164	Diamond-Blackfan anemia 15 with mandibulofacial dysostosis	RPS28 (6234)
ORPHA:246	Postaxial acrofacial dysostosis	DHODH (1723)
ORPHA:1988	Femoral-facial syndrome	
OMIM:245600	Multiple joint dislocations, short stature, craniofacial dysmorphism, and congenital heart defects	B3GAT3 (26229), CHST3 (9469)
OMIM:606156	Sener syndrome	
OMIM:248910	Cutaneous mastocytosis, conductive hearing loss, and microtia	
ORPHA:3429	Verloove Vanhorick-Brubakk syndrome	
ORPHA:1642	Distal monosomy 9p	
OMIM:139210	Myhre syndrome	SMAD4 (4089)
ORPHA:3216	Conductive deafness-malformed external ear syndrome	
ORPHA:90024	Deafness with labyrinthine aplasia, microtia, and microdontia	FGF3 (2248)
ORPHA:2547	Microphthalmia-microtia-fetal akinesia syndrome	
OMIM:300373	Osteopathia striata with cranial sclerosis	AMER1 (139285)
OMIM:614083	Fanconi anemia, complementation group l	FANCL (55120)
OMIM:614851	Seckel syndrome 7	NIN (51199)
ORPHA:293939	Distal xq28 microduplication syndrome	
OMIM:613603	Chromosome 4q32.1-q32.2 triplication syndrome	
OMIM:236670	Muscular dystrophy-dystroglycanopathy (congenital with brain and eye anomalies), type a, 1	POMT2 (29954), POMT1 (10585), FKTN (2218), FKRP (79147), LARGE1 (9215)

(continued)

Table 4.1 (continued)

Disease ID	Disease name	Associated genes
OMIM:609654	Short stature and facioauriculothoracic malformations	
OMIM:600123	Atrioventricular septal defect with blepharophimosis and anal and radial defects	
OMIM:616462	Acrofacial dysostosis, Cincinnati type	POLR1A (25885)
ORPHA:709	Peters plus syndrome	B3GLCT (145173)
OMIM:602562	Mandibulofacial dysostosis with macroblepharon and macrostomia	
OMIM:300712	Craniofacioskeletal syndrome	
OMIM:611863	Microtia, eye coloboma, imperforation of the nasolacrimal duct	
OMIM:122780	Coxoauricular syndrome	
OMIM:123560	Cryptomicrotia-brachydactyly syndrome	
ORPHA:920	Ablepharon macrostomia syndrome	TWIST2 (117581)
ORPHA:1788	Acrofacial dysostosis, Rodríguez type	
ORPHA:1926	Diabetic embryopathy	
OMIM:606155	Fryns-Aftimos syndrome	
OMIM:227280	Faciocardiorenal syndrome	
OMIM:608624	Midface hypoplasia, obesity, developmental delay, and neonatal hypotonia	
ORPHA:138	Charge syndrome	CHD7 (55636), SEMA3E (9723)
OMIM:156200	Mental retardation, autosomal dominant 1	MBD5 (55777)
OMIM:607872	Chromosome 1p36 deletion syndrome	
OMIM:613803	Meier-Gorlin syndrome 3	ORC6 (23594)
OMIM:146510	Pallister-Hall syndrome	GLI3 (2737)
OMIM:214800	CHARGE syndrome	CHD7 (55636), SEMA3E (9723)
OMIM:138770	GMS syndrome	
OMIM:616734	Skin creases, congenital symmetric circumferential, 2	MAPRE2 (10982)
OMIM:601390	Van Maldergem syndrome 1	DCHS1 (8642)
OMIM:608013	Gaucher disease, perinatal lethal	GBA (2629)
OMIM:181270	Scalp-ear-nipple syndrome	KCTD1 (284252)
OMIM:616006	Hennekam lymphangiectasia-lymphedema syndrome 2	FAT4 (79633)
OMIM:615546	Van Maldergem syndrome 2	FAT4 (79633)
OMIM:210710	Microcephalic osteodysplastic primordial dwarfism, type 1	RNU4ATAC (100151683)
OMIM:611717	Spondyloepiphyseal dysplasia-brachydactyly and distinctive speech	
ORPHA:79113	Mandibulofacial dysostosis-microcephaly syndrome	EFTUD2 (9343)

Table 4.1 (continued)

Disease ID	Disease name	Associated genes
OMIM:610706	Deafness, congenital, with inner ear agenesis, microtia, and microdontia	FGF3 (2248)
ORPHA:436003	Contractures-developmental delay-Pierre Robin syndrome	
OMIM:143095	Spondyloepiphyseal dysplasia with congenital joint dislocations	CHST3 (9469)
OMIM:222470	Trichohepatoenteric syndrome 1	TTC37 (9652)
OMIM:218649	Craniosynostosis-mental retardation syndrome of Lin and Gettig	
OMIM:129900	Ectrodactyly, ectodermal dysplasia, and cleft lip/palate syndrome1	
OMIM:601088	Ayme-Gripp syndrome	MAF (4094)
OMIM:239800	Hypertelorism, microtia, facial clefting syndrome	
OMIM:608149	Kagami-Ogata syndrome	
OMIM:604292	Ectrodactyly, ectodermal dysplasia, and cleft lip/palate syndrome3	TP63 (8626)
OMIM:243440	Isotretinoin embryopathy-like syndrome	
OMIM:164210	Hemifacial microsomia	
OMIM:210720	Microcephalic osteodysplastic primordial dwarfism, type 2	PCNT (5116)
OMIM:277380	Methylmalonic aciduria and homocystinuria, cblF type	LMBRD1 (55788)
OMIM:164220	Schilbach-Rott syndrome	
ORPHA:2994	Short stature-craniofacial anomalies-genital hypoplasia syndrome	
OMIM:211910	Camptodactyly syndrome, Guadalajara, type 1	
OMIM:600674	Microtia-anotia	
OMIM:200110	Ablepharon-macrostomia syndrome	TWIST2 (117581)
ORPHA:2983	Disorder of sex development-intellectual disability syndrome	
ORPHA:939	3-Hydroxyisobutyric aciduria	
OMIM:261540	Peters plus syndrome	B3GLCT (145173)
ORPHA:861	Treacher Collins syndrome	TCOF1 (6949), POLR1D (51082), POLR1C (9533)
OMIM:613309	Diamond-Blackfan anemia 10	RPS26 (6231)
ORPHA:261295	20p12.3 microdeletion syndrome	BMP2 (650)
OMIM:300946	Diamond-Blackfan anemia 14 with mandibulofacial dysostosis	TSR2 (90121)
OMIM:227330	Faciodigitogenital syndrome, autosomal recessive	
OMIM:147770	Johnson neuroectodermal syndrome	

(continued)

Table 4.1 (continued)

Disease ID	Disease name	Associated genes
OMIM:171480	Phocomelia-ectrodactyly, ear malformation, deafness, and sinus arrhythmia	
OMIM:612290	Microtia, hearing impairment, and cleft palate, microtia with or without hearing impairment, included	HOXA2 (3199)
ORPHA:1352	Atrioventricular defect-blepharophimosis-radial and anal defect syndrome	
OMIM:309580	Mental retardation-hypotonic facies syndrome, X-linked, 1	ATRX (546)
OMIM:113650	Branchio-oto-renal syndrome 1	EYA1 (2138), SIX1 (6495)
ORPHA:2549	Oculo-auriculo-vertebral spectrum with radial defects	
OMIM:141300	Hemifacial atrophy, progressive	
ORPHA:1770	XY-type gonadal dysgenesis-associated anomalies syndrome	
OMIM:613804	Meier-Gorlin syndrome 4	CDT1 (81620)
ORPHA:2878	Phocomelia-ectrodactyly-deafness-sinus arrhythmia syndrome	
OMIM:113620	Branchio-oculo-facial syndrome	TFAP2A (7020)
OMIM:602588	Branchiootic syndrome 1	EYA1 (2138)
OMIM:190685	Down syndrome trisomy 21, included	GATA1 (2623)
ORPHA:245	Nager syndrome	SF3B4 (10262)
ORPHA:280	Wolf-Hirschhorn syndrome	LETM1 (3954), NSD2 (7468), NELFA (7469)
ORPHA:1597	Distal monosomy 17q	
OMIM:251800	Microtia with meatal atresia and conductive deafness	
ORPHA:261112	Monosomy 9p	
ORPHA:171839	Craniosynostosis-hydrocephalus-Arnold-Chiari malformation type 1-radioulnar synostosis syndrome	
OMIM:275630	Chanarin-Dorfman syndrome	ABHD5 (51099)
OMIM:613800	Meier-Gorlin syndrome 2	ORC4 (5000)
ORPHA:93	Aspartylglucosaminuria	AGA (175)
ORPHA:794	Saethre-Chotzen syndrome	FGFR3 (2261), FGFR2 (2263), TWIST1 (7291)
OMIM:612138	Epidermolysis bullosa simplex with pyloric atresia	PLEC (5339)
OMIM:601353	Brachycephaly, deafness, cataract, microstomia, and mental retardation	
OMIM:301040	Alpha-thalassemia/mental retardation syndrome, X-linked	ATRX (546)
ORPHA:3301	Tetraamelia-multiple malformations syndrome	WNT3 (7473)

Table 4.1 (continued)

Disease ID	Disease name	Associated genes
OMIM:249620	Mental retardation, congenital heart disease, blepharophimosis, blepharoptosis, and hypoplastic teeth	
OMIM:260660	Cousin syndrome	TBX15 (6913)
ORPHA:1703	Mosaic trisomy 14	
OMIM:236410	Humeroradial synostosis with craniofacial anomalies	
OMIM:614813	Short stature, onychodysplasia, facial dysmorphism, and hypotrichosis	POC1A (25886)
OMIM:107480	Townes-Brocks syndrome	SALL1 (6299)
ORPHA:268249	Mycophenolate mofetil embryopathy	
ORPHA:1914	Embryofetopathy due to oral anticoagulant therapy	
ORPHA:2145	Craniosynostosis, Herrmann-Opitz type	
OMIM:269870	Short stature-obesity syndrome	
ORPHA:1508	Coxoauricular syndrome	
OMIM:616723	Spondyloepimetaphyseal dysplasia, Faden-Alkuraya type	RSPRY1 (89970)
ORPHA:1834	Axial mesodermal dysplasia spectrum	
ORPHA:374	Goldenhar syndrome	
OMIM:305450	Opitz-Kaveggia syndrome	MED12 (9968)
ORPHA:2135	Hennekam-Beemer syndrome	
OMIM:612530	Chromosome 1q41-q42 deletion syndrome	
ORPHA:1606	1p36 deletion syndrome	SKI (6497), KCNAB2 (8514), GABRD (2563), PRDM16 (63976), RERE (473)
OMIM:141400	Hemifacial microsomia with radial defects	
OMIM:613320	Spondylometaphyseal dysplasia, Megarbane-Dagher-Melki type	PAM16 (51025)
ORPHA:139450	Microtia-eye coloboma-imperforation of the nasolacrimal duct syndrome	
OMIM:616580	Au-Kline syndrome	HNRNPK (3190)
ORPHA:1327	Camptodactyly syndrome, Guadalajara type 1	
OMIM:101400	Saethre-Chotzen syndrome	FGFR2 (2263), TWIST1 (7291)
OMIM:610536	Mandibulofacial dysostosis, Guion-Almeida type	EFTUD2 (9343)
OMIM:224690	Meier-Gorlin syndrome 1	ORC1 (4998)

perspective of the overall care of the patient. Although the majority of cases of external ear anomalies have no other associated defects, approximately 20–40% will have some recognizable syndrome [8, 9]. However, a discussion of associated syndromes naturally leads to the management of external ear anomalies. The most common associated defect is conductive and sensorineural hearing loss. Thus, all children with an external ear anomaly should have an audiologic evaluation [10]. The rate of hearing loss may be low but can have a profound impact on children, with numbers ranging from 0% to 16% [6, 11–13]. There is also a reported association between microtia and cervical spine fusion, independent of the OAV spectrum. Thus cervical spine imaging should be considered in children with isolated microtia in order to exclude vertebral anomalies. Another association that has been touted is between the kidneys and the ear. In the normal child with isolated microtia/anotia and no inner or middle ear abnormalities, there are no conclusive epidemiologic data that point to a link between external ear anomalies and renal problems necessitating a urologic evaluation [14–16].

Oculo-auriculo-vertebral Spectrum (OAVS)

The OAVS is a spectrum of conditions that affect similar structures, with Goldenhar being the most severe, hemifacial microsomia being less severe, and milder cases still included in the OAV spectrum [9]. First described by Gorlin [17], the clinical features involve first and second branchial arch derivatives [18] and typically affect the external ear, middle ear, mandible, temporomandibular joint, facial soft tissue and musculature, as well as the orbit, cranium, and neck. There may be defects of the cardiac, vertebral, and central nervous systems, with phenotypic expression being highly variable. Craniofacial abnormalities involve mild to severe ear anomalies (peri-auricular pits and tags, dysplasia, microtia, anotia) with or without conductive and/or sensorineural healing loss, ocular defects (epibulbar dermoids, microphthalmia, coloboma of upper eyelid), regional cranial nerve palsies (facial nerve, trigeminal nerve anesthesia, impaired palatal motion, impaired extraocular motion), cleft palate, macrostomia, and vertebral anomalies (Figs. 4.1 and 4.2).

The variability in the disease, coupled with the disparate locations it affects, has led to multiple descriptions of the same or similar spectrum. These include hemifacial macrosomia, oculo-auriculo-vertebral dysplasia [17], Goldenhar syndrome [19], Goldenhar-Gorlin syndrome [20], first arch syndrome [21], first and second branchial arch syndrome [22], familial facial dysplasia [23], and unilateral craniofacial macrosomia [24], to name a few. The overlaps in earlier descriptions of these were first noted and described as a spectrum [9]. The heterogeneity in presentation and variable genetic expression has led to multiple naming conventions. However, detailed analyses of familial cases of Goldenhar syndrome point to Goldenhar, hemifacial macrosomia, and "isolated" microtia/anotia as part of a continuum [25, 26]. The etiology of OAVS is still poorly described without an obvious genetic locus [27, 28]. Multiple familial analyses have demonstrated the variable phenotypic expression and the possibility that there is an autosomal dominant mode of inheritable with reduced penetrance [8, 25, 26, 29, 30]. Because of these issues, the reported estimates range from 1/3000 to 1/40,000 live births.

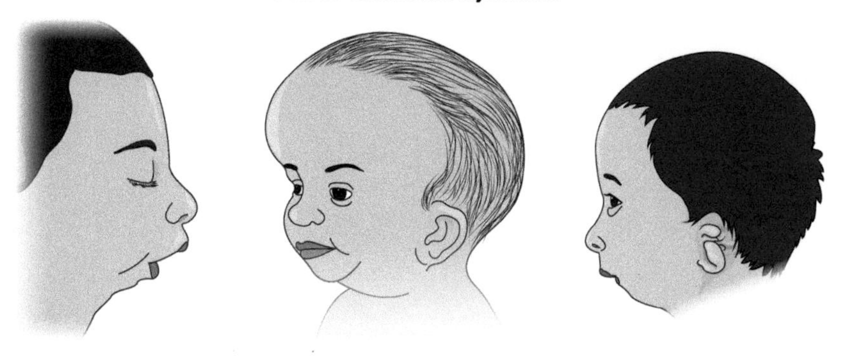

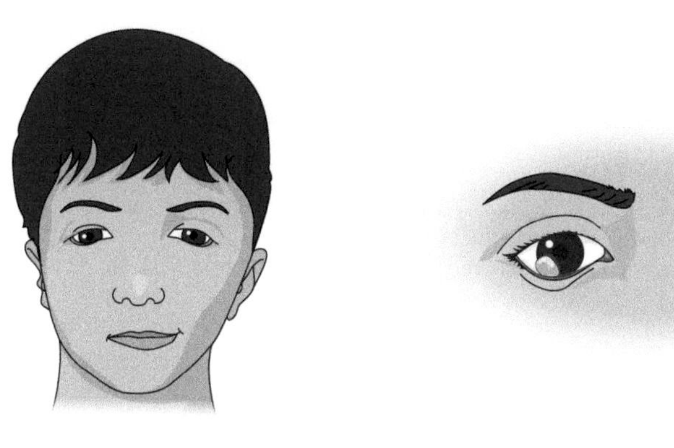

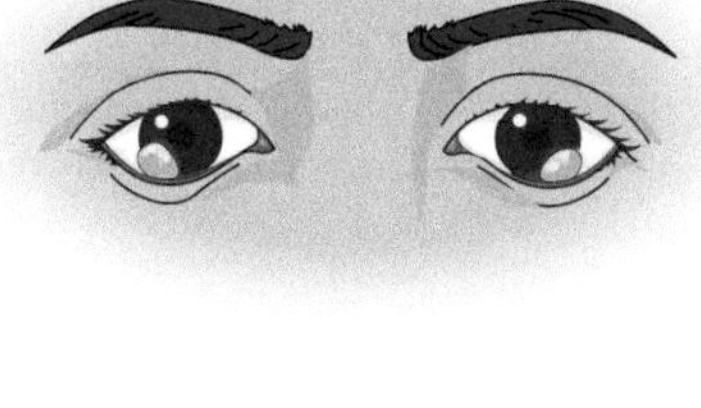

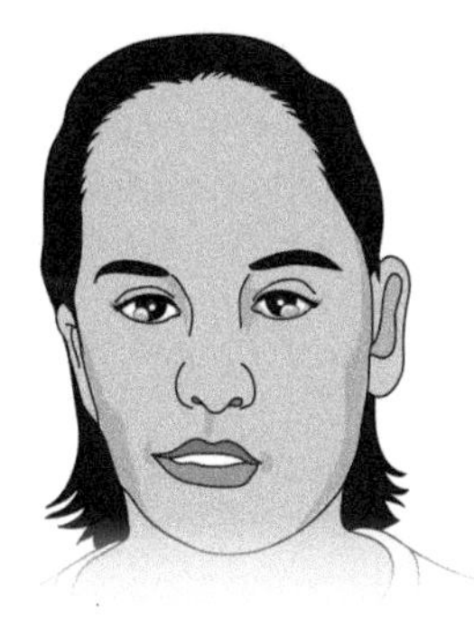

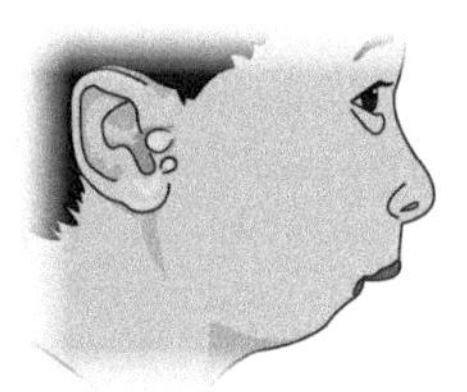

Fig. 4.1 Illustrated manifestations of Goldenhar syndrome

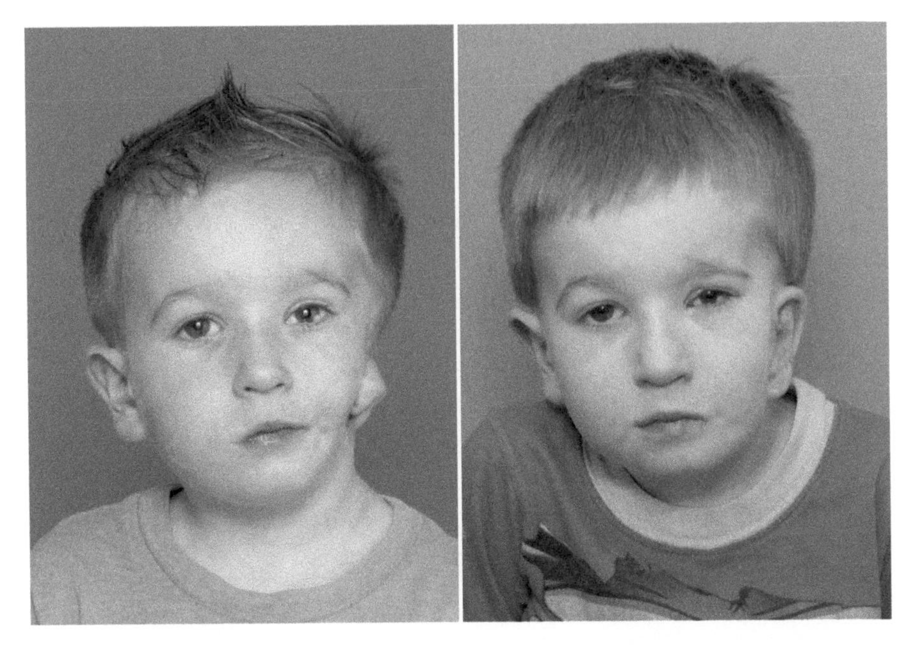

Fig. 4.2 A 3-year-old boy with Goldenhar syndrome. Note the left-sided epibulbar dermoid, mandibular hypoplasia, and microtia. He underwent left-sided ear reconstruction with porous high-density polyethylene ear implant as well as fat grafting. (Courtesy of Dr. Reinisch and Dr. Tahiri)

Treacher Collins Syndrome (TCS)

TCS is a congenital disorder described by Edward Treacher Collins in 1900 and subsequently expanded the phenotype and called it mandibulofacial dysostosis [31, 32]. It has also been called the Franceschetti-Klein syndrome [33]. It is associated with craniofacial anomalies involving the ears, eyes, and facial bones (zygoma, maxilla, mandible). These manifest as micrognathia, negative canthal vector, hypoplastic zygoma, lower lid colobomas, cleft palate, malocclusion, conductive hearing loss, preauricular displacement of hair onto cheeks, and microtia/anotia (Figs. 4.3a, b, 4.4, 4.5, 4.6, and 4.7). Afflicted patients are of normal intelligence [34].

It is estimated to affect 1/50,000 people and occurs from mutations in the TCOF1, POLR1C, and POLR1D genes [35]. These genes play important roles in ribosomal RNA function. The defect causes apoptosis of cells within the craniofacial skeleton, but it is unclear as to why it is limited in that fashion. Interestingly, 60% of TCOF1 and POLR1D mutations are new and not transmitted from parent. These are the autosomal dominant mutations, while POLR1C is recessively transmitted. TCOF1 is responsible for 81–93% or all mutations [34].

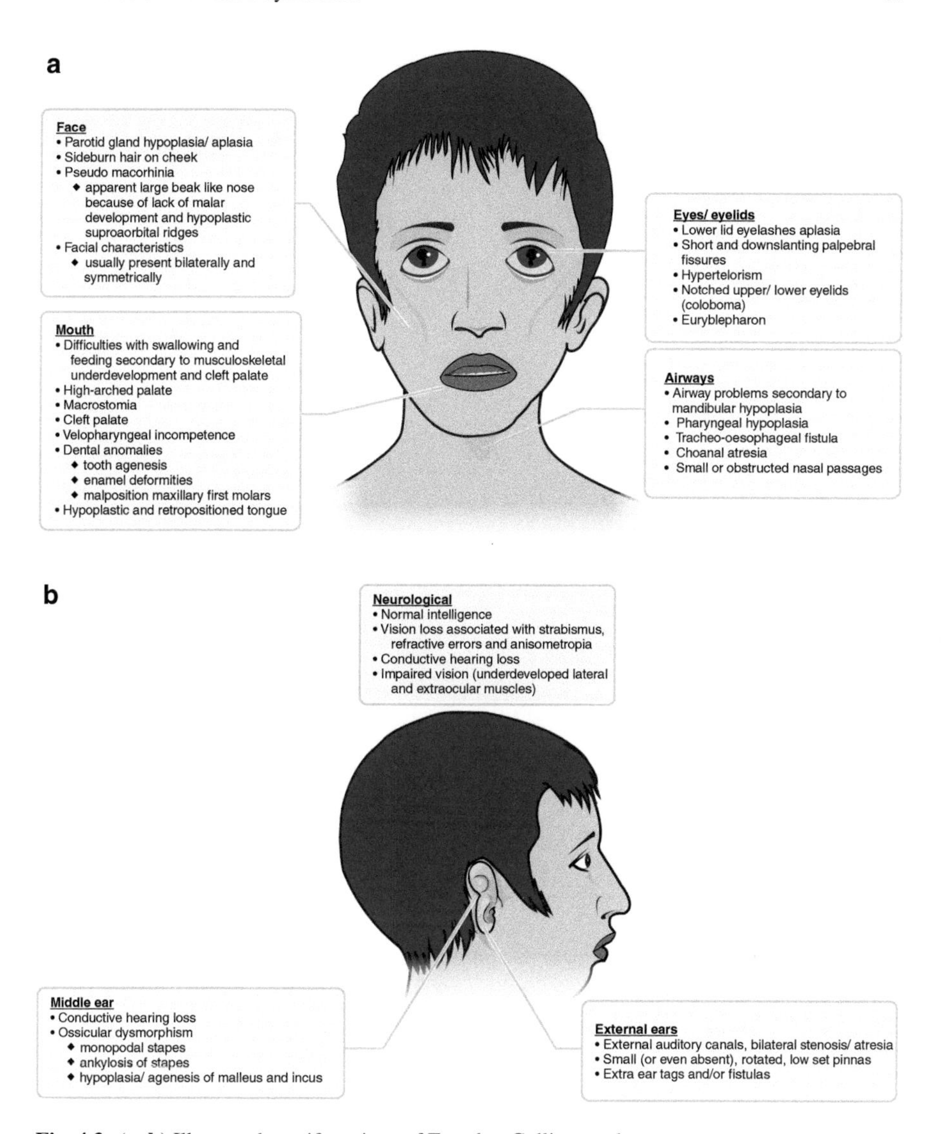

Fig. 4.3 (**a**, **b**) Illustrated manifestations of Treacher Collins syndrome

Charge

CHARGE syndrome is a mnemonic for a rare disorder that affects certain organ systems [36]. It is defined by (C) colobomas and cranial nerve defects, (H) heart defects, (A) atresia of the choanae, (R) retardation of growth, (G) genital underdevelopment due to hypogonadotropic hypogonadism, and (E) ear abnormalities and sensorineural healing loss [37]. The ear abnormalities are not in the microtia/anotia spectrum but are rather very specific and recognizable as a "CHARGE ear" [38].

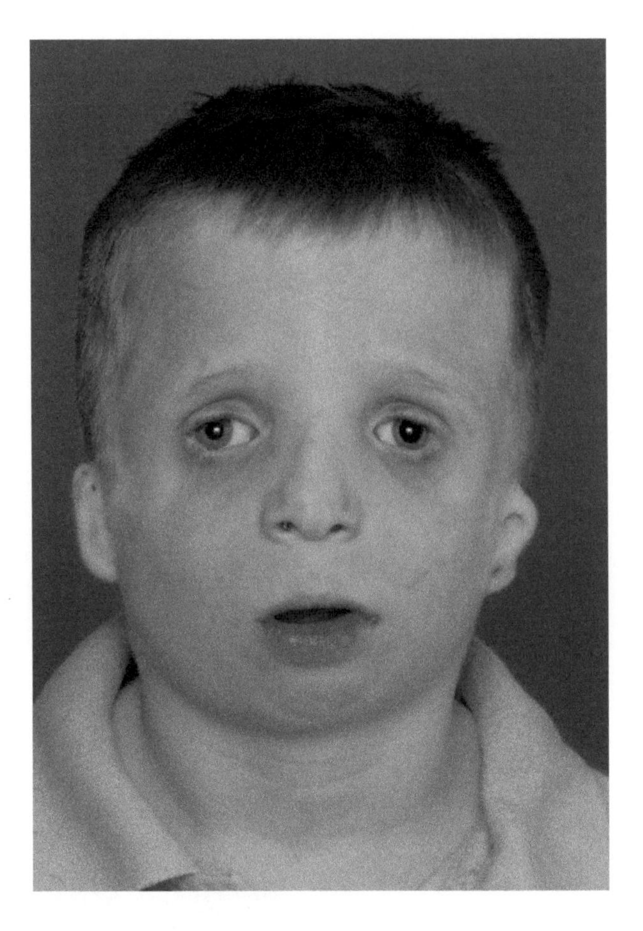

Fig. 4.4 A 7-year-old boy with Treacher Collins syndrome. Note the bilateral microtia, hypoplastic zygomas, lower eyelid colobomas, downslanting palpebral fissures and micrognathia. (Courtesy of Dr. Reinisch and Dr. Tahiri)

These include short wide cupped asymmetrical pinnae, distinctive triangular concha, discontinuity between the antihelix and antitragus, and "snipped-off" portions of the helical folds (Fig. 4.8a–d). CHARGE is usually caused by a new mutation in the CHD7 gene which is an important component of the neural crest transcriptional circuitry. This leads to defects in organ systems that contain neural crest derivatives. It occurs in 0.1–1.2/10,000 live births.

Nager Syndrome

Nager syndrome is a prototype for a cluster of disorders termed the acrofacial dysostoses (AFD) [39]. It was first described by Nager in 1948 and is characterized by negative canthal vector, malar hypoplasia, high basal bridge, micrognathia, external ear defects, preauricular hair, lid colobomas, and cleft palate and temporomandibular anomalies [40] (Figs. 4.9 and 4.10a, b). In this way it is very similar to TCS but differentiated by preaxial limb anomalies (hypoplastic or absent thumbs and/or

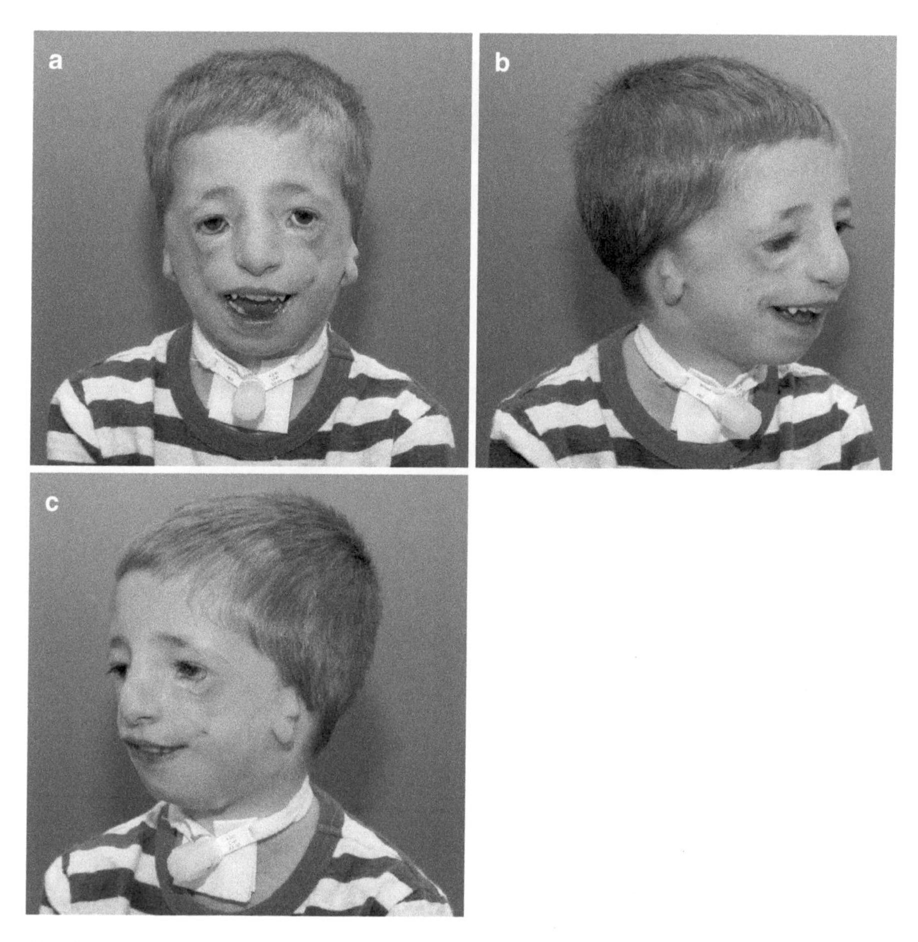

Fig. 4.5 (**a–c**) Another example of a patient with Treacher Collins syndrome. This patient had severe upper airway obstruction (due to the micrognathia) and required a tracheostomy. (Courtesy of Dr. Reinisch and Dr. Tahiri)

radii) and proximal radioulnar synostosis. The exact incidence and prevalence of the disease are unknown, but there are over 100 case reports in the literature. Chromosomal mapping and molecular cytogenetic studies demonstrate that it may be due to haploinsufficiency of SF3B4 [41].

Branchio-oto-renal Syndrome

Branchio-oto-renal (BOR) syndrome is a rare autosomal dominant trait characterized by ear pits or tags, branchial cysts, branchial fistulas (Fig. 4.11a–d), hearing loss, and renal abnormalities [42–44]. It affects approximately 1/40,000 people and

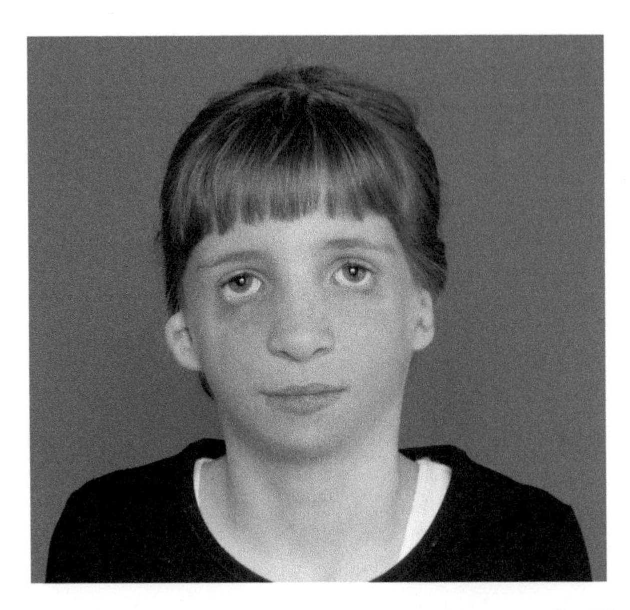

Fig. 4.6 A 8 year-old-female with Treacher Collins syndrome. Please note the difference in severity between this patient and the patient depicted in Fig. 4.5. (Courtesy of Dr. Reinisch and Dr. Tahiri)

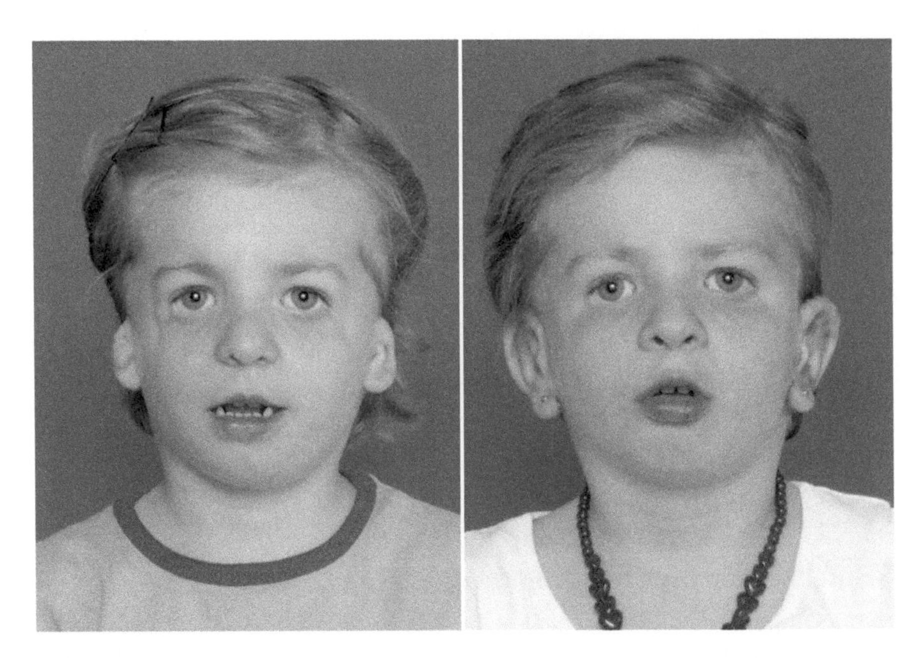

Fig. 4.7 A 4-year-old female with Treacher Collins syndrome and bilateral microtia. She underwent bilateral ear reconstruction with porous high-density polyethylene ear implant. (Courtesy of Dr. Reinisch and Dr. Tahiri)

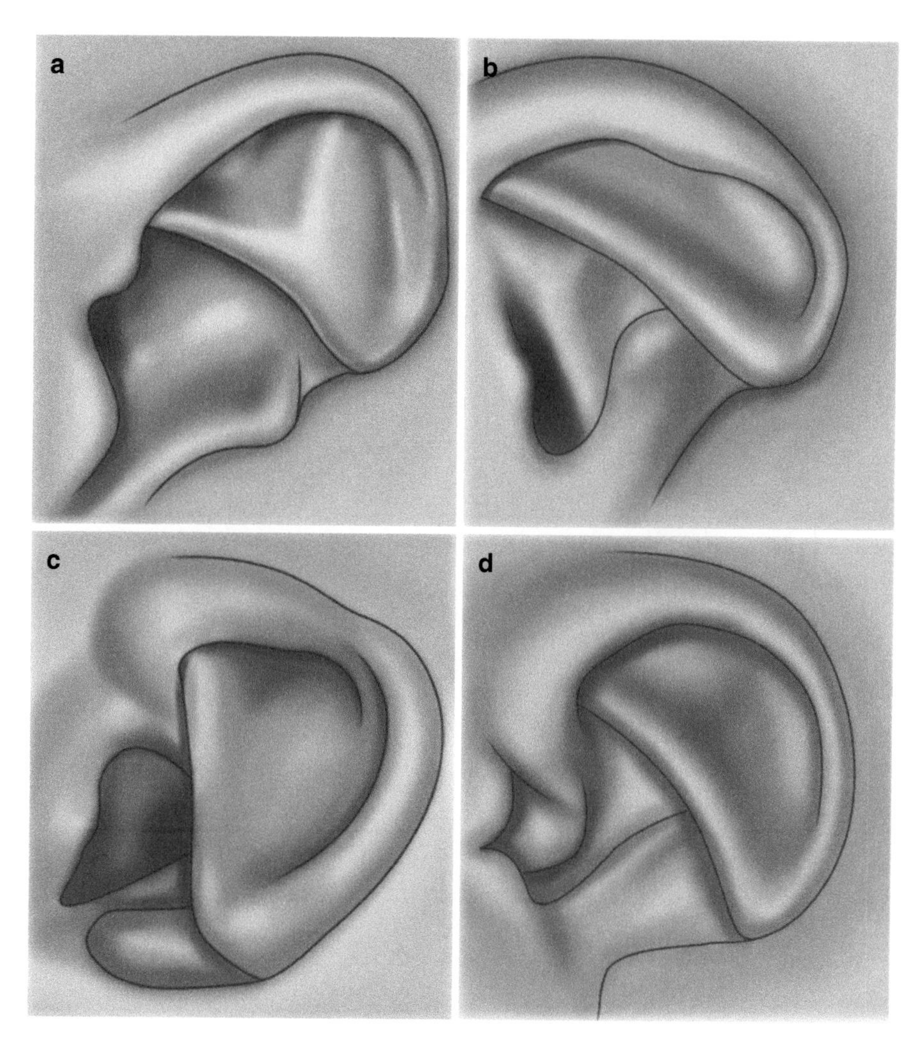

Fig. 4.8 (**a–d**) Manifestations of CHARGE syndrome: External ear anomalies present in the CHARGE ear, stylized to show similarities. The helical fold can be thin, "clipped off," or absent along the inferior edge. The antihelix may extend out to the helical rim without connection to the antitragus, which may be present but attenuated. The conchal bowl takes on a more triangular appearance due to the disruption of the posterior rim from the disconnection of antitragus and antihelix. The lobule is also frequently small or absent

occurs from mutation of EYA1, SIX1, or SIX5 genes [45, 46]. The majority (40%) of mutations occur in EYA1.

The external ear malformation is not usually associated with other malformations, but this should not lead to a delay in the diagnosis of these syndromes. Such malformations should prompt an audiologic evaluation, which in the infant to preschool years can be performed with brainstem evoked response or impedance audiometry. If abnormal, a high-resolution computed tomography is useful to delineate

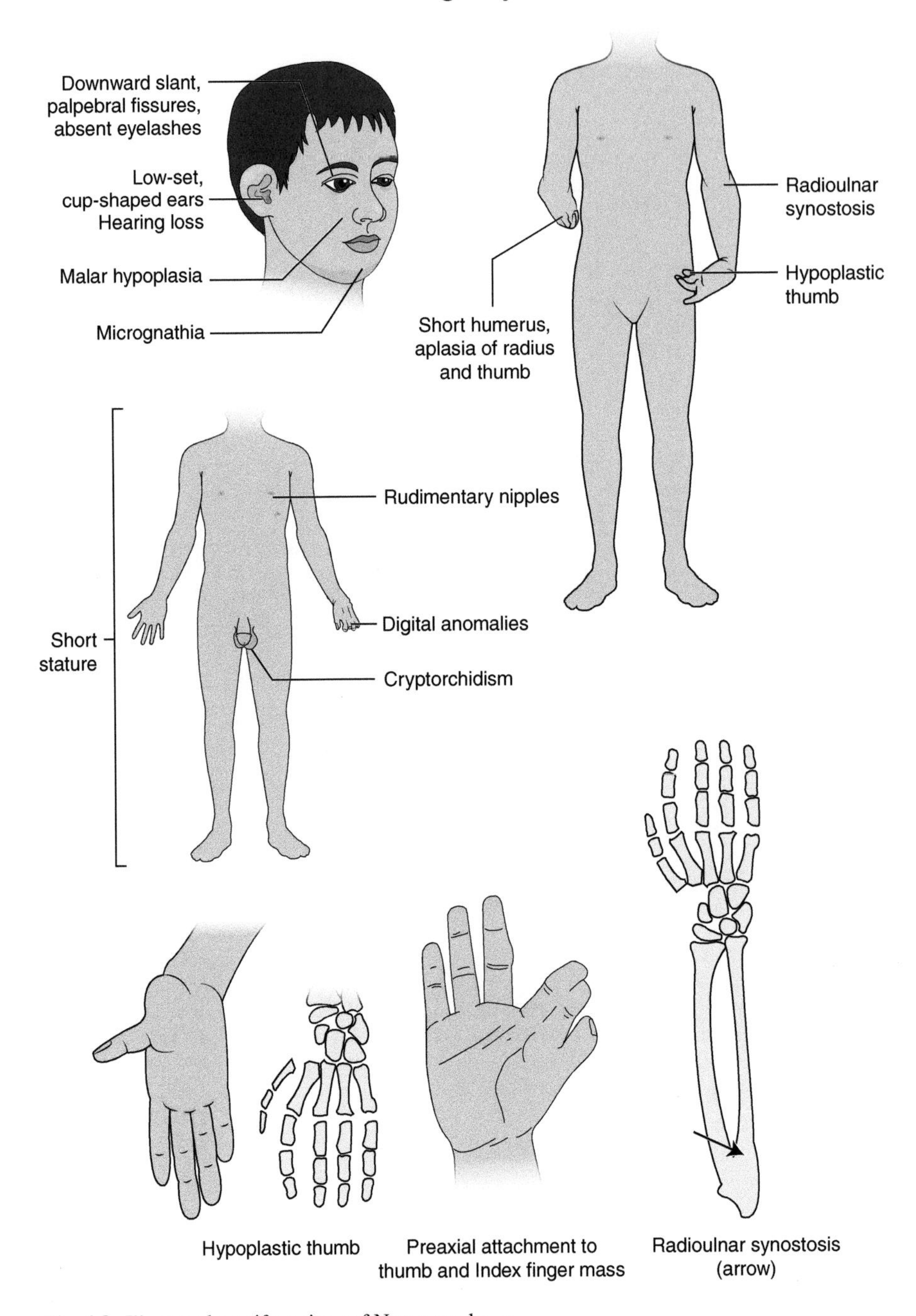

Fig. 4.9 Illustrated manifestations of Nager syndrome

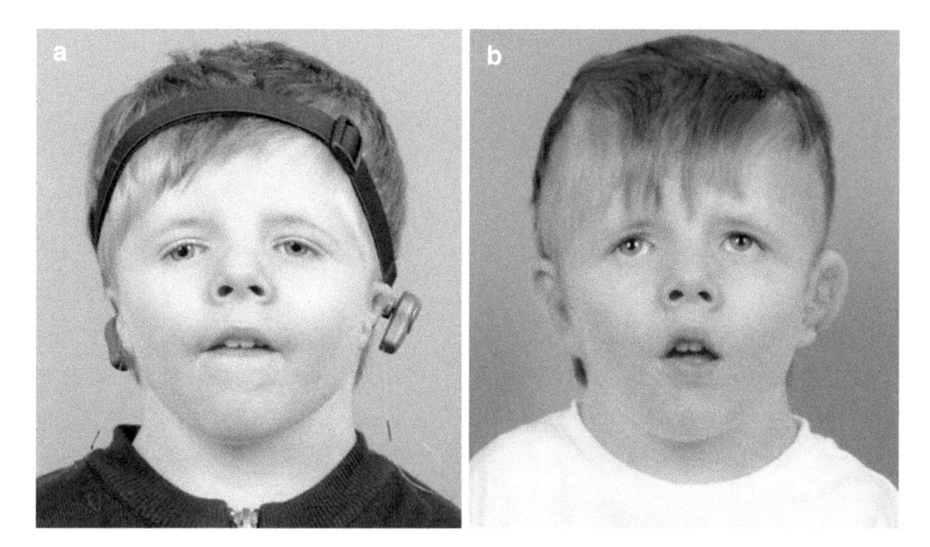

Fig. 4.10 (**a**, **b**) A 4-year-old boy with Nager syndrome. He underwent ear reconstruction with high-density polyethylene ear implants. He is shown 6 months following the right reconstruction and 4 weeks following the left reconstruction. (Courtesy of Dr. Reinisch and Dr. Tahiri)

middle and inner ear anatomy that may be reconstructable by the pediatric otolaryngologist. Other anomalies should be evaluated by their cognate specialities. The ones most commonly encountered are facial and spinal abnormalities. The inability to fully move the face and skull at the neck should prompt a spinal radiologic evaluation. Ear anomalies can commonly be associated with mandibular hypoplasia, which should prompt an airway evaluation, especially in the presence of feeding or breathing difficulties. Other issues that are related to soft tissues are macrostomia and facial nerve paralysis, which should also be evaluated in a multidisciplinary clinic.

Conclusion

Although these are the most common defects that account for most syndromic cases of microtia, this is not a comprehensive list, as new syndromes are being discovered and added, and previously distinct entities are discovered to be related via molecular cytogenetics. Ultimately, the overall care of the patient with a surgically reconstructable ear should be of utmost importance, and recognition of associated signs of syndromes facilitates the care of these patients via specialists. The most common location for this care is a multidisciplinary cleft and craniofacial unit, as many of the specialists needed for the care of these children are already assembled for other diseases.

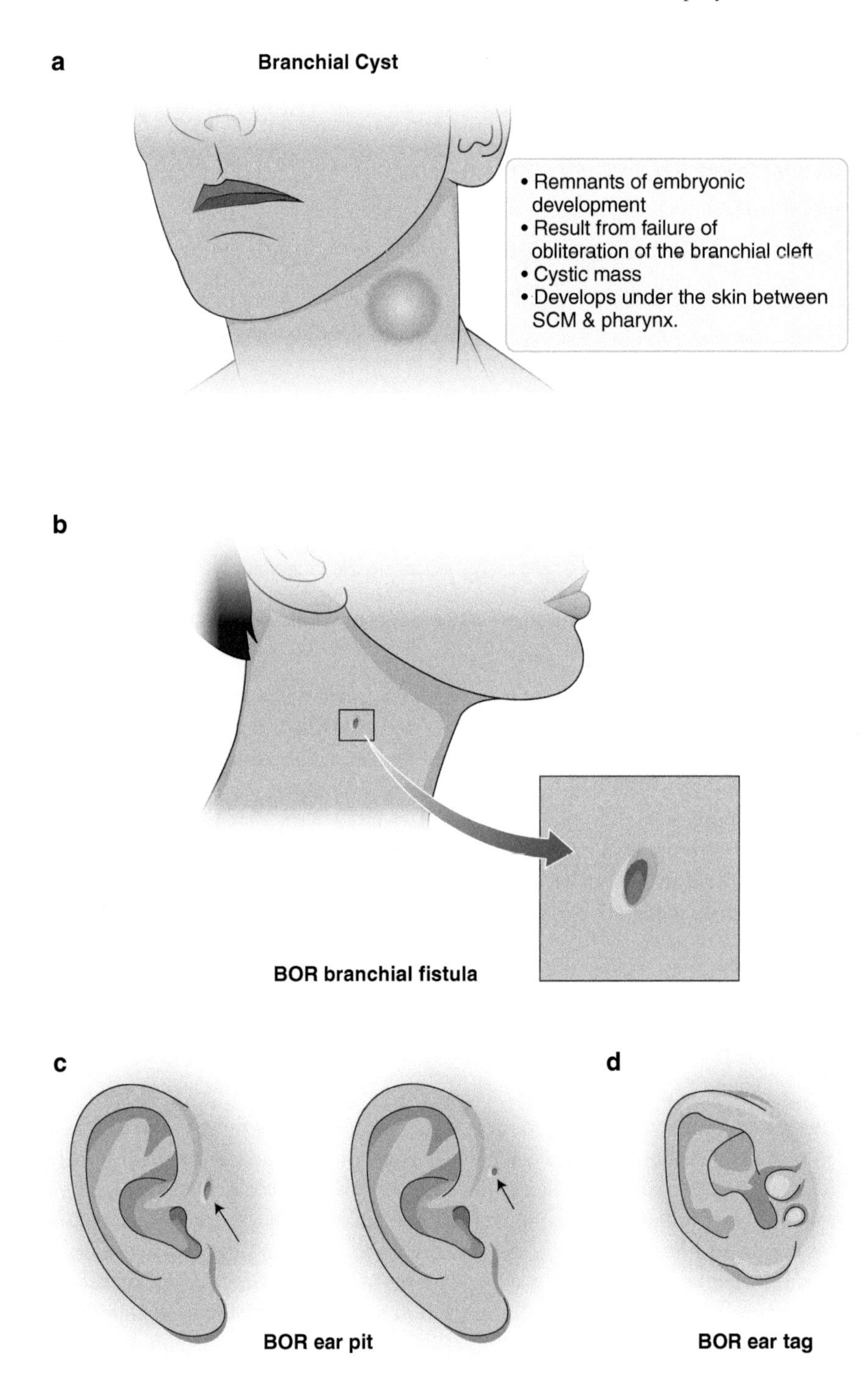

Fig. 4.11 (**a**–**d**) Branchio-oto-renal syndrome: Illustrated otological Manifestations

References

1. Nishimura Y, Kumoi T. The embryologic development of the human external auditory meatus. Acta Otolaryngol. 1992;112(3):496–503.
2. Wood-Jones F, Wen I. The development of the external ear. J Anat. 1934;68(Pt 4):525.
3. Streeter GL. Development of the auricle in the human embryo. Contrib Embryol. 1922;69:111.
4. Schoenwolf GC, Bleyl SB, Brauer PR, Francis-West PH. Development of the ears. In: Larsen's human embryology. 5th ed. New York: Churchill Livingstone; 2015.
5. Noden DM, Trainor PA. Relations and interactions between cranial mesoderm and neural crest populations. J Anat. 2005;207(5):575–601.
6. Mastroiacovo P, Corchia C, Botto LD, Lanni R, Zampino G, Fusco D. Epidemiology and genetics of microtia-anotia: a registry based study on over one million births. J Med Genet. 1995;32(6):453–7.
7. Harris J, Källén B, Robert E. The epidemiology of anotia and microtia. J Med Genet. 1996;33(10):809–13.
8. Kaye CI, Rollnick BR, Hauck WW, Martin AO, Richtsmeier JT, Nagatoshi K. Microtia and associated anomalies: statistical analysis. Am J Med Genet. 1989;34(4):574–8.
9. Cohen MM Jr, Rollnick BR, Kaye CI. Oculoauriculovertebral spectrum: an updated critique. Cleft Palate J. 1989;26(4):276–86.
10. Roth DA-E, Hildesheimer M, Bardenstein S, Goidel D, Reichman B, Maayan-Metzger A, et al. Preauricular skin tags and ear pits are associated with permanent hearing impairment in newborns. Pediatrics. 2008;122(4):e884–e90.
11. Jaffe BF. Pinna anomalies associated with congenital conductive hearing loss. Pediatrics. 1976;57(3):332–41.
12. Bassila MK, Goldberg R. The association of facial palsy and/or sensorineural hearing loss in patients with hemifacial microsomia. Cleft Palate J. 1989;26(4):287–91.
13. Naunton RF, Valvassori GE. Inner ear anomalies: their association with atresia. Laryngoscope. 1968;78(6):1041–9.
14. Kugelman A, Tubi A, Bader D, Chemo M, Dabbah H. Pre-auricular tags and pits in the newborn: the role of renal ultrasonography. J Pediatr. 2002;141(3):388–91.
15. Deshpande SA, Watson H. Renal ultrasonography not required in babies with isolated minor ear anomalies. Arch Dis Child Fetal Neonatal Ed. 2006;91(1):F29–30.
16. Wang RY, Earl DL, Ruder RO, Graham JM. Syndromic ear anomalies and renal ultrasounds. Pediatrics. 2001;108(2):e32–e.
17. Gorlin RJ, Jue KL, Jacobsen U, Goldschmidt E. Oculoauriculovertebral dysplasia. J Pediatr. 1963;63:991–9.
18. Poswillo D. The pathogenesis of the first and second branchial arch syndrome. Oral Surg Oral Med Oral Pathol. 1973;35(3):302–28.
19. Goldenhar M. Associations malformatives de l'oeil et de l'oreille: en particulier le syndrome dermoide epibulbaire-appendices auriculaires-fistula auris congenita et ses relations avec la dysostose mandibulo-faciale: Médecine et Hygiène; 1952.
20. Aleksic S, Budzilovich G, Reuben R, Feigin I, Finegold M, McCarthy J, et al. Congenital trigeminal neuropathy in oculoauriculovertebral dysplasia-hemifacial microsomia (Goldenhar-Gorlin syndrome). J Neurol Neurosurg Psychiatry. 1975;38(10):1033–5.
21. McKenzie J. The first arch syndrome. Arch Dis Child. 1958;33(171):477–86.
22. Grabb WC. The first and second branchial arch syndrome. Plast Reconstr Surg. 1965;36(5):485–508.
23. Ide CH, Miller GW, Wollschlaeger PB. Familial facial dysplasia. Arch Ophthalmol. 1970;84(4):427–32.
24. Grayson BH, Boral S, Eisig S, Kolber A, McCarthy JG. Unilateral craniofacial microsomia: part I. mandibular analysis. Am J Orthod. 1983;84(3):225–30.
25. Rollnick BR, Kaye CI. Hemifacial microsomia and variants: pedigree data. Am J Med Genet. 1983;15(2):233–53.

26. Rollnick BR, Kaye CI, Nagatoshi K, Hauck W, Martin AO. Oculoauriculovertebral dysplasia and variants: phenotypic characteristics of 294 patients. Am J Med Genet. 1987;26(2):361–75.
27. Beleza-Meireles A, Clayton-Smith J, Saraiva JM, Tassabehji M. Oculo-auriculo-vertebral spectrum: a review of the literature and genetic update. J Med Genet. 2014;51(10):635–45.
28. Kelberman D, Tyson J, Chandler D, McInerney A, Slee J, Albert D, et al. Hemifacial microsomia: progress in understanding the genetic basis of a complex malformation syndrome. Hum Genet. 2001;109(6):638–45.
29. Kaye CI, Martin AO, Rollnick BR, Nagatoshi K, Israel J, Hermanoff M, et al. Oculoauriculovertebral anomaly: segregation analysis. Am J Med Genet. 1992;43(6):913–7.
30. Kaye CI, Rollnick BR, Pruzansky S. Malformations of the auricle: isolated and in syndromes. IV. Cumulative pedigree data. Birth Defects Orig Artic Ser. 1979;15(5C):163–9.
31. Beighton G. The person behind the syndrome: Springer Science & Business Media; 2012.
32. Dixon MJ. Treacher Collins syndrome. Hum Mol Genet. 1996;5:1391–6.
33. Franceschetti A, Klein D. The mandibulofacial dysostosis; a new hereditary syndrome. Acta Ophthalmol. 1948;27(2):143–224.
34. Katsanis S, Jabs E. Treacher Collins Syndrome. 2004 Jul 20 [Updated 2012 Aug 30]. GeneReviews™[Internet] Seattle: University of Washington, Seattle; 2014.
35. Wise CA, Chiang LC, Paznekas WA, Sharma M, Musy MM, Ashley JA, et al. TCOF1 gene encodes a putative nucleolar phosphoprotein that exhibits mutations in Treacher Collins Syndrome throughout its coding region. Proc Natl Acad Sci. 1997;94(7):3110–5.
36. Pagon RA, Graham JM, Zonana J, Yong S-L. Coloboma, congenital heart disease, and choanal atresia with multiple anomalies: CHARGE association. J Pediatr. 1981;99(2):223–7.
37. Lalani S, Hefner M, Belmont J, Davenport S. CHARGE Syndrome. 2006 Oct 2 [Updated 2012 Feb 2]. GeneReviews™[Internet] Seattle (WA): University of Washington, Seattle; 2014.
38. Davenport SLH, Hefner MA, Thelin JW. CHARGE syndrome. Part I. external ear anomalies. Int J Pediatr Otorhinolaryngol. 1986;12(2):137–43.
39. Chemke J, Mogilner BM, Ben-Itzhak I, Zurkowski L, Ophir D. Autosomal recessive inheritance of Nager acrofacial dysostosis. J Med Genet. 1988;25(4):230–2.
40. McDonald MT, Gorski JL. Nager acrofacial dysostosis. J Med Genet. 1993;30(9):779–82.
41. Bernier FP, Caluseriu O, Ng S, Schwartzentruber J, Buckingham KJ, Innes AM, et al. Haploinsufficiency of SF3B4, a component of the pre-mRNA spliceosomal complex, causes Nager syndrome. Am J Hum Genet. 2012;90(5):925–33.
42. Chen A, Francis M, Ni L, Cremers CW, Kimberling WJ, Sato Y, et al. Phenotypic manifestations of branchio-oto-renal syndrome. Am J Med Genet. 1995;58(4):365–70.
43. Fitch N, Srolovitz H. Severe renal dysgenesis produced by a dominant gene. Am J Dis Child (1960). 1976;130(12):1356–7.
44. Fraser FC, Ling D, Clogg D, Nogrady B. Genetic aspects of the BOR syndrome--branchial fistulas, ear pits, hearing loss, and renal anomalies. Am J Med Genet. 1978;2(3):241–52.
45. Abdelhak S, Kalatzis V, Heilig R, Compain S, Samson D, Vincent C, et al. A human homologue of the Drosophila eyes absent gene underlies branchio-oto-renal (BOR) syndrome and identifies a novel gene family. Nat Genet. 1997;15(2):157–64.
46. Kochhar A, Fischer SM, Kimberling WJ, Smith RJ. Branchio-oto-renal syndrome. Am J Med Genet A. 2007;143a(14):1671–8.

Chapter 5
Autologous Ear Reconstruction

Sabrina Cugno and Neil Bulstrode

History of Autologous Reconstruction

Although Gillies [1] is credited as the first to propose the use of autogenous costal cartilage for auricular framework fabrication, the modern era of ear reconstruction began in 1959, when Tanzer [2] reintroduced the use of rib cartilage for autologous microtia reconstruction, which is still recognized as the gold standard reconstructive option. In his original description, Tanzer noted that "the principal difficulties in producing an acceptable surgical substitute for a missing ear fall into four general categories; namely, the furnishing of skin in adequate amounts and of matching quality, the production of a framework which will remain permanently and inertly in its bed, the creation of delicacy and contour, and the proper and permanent positioning of the restored ear to furnish a symmetrical counterpart to the opposite appendage" [2].

Tanzer described the ear as composed of four separate planes, consisting of the conchal floor, the posterior conchal wall, the anti-helix-scapha complex and the helix, each separated by the series of right angles [3]. Tanzer proposed a six-stage technique for autologous microtia reconstruction, wherein the first stage consisted of repositioning a useable auricular remnant to a proper location based on the predetermined position of the reconstructed ear [4]. The second stage consisted of

S. Cugno (✉)
Department of Plastic and Reconstructive Surgery, Montreal Children's Hospital, Shriners Hospital for Children, CHU Sainte-Justine, Montreal, QC, Canada
e-mail: microtia@drcugno.com

N. Bulstrode
Department of Plastic and Reconstructive Surgery, Great Ormond Street Hospital, London, UK
e-mail: neilbulstrode@doctors.org.uk

© Springer Nature Switzerland AG 2019

J. F. Reinisch, Y. Tahiri (eds.), *Modern Microtia Reconstruction*,
https://doi.org/10.1007/978-3-030-16387-7_5

framework fabrication from the *contralateral* sixth, seventh, and eighth costal cartilages, which were harvested in a *sub*perichondrial fashion. The base of the framework, consisting of the scapha and anti-helix, was fashioned from the sixth and seventh cartilage segments, including the adjoining synchondrosis. The eighth costal cartilage was used to form the helix and was fixed to the base block with wire sutures. The framework was then introduced through the vertical scar at the original position of the lobule into a subcutaneous pocket in the mastoid region. Adherence of the skin envelope to the underlying framework was ensured by use of through-and-through mattress sutures tied over gauze. Alternatively, if the skin envelope was insufficient, Tanzer proposed to displace the skin posteriorly, fixing the edge to the anti-helix and covering the conchal cavity with a full thickness skin graft harvested from the contralateral retro-auricular sulcus. Adhesion of the skin envelope to the framework was bolstered by the creation of multiple small perforations through the cartilage along the helical sulcus and in the triangular fossa [3]. In the third stage, the retro-auricular sulcus was fashioned in a *valise handle* fashion, with the superior, posterior, and inferior conchal walls constructed sequentially in three stages using a retro-auricular skin flap and skin graft (the third stage was later modified by Tanzer to formulate a four-stage repair) [5]. Tanzer also subsequently proposed a cartilage graft to further augment projection [3]. However, Tanzer suggested that the reconstructed ears are less conspicuous if not appreciably elevated from the side of the head. Rather, he recommended a reduction in the projection of the opposite ear, perhaps a reflection of the modest results achieved. The final stage of reconstruction consisted of the formation of the tragus and deepening of the conchal floor. The conchal floor was constructed by the method of Kirkham [6], where an anteriorly based flap is elevated from the concha, folded onto itself to produce the tragus, and a graft is placed in the denuded conchal defect. Tanzer later evolved his technique to combine the first and second stages for a three-stage method of reconstruction [7].

Brent's Technique

Following the original precepts of Tanzer, Brent refined autogenous reconstruction with the introduction of his four-stage technique [8–11]. The primary advance contributed by Brent was the placement of the cartilaginous framework in ideal position *prior to transposition of the lobule*, which is the reverse of Tanzer's sequence. When the lobular remnant is transposed at the first stage, the placement of the ear construct must be adapted to the lobe with a compromise on ideal location. Brent began reconstruction as early as age 6, although favored age 8 years. Through a small pre-auricular incision (anterior to the vestige), the deformed fibrocartilage was removed, the cutaneous pocket created, and the framework was placed. Brent, applying a method introduced by Cronin for Silastic frameworks [12, 13], inserted two silicone catheters beneath and behind the framework to co-apt the skin envelope to the framework and ensure hemostasis by means of vacuum tube suction. The ear construct was fashioned in a manner akin to that of Tanzer; however, cartilage harvest was performed in an *extra*-perichondrial manner. Over the years, Brent advocated preservation of a superior margin of the sixth costal cartilage in order to retain a tether to the sternum and maintain chest wall integrity. He contended that maintenance of the costal margin prevented outward flaring of the ribs during adolescent growth. In his initial reconstructions, Brent utilized wire sutures for fabrication of the framework; however, wire extrusion later prompted a change to use of clear nylon [11, 14]. While Brent advocated attainment of adequate projection at the time of framework fabrication by exaggerating the helical height in lieu of release of the framework and creation of an auriculocephalic sulcus, in cases where increased projection and/or sulcus formation was desired, the latter were created as described by Tanzer. More specifically, a peripheral incision was made around the margin of the framework, and the construct was elevated with preservation of a layer of vascularized connective tissue on the posterior surface of the cartilaginous framework. The retro-auricular skin was advanced toward the sulcus and the denuded areas skin grafted. Under appropriate circumstances, lobule transposition was combined with an elevation procedure [14]. In cases where a more complex vestige existed, Brent first converted the vestige to a classic lobular-type microtia as a preliminary stage by removing the dysmorphic cartilage prior to the creation of a pocket and framework insertion [10]. The final stage of reconstruction combined construction of the tragus, conchal excavation, and if indicated, contralateral prominent ear correction. Brent favored combining these procedures as the contralateral auricle served to furnish the crescentic chondrocutaneous composite graft from the anterolateral surface of the concha, used for tragal construction. In like manner, a composite graft from the scapha was used in cases of contralateral reduction for a macrotic ear [11]. The chondrocutaneous composite graft was affixed to the under-surface of a flap created through a J-shaped incision placed at the proposed location of the posterior tragal margin and inter-tragal notch. The conchal floor defect created following flap elevation was covered by advancing the skin in the concha or resurfaced with a skin graft harvested from the posterior surface of the contralateral earlobe. If the contralateral ear was not prominent, then the defect in the concha was skin grafted, and in cases of bilateral microtia, a modified Kirkham method as described by Tanzer was considered for tragus construction. Alternatively, remnants of the microtic vestige, particularly a diminutive malpositioned lobule, were used to simulate a tragus. Later, Brent reconstructed the tragus at the time of the initial framework fabrication with a tragal strut [14], perhaps influenced by his contemporary, Satoru Nagata. The cartilage segment was fixed to the frame creating the anti-tragal eminence, curved, and its distal tip was sutured to the crus of the helix. However, Brent maintained a preference for the use of a composite graft for tragus construction, stating that a more delicate and natural result was achieved [15].

Nagata's Technique

In 1993, Nagata published his modified *two*-stage approach to autologous microtia reconstruction [16], wherein the lobule is transposed *in the same stage* as framework fabrication (including tragus construction) and placement. Thus, Nagata's first stage combines the first, second, and final stages of Brent's technique. In addition, both authors proposed their own respective classification systems to describe the variable appearance of the microtia deformity. While Brent acknowledged the possibility of simultaneous lobule transposition and framework placement, and submitted to the superior appearance of the tragus with this technique, he maintained that lobule transposition was better reserved as a secondary procedure. Both Nagata [16] and Firmin (initially) [17] transpose the lobule and use the posterior surface of the lobe to line the tragal strut of the framework at the first stage. Indeed, *construction of the tragus and inter-tragal notch* was a fundamental improvement advanced by Nagata.

In the technique presented by Tanzer, an incision was employed, which extended from the posterior surface of the lobule to the mastoid surface in a V-shaped manner, and the lobule was transposed posteriorly. Modifications to the line of incision presented by Nagata evolved from this original V-shaped incision to a large W-shaped incision, as illustrated in Fig. 5.1a and b, thereby creating four skin flaps. The points *A* and *B*, located 1 cm from the central portion of the W-shaped incision, are sutured together to create an inverted cone of skin to line the recess of the inter-tragal notch. The central portion of the skin flap formed by the W-shaped skin incision serves as a subcutaneous pedicle. Nagata advocated the preservation of a subcutaneous pedicle to augment the vascularity of the distal extent of the mastoid flap [18], which will cover the concha and posterior surface of the tragus. On the anterior surface of the lobule, Tanzer employed a straight-line incision for lobule transposition. Nagata modified the line of incision to form the anterior lobule skin flap and anterior skin flap of the tragus. Thus, anterior and posterior skin flaps of the lobule are formed, an anterior tragal flap, and a mastoid skin flap. A small circular incision (2 mm) at the

→

Fig. 5.1 Nagata W-shaped skin incision, evolution from Tanzer V-shaped skin incision. (**a**) First stage operation for lobular-type microtia. (i) Outline for the construction of ear; skin incisions for lateral portion of lobule, mastoid surface. (ii) Skin incisions for anterior skin flap of tragus, for inter-tragal notch. (iii) Outline for W-shaped skin incision. (iv) Mastoid, posterior skin flap created by W-shaped skin incision. (v) Skin incision for anterior part of lobule; anterior skin flaps of tragus, lobule formed. S = subcutaneous pedicle. (vi, vii) Ear cartilage remnant completely removed. (viii) Skin undermined additional 1.5 cm from outline in 1; subcutaneous pedicle left. (ix) Skin pocket created for insertion of frame. Points A and B (shown in iv) are sutured to create inter-tragal notch. (**b**) First stage operation for conchal-type microtia. (i) Outline for construction of ear; skin incisions for mastoid surface, lateral portion of lobule. (ii) Skin incision for anterior portion of ear. (iii) Plot of modified W-shaped skin incision. (iv) Skin flaps prior to removal of ear cartilage remnant. (v) Subdermal layers detached from ear cartilage remnant. (vi) Upper portion only of ear cartilage remnant removed. (vii) Skin flaps following removal of ear cartilage remnant. (viii) Modified frame used for conchal-type microtia. (ix) Ear at the end of the first stage of reconstruction

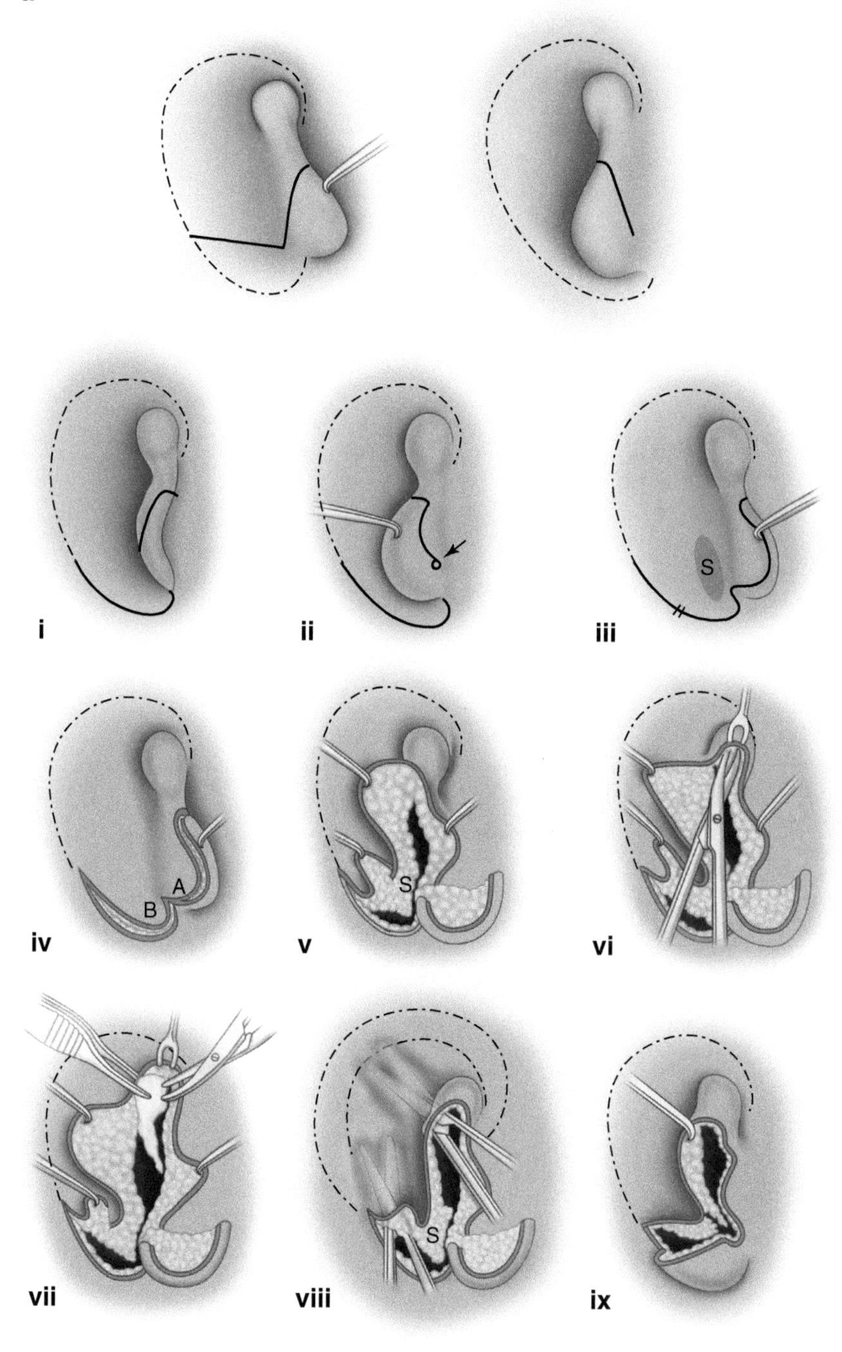
a
S
i
ii
iii
A
B
iv
S
v
vi
vii
S
viii
ix

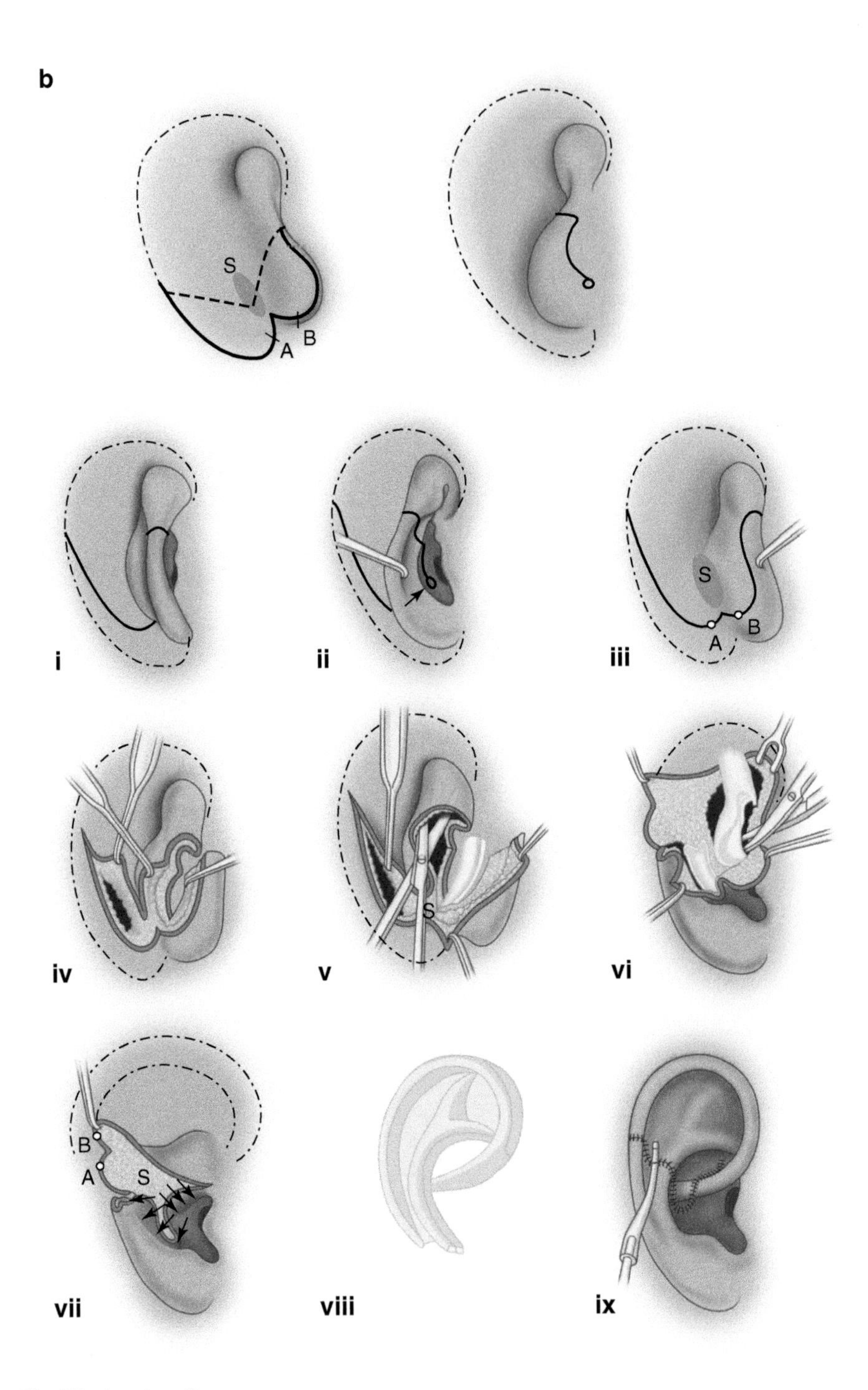

Fig. 5.1 (continued)

base of the lobule transposition flap forms a point of attachment for the inter-tragal notch. The V-shaped incision utilized by Tanzer resulted in transposition of the lobule. The skin of the posterior surface of the lobule and adjacent mastoid were not used to advantage, and skin grafting of the concha was required. Thus, a fundamental contribution to management of the skin envelope by Nagata was *increasing the surface area of skin available to cover the cartilaginous construct* by lowering the line of a W-shaped incision and using the posterior skin flaps to cover the anterior portion of the framework, thereby resulting in elimination of the use of skin grafts in the first stage [19].

For conchal-type microtia, the same posterior incision is used as for lobular-type microtia, with modification to the incision along the anterior surface of the vestige. The line of incision for the anterior surface extends from the helix posteriorly along the indentation of the small concha. The terminal portion of the incision (inferior portion of the tragus) is removed in a circular fashion with a diameter of 2 mm to construct a U-shaped inter-tragal notch. The indentation of the small concha, following complete removal of remnant cartilage, is elevated and protruded for coverage of the anterior surface of the tragus [20, 21]. Brent argued that the downside of the Nagata technique is a less natural-looking lobule, as the greater part of the posterior lobe is used to line the concha and posterior aspect of the tragus [22].

Nagata's technique has been adopted as the foremost technique for autologous microtia reconstruction. However, this technique necessitates a detailed understanding of the three-dimensional architecture of the normal ear. Once thorough comprehension of the morphologic features of the auricle is acquired, results are reproducible and mimic the normal ear. Fundamental contributions to framework fabrication were features such as the inter-tragal notch, tragus, and crus helicis with associated cymba and cavum conchae. For framework fabrication, the *ipsilateral* sixth through ninth costal cartilage segments are harvested leaving the *posterior* perichondrium in situ. The base block of the framework is constructed from the seventh and eighth costal cartilages, while the remaining portions of these two costal cartilage segments are used to form the anti-helix and inferior and superior crura, as well as the tragus and inter-tragal notch. Thus, Nagata produced the anti-helical complex from *additional* rib cartilage and fixed it to the framework base block, rather than carving the anti-helix into the base frame as in the Brent technique. This resulted in significantly improved definition of the anti-helix. Moreover, with the Brent framework, in cases where the anti-helix is carved in the area of synchondrosis, a depression is often observed at the synchondrosis secondary to soft tissue resorption [17]. The helix and crus helicis units are constructed from the ninth costal cartilage. The crus helicis is extended to the posterior surface of the anti-helix of the base frame, rather than terminating in a floating manner, thereby defining the cavities of the cymba and cavum concha. The latter remains a shortcoming of Brent's technique, where the crus helicis is incomplete and there is no separation of the components of the conchal cavity and an ill-defined disjunction between helical root and tragus. The individual units of the framework are fixed together with 38-gauge wire at 3 mm intervals. A segment from the sixth costal cartilage is banked under the chest skin for use during the second stage of reconstruction. The framework is introduced into the skin pocket around the subcutaneous pedicle. The skin envelope is meticulously adapted to the framework with the use of compression bolster sutures. Initially, Nagata placed drainage holes in the base of the framework in the triangular fossa and scapha and later abandoned this practice [23]. The more complex three-dimensional framework with Nagata's technique necessitates more cartilage for fabrication, and thus reconstruction is performed after age 10 years, provided the chest circumference at the level of the xiphoid process is at least 60 cm. Cartilage harvest was later refined, preserving the *entire* perichondrium at the donor site and filling the perichondrial envelope with remaining cartilage fragments [24]. Nagata credits conservation of the entire perichondrium as integral to the prevention of chest wall deformity. The latter method proved to result in regeneration of the cartilage, providing suitable material for secondary reconstruction or in cases of bilateral microtia [25].

The second stage, retro-auricular sulcus formation, is performed 6 months following framework fabrication and placement [23]. An incision is made along the periphery of the construct, 5 mm from the border of the helical rim. While Nagata originally performed elevation of the construct in a manner reminiscent of the method used by Brent, namely, skin grafting to the posterior surface of the framework, he later added the use of a semi-lunar and most recently concave costal cartilage block fixed with 4-0 nylon sutures to the posterior surface of the framework at the level of the posterior conchal wall. The latter was covered with a temporoparietal fascial flap and skin graft. The fascial flap is harvested through a zig-zag skin incision with care not to injure the hair follicles. The fascial flap is then passed through a subcutaneous tunnel to the posterior surface of the reconstructed ear. The retro-auricular skin is advanced toward the sulcus, and a full thickness skin graft was used to cover the remaining surfaces [23]; later, Nagata modified his technique and resurfaced the temporoparietal fascial flap with a split-thickness skin graft harvested from the ipsilateral scalp. Most recently, Chen and colleagues [26] described a modification to Nagata's second stage, where a split-thickness skin graft is raised in continuity with the full thickness skin over the anterior surface of the reconstructed ear to surface the retro-auricular area and create continuous cutaneous coverage of the ear.

Nagata's technique for the second stage of autologous auricular reconstruction presented many important improvements over Tanzer and Brent's approach to retro-auricular sulcus formation. Brent proposed elevation of the ear and coverage with a split-thickness skin graft. However, notable retraction (effacement) of the sulcus and resultant loss of auricular projection was ensured. Nagata advanced the concept of placement of a segment of cartilage graft along the posterior surface of the anti-helix to augment the posterior wall of the concha thereby contributing to the projection of the ear and preventing the retraction of the retro-auricular sulcus. Brent recognized the considerable advantage of this technique; however, preferring to reserve the temporoparietal fascial flap for secondary reconstructions, he favored harvest the occipitalis (mastoid) fascia. The cartilage graft was banked at the time of the first stage under the chest incision or beneath the scalp posterior to the construct [22].

Modifications by Firmin

While advances in skin approach, framework fabrication and formation of the retro-auricular sulcus presented by Nagata were significant; based on the morphology of the microtia, Firmin proposed a classification system for the type of skin incision required for framework placement, perhaps more useful than those of her contemporaries [27–29] (Fig. 5.2). Indeed, once facility with framework fabrication is achieved, the reconstructive ear surgeon will attest that management of cutaneous cover remains the principal challenge.

The *type 1 skin incision* is the skin approach classically described by Brent and Nagata and was originally used for typical lobular microtia, where the lobule is in an ideal position. However, unlike Nagata, a subcutaneous pedicle was not retained in the posterior mastoid flap, as Firmin was not convinced that maintenance of a subcutaneous pedicle augmented the vascularity of the flap. More specifically, this skin approach is a Z-plasty incision where one flap includes the lobule that is subsequently transposed posteriorly, and the other flap the mastoid skin. The anterior limb of the Z-plasty is placed on the future anterior surface of the lobule and is drawn in a curved fashion, including most of the lobule. The adjacent limb is drawn just above the free border of the lobule, and the posterior limb is then extended onto the retro-auricular skin at the level where the lobule should be placed. However, Firmin has now abandoned this skin approach in favor of a type 2 skin incision. This technical adaptation came from observation of tenuous vascularity of the posterior (mastoid) skin flap and difficulty in setting the lobule in the correct location with transposition. A type 1 approach is limited to cases where the lobule is suitably positioned. In those circumstances where a type 1 approach is not appropriate, type 2 or 3b approaches should be considered. *Type 2 transfixion incision* describes a full-thickness transverse incision on the remnant auricle that is extended posteriorly onto the mastoid skin to permit adhesion of the microtia ear remnant to the retro-auricular skin and creation of a skin pocket for insertion of the framework. The posterior skin edge of the remnant is sutured to the inferior skin edge of a corresponding transverse incision in the mastoid skin, and the anterior skin edge is sutured to the edge of the superiorly based skin flap that covers the cartilage framework. Depending on the remnant, either a superior or more commonly inferior transfixion incision is made. The transfixion incision is indicated for both lobular- and conchal-type microtia, where the inferior (or superior) portion of the auricle is sufficiently developed to accept the lower (or upper) extremity of the framework. The position of the incisions are determined by pulling the remnant posteriorly to reach the outline of framework placement [30]. *Type 3 incision* is a simple skin incision to create a skin pocket for framework placement and has been subclassified into types 3A and 3B. *Type 3A* is used when the ear is malformed but comparable in size to the contralateral normal side, such that the deformed cartilage can be dissected from the skin envelope and the framework placed into the cutaneous pocket created. As the sulcus is preserved, this skin approach achieves single-stage reconstruction. For type 3A incision, the skin

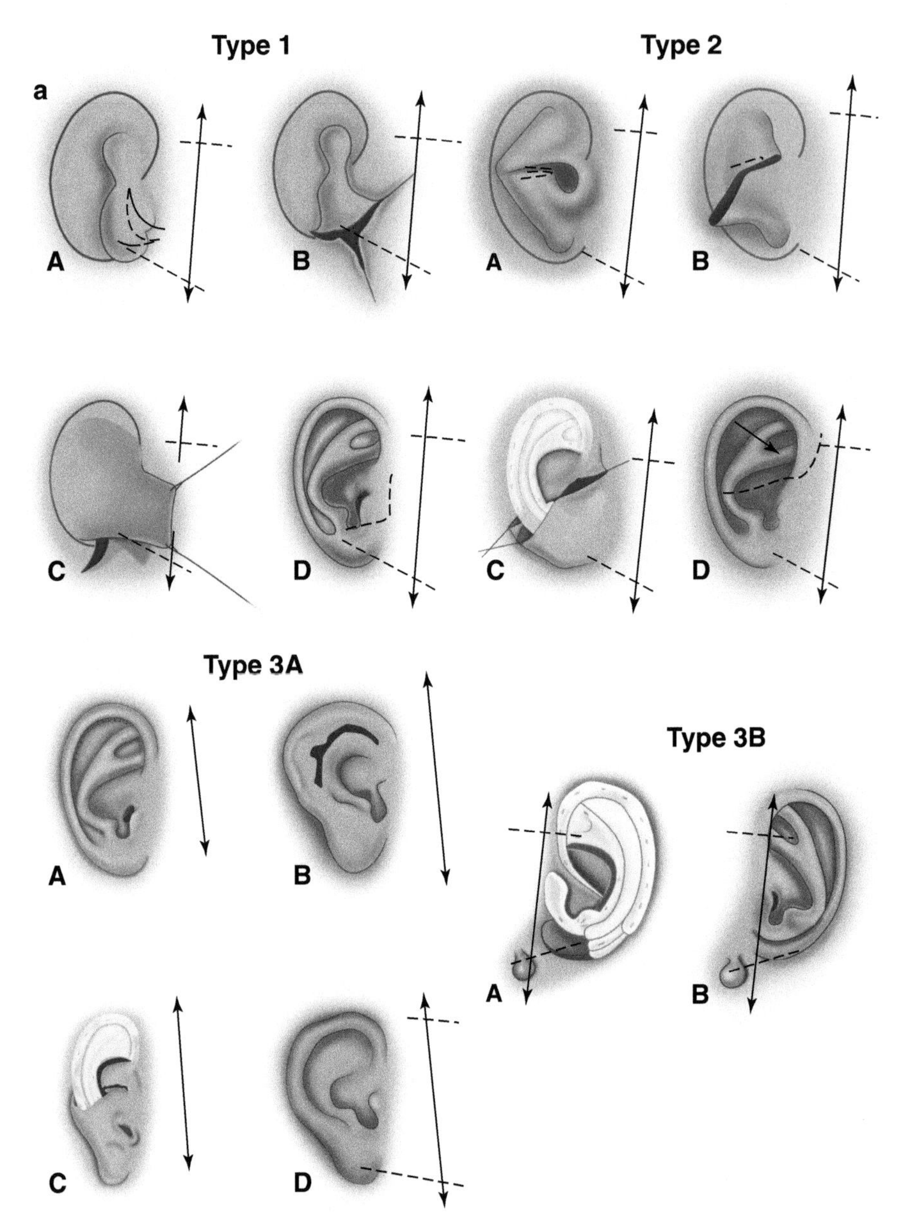

Fig. 5.2 Firmin types 1–3 skin incisions. Type 1 skin approach: Placement of the incision (Z-plasty), elevation of the flaps, exchange of the skin flaps, and aspect at the end of the procedure. Type 2 skin approach: Transfixion incision of the remnants. Adhesion of the posterior edge of the transfixion incision to the inferior edge of the back cut. The inferior part of the framework is introduced into the lobule. The superior part of the framework is covered with a retro-auricular skin flap. Type 3A skin approach (can only be performed in 1 stage): The skin incision gives access to the deformed fibrocartilage. Through removal of the fibrocartilage, a skin pocket has been created to receive the framework. The framework is introduced into the skin pocket, replacing the deformed fibrocartilage. The anterior and posterior surfaces of the framework are covered with skin. Type 3B skin approach: As there are no remnants to remove, the skin incision is only used to prepare the skin pocket. The framework is introduced into the skin pocket, and the small ectopic remnant will be removed during the second stage (i.e., elevation of the framework)

envelope of upper pole of the ear must be of appropriate size to accommodate the cartilaginous framework. If the superior pole is deemed of insufficient size, then a type 2 incision is used, and the reconstruction is performed in two stages. *Type 3B* is implemented for cases of anotia (absent remnant) or where the microtic remnant cannot be used (e.g., significant auricular dystopia relative to the ideal position of the reconstructed ear), and the incision is simply used for pocket dissection. When a type 3B skin approach is selected, the lobule will be formed during the second stage when the ear is elevated. In patients with severe hemi-facial microsomia, the microtia remnant, irrespective of the size or morphology, is often in an ectopic location, such that it is disregarded and a type 3B skin incision is preferred. In cases where no remnant exists (anotia), the incision can be placed in the hairline. With practice, consistent appropriate selection of skin approach can be realized.

Firmin has also presented classification systems for the type of frameworks required based on the microtic vestige, as well as for the second stage of reconstruction, which includes the techniques for ear elevation popularized by her predecessors [29, 30]. Firmin also described two complementary cartilage segments that are often adjoined to the framework, namely, *projection pieces I and II* [30]. The former is a strut that is placed behind the root of the helix, with or without extension to the tragus. This projection piece provides stability and projection to the crus helicis and tragus, and can be used to fix the root of the helix as an alternative to Nagata's technique where the crus is secured to the posterior conchal wall. Firmin's projection piece II, previously described by Brent [9], is positioned on the posterior surface of the anti-helix similar to the placement of the cartilage block at the second stage of reconstruction, in order to increase projection of the ear by augmenting the posterior wall of the concha (enhancing the depth of the concha). However, the addition of this cartilage segment is predicated on a well-vascularized skin envelope with sufficient laxity in the middle third of the ear, as the resultant increased thickness of the framework can pose undue tension on the cutaneous cover. The addition of this projection piece often precludes placement of a cartilage block for enhanced projection in the second stage. Indeed, the addition of projection pieces at the first stage results in satisfactory projection such that in many cases, the second stage is not performed. If a second stage is done, for creation of a retro-auricular sulcus, the method popularized by Brent (elevation and placement of a skin graft) can be used. A common criticism of the second stage of autologous reconstruction is loss of definition, and so this more aggressive approach in the first stage results in an overall superior result. If adequate projection was achieved in the middle third of the ear after the first stage, but additional projection is required in the upper and lower thirds of the reconstruction, Firmin described a modification to the Brent technique for elevation of the ear [30]. In this case, the reconstructed ear is similarly elevated with vascularized tissue along its posterior surface, but a tunnel is fashioned between the framework and retro-auricular soft tissue to permit placement of a cartilage graft beneath the crura of the anti-helix or anti-tragus for additional projection of the superior portion of the framework or lobule, respectively. The latter projection piece is designated *projection piece III*.

Authors' Technique

In the authors' practice, auricular reconstruction is realized as a two-stage procedure, as initially described by Nagata and later modified by Firmin [31]. Autologous reconstruction is offered at the minimum age of 9 years, depending on the physical and psychological maturity of the child. At this age, there is usually sufficient costal cartilage for framework fabrication and most children have the requisite level of understanding to be an active member in the treatment plan and postoperative rehabilitation and care. The benefits of the child's participation in the discussion when they reach competence appreciably outweighs the unproven benefit of operating on younger children who are unable to dialogue in an appropriate fashion, and it is our contention that early intervention abates parental anxiety rather than the child's suffering. Moreover, auricular growth is principally complete at age 10 years and thus the contralateral normal ear on which a template for the reconstruction is fabricated. For patients older than 20 years, preoperative imaging of the thorax should be considered prior to auricular reconstruction for assessment of ossification of the cartilage.

For the first stage of reconstruction, following induction of general anesthesia, preoperative markings are made (Fig. 5.3a and b) [27]. On frontal view, the position of the most inferior point of the lobule relative to the contralateral side is determined. On the unaffected side, two distances are outlined and transposed onto the side with microtia: the distance between the lateral canthus to the most anterior point of the helix and between the lateral commissure to the lowest point of the lobule. The latter two measures determine the anterior- and inferior-most points for placement of the reconstructed ear. Next, the angle between the axis of the nasal dorsum and the normal ear is ascertained, and the former two are marked on the abnormal side and used to determine the inclination of the ear construct. Finally, the course of the superficial temporal artery is marked using a Doppler probe. An outline of the contralateral normal ear is drawn onto X-ray film, which serves as the template for fabrication of the auricular framework. A stencil for the base of the framework is then adapted from the template of the ear, and a second pattern is drawn several millimeters smaller in all dimensions to account for the thickness of

Fig. 5.3 (**a**) Preoperative measurements and markings for the assessment of ideal location for the reconstructed ear. In the frontal view, the position of the lobule is compared to the normal side. On the unaffected side, the distance between the lateral canthus and the most anterior point of the helix, and between the lateral commissure and lowest point of the lobule are outlined. Lines parallel to the axis of the ear and nose are drawn, and the angle between these measures is calculated. These measurements are transferred to the abnormal side. (**b**) Three representative cases are shown: the first row illustrates the compromise to the location of the reconstructed ear that is made in the horizontal plane in a case of hemifacial microsomia; the second row shows the proposed location of the reconstructed ear relative to the dystopic auricular remnant with external auditory canal; the third row shows determination of framework placement in a case of bilateral microtia, for which there is no contralateral reference. (**b**: Used with permission of John Wiley and Sons from Cugno and Bulstrode [31])

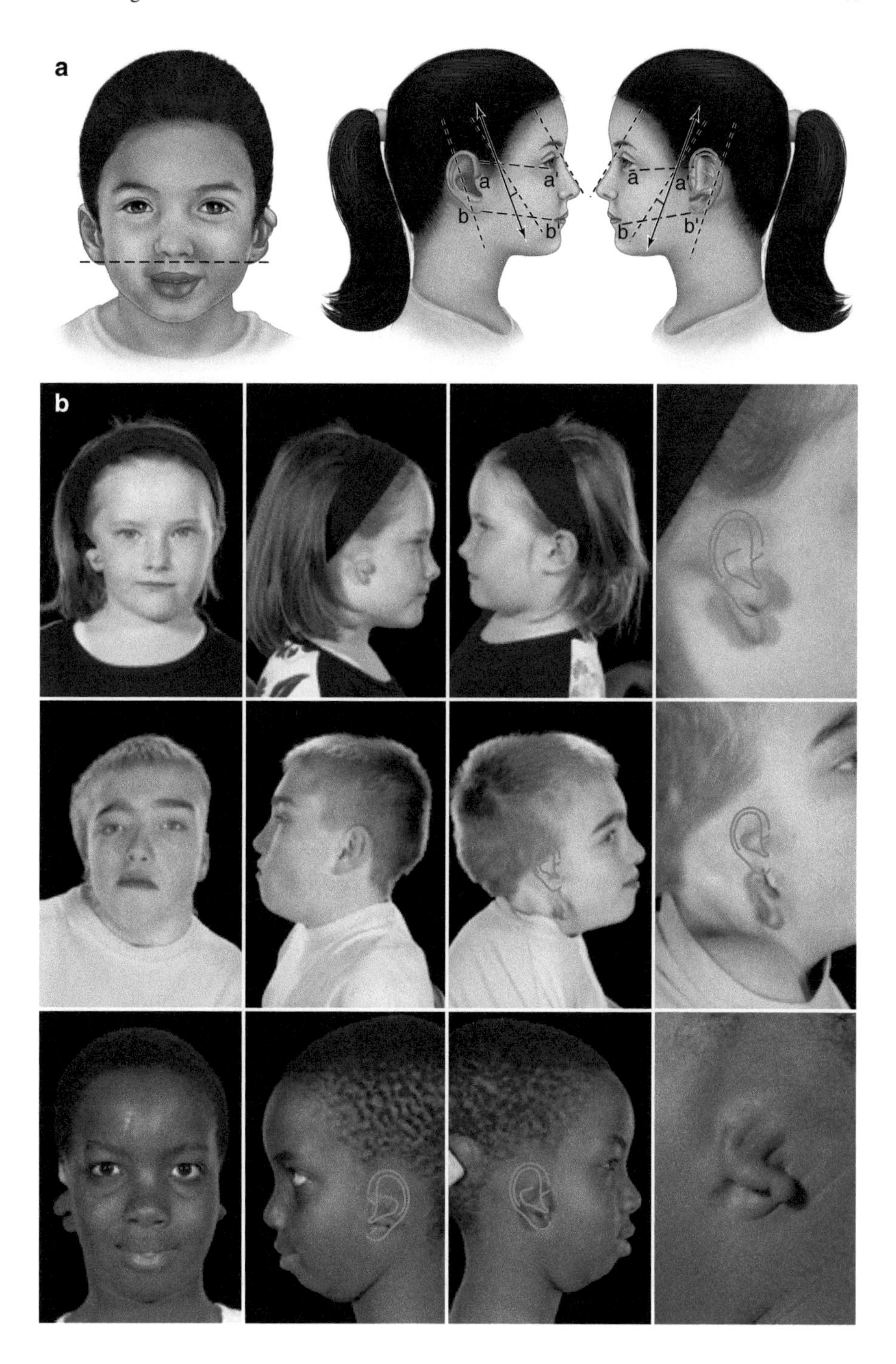
a
a
a'
b
b'
a
a'
b
b'
b

the skin envelope. In cases of bilateral microtia, the template for framework fabrication is based on a parent. Once the ideal location of the future ear on the abnormal side is determined, the outline of the normal ear is drawn, potential adaptations of the microtic remnants are assessed, and then the appropriate skin approach is selected.

Precise placement of the reconstructed ear is the first and foremost step in auricular reconstruction, and should never be compromised, even in the presence of large remnant or external auditory meatus and/or canal, as even the most impressive reconstruction will be considered unsatisfactory if in an ectopic location. In patients of severe hemifacial microsomia, determination of the position of the reconstructed ear remains a challenge. However—as the ear is sited posterior to the temporomandibular joint and ramus of the mandible, projecting over the mastoid process of the temporal bone of the *cranium* and is not located on the face per se—positioning of the framework can be ascertained despite a background of considerable facial asymmetry. On the affected side, the distance between the lateral canthus and the auricular area is often shorter, and mandibular hypoplasia begets a perceived asymmetry of the inferior part of the ear. Thus, it is often necessary to accept a compromise in location of the auricle in the anteroposterior (horizontal) plane as the two facial profiles are never observed simultaneously. However, framework placement in the *vertical* plane (as well as the axis of the ear) must be precisely determined as disparity in the position of the two ears would be noted on frontal (and posterior) view [32]. Interestingly, Firmin noted an absence of the pre-auricular sideburn as a consistent finding in patients with hemifacial microsomia, even in the absence of any discernible facial asymmetry, and thus this valuable facial landmark cannot be used to advantage in determining the position for the reconstructed ear. Other issues in microtia reconstruction particular to these patients include a low hairline, anomalous trajectory of the branches of the superficial temporal artery, aberrant location of the frontal branch of the facial nerve, significant hypoplasia of the auricular region including atrophic skin, and eccentric positioning of microtic remnants, including if present, dystopic external auditory meatus [32]. In cases of an ectopic meatus with external auditory canal, the surrounding fibrocartilage can be excised allowing the transposition of the meatus to a more appropriate position. Nagata described the transposition of an aberrantly positioned external auditory canal and meatus to its proper anatomic location as a subcutaneous pedicled flap [33]. Park also addressed management of auricular reconstruction in dystopic microtia with the presence of an external auditory canal, where a skin incision is made around the vestige and the cartilaginous portion of the meatal canal is dissected from the bone preserving superior attachments to the temporoparietal fascia and suspended to the periosteum of the temporal bone [34].

The authors' decision on type of skin approach is based on the principles characterized by Firmin, as previously described, and depends on the position of the microtic remnant and the location of any existing scars. Once the appropriate skin incision is made and the amorphous remnant fibrocartilage is removed, the auricular pocket is dissected in the plane deep to the subdermal vascular plexus, with dissection extended at least 1 cm beyond the limits of intended framework placement (marked auricular outline) to recruit sufficient skin to adequately cover the contours of the construct without undue tension. In cases of hemifacial microsomia, dissection of the subcutaneous pocket and removal of remnant cartilage should be performed judiciously to avoid inadvertent injury to the facial nerve branches [32]. The cartilage framework is placed in the subcutaneous pocket over two suctions drains, as described by Brent.

The xiphoid process and costal margin along the ipsilateral chest are outlined. A first (eighth) floating costal cartilage segment is palpated, and a 5 cm oblique incision is marked between xiphoid and distal tip of the eighth rib (Fig. 5.4a–c). The rectus abdominis fascia is incised, and the lateral border of the muscle is identified and retracted medially to localize the costal cartilage. The cartilage segments of ribs six to eight (and occasionally nine) are harvested, preserving the *posterior* perichondrium in situ (except for the eighth costal cartilage, which is harvested with the complete perichondrial sleeve). The junction of costal cartilage and bone is readily identified as a white-gray junction. The reconstructed framework is made several millimeters smaller in all dimensions than the template of the normal ear to account for skin thickness. The components of the framework are fixed together with wire sutures, as popularized by Nagata, and wires are embedded into the cartilage to avoid risk of exposure. The cartilaginous base block is fashioned from the synchondrosis of ribs 6 and 7 with cartilage sculpting effected on the surface denude of perichondrium (as the perichondrial surface ensures cohesion of the cartilaginous block to the recipient bed, as well as continuity of the synchondrosis and adhesion of the two segments of the base block). Thus, the posterior surface of the harvested cartilage becomes the anterior surface of the reconstructed ear. Occasionally, perforations are made through the cartilage base along the scapha and in the triangular fossa, as originally described by Tanzer [3], to augment adherence of the skin to the framework. In cases of anotia, where there is no microtic vestige to replicate the lobule, the framework is necessarily extended in this inferior portion and the lobule defined at the time of the second stage. Even in cases of lobular microtia, the framework is fabricated such that the cartilage base extends into the lobule, which assists in maintaining the lobule in the desired position. The cartilage can be removed later or at the time of ear piercing, if subsequently performed. Occassiaonally, for female patients, a large perforation is placed in the lobule of the framework to facilitate subsequent ear piercing. The helix and anti-helix are shaped from the eighth rib. For the formation of the helical rim, the outer convex surface of the eighth rib is thinned to instigate warping of the cartilage in order to recreate the arch of the helix [35]. If the eighth rib is too short to form the complete length of the helix, an additional piece of cartilage can be adjoined beyond the point of curvature (i.e., along the straight posterior border of the framework). Great care must be taken to ensure that the join is graded and smooth in order to avoid notching once the reconstruction has matured. If the eighth rib is deficient, then the ninth rib can be used for anti-helix formation. When carving the anti-helix, the morphology of the superior and inferior crura should be appreciated and correctly reproduced, with a sharp inferior crus that extends deep to the helical rim and a wide ill-defined superior crus that fades into the scaphoid fossa. The tragus, anti-tragus, and cartilage block used to reconstruct

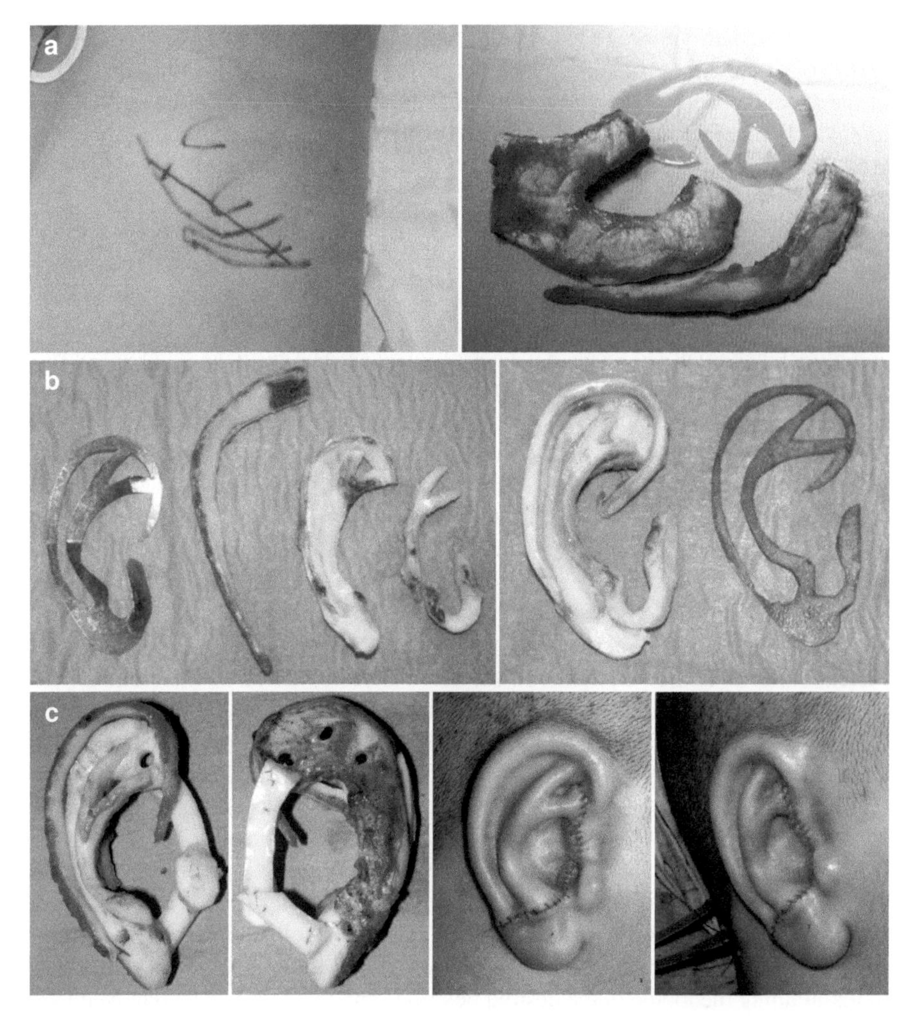

Fig. 5.4 Framework fabrication. (**a**) A 5 cm oblique incision is marked along the costal margin ipsilateral to the side to be reconstructed. The cartilage segments of ribs 6–8 are harvested and the framework fashioned as described. (**b**) The senior author has modified framework fabrication and no longer sculpts the anti-helix, tragus, and anti-tragus segments as a single unit. Instead, the anti-helix and anti-tragus are shaped as a single component and a cartilaginous strut is made to span the base block, onto which the tragus is placed. (**c**) Intraoperative result at the end of the first stage of reconstruction. (**a**–**c**: Used with permission of John Wiley and Sons from Cugno and Bulstrode [31])

the posterior wall of the concha during the second stage (framework elevation) are carved from remaining cartilaginous segments. Initially, the tragus-anti-tragus was carved as a unit, and ideally from the medial portion of the sixth or seventh rib, where the cartilage is the thickest [30]. More recently, the senior author has modified his technique for framework fabrication and no longer sculpts the tragus and anti-tragus segments as a single unit. Instead, the anti-helix and anti-tragus are shaped as a single piece, and a *cartilaginous strut* is made to span the base block (extending from the root of the helix to the distal extent of the base of the framework), onto which the tragus (separate piece) is placed, as shown in Fig. 5.4a–c. The disjunction between anti-tragus and tragus allows the cutaneous cover to drape within this recess creating the semblance of the inter-tragal notch. This strut is essentially a combination of Firmin's projection pieces I and III, and can be formed from one or two pieces of cartilage. If two pieces are used, they are joined in overlapping fashion at the under-surface of the tragus.

For adult microtia reconstruction, particular consideration in fabrication of the framework must be made. Rib cartilage differentiates into bone as we age and thus presents a greater challenge for carving the framework. In the presence of significant ossification, the contours of anti-helix are carved from the base frame, as originally proposed by Tanzer and Brent. In like manner, the helix can be sculpted from the base block or added as an additional piece. In insufficient helical projection is achieved with carving the framework in one piece and the cartilage remains too ossified to adequately sculpt the curve of the helix without inadvertent fracture, Brent proposed a technique where the helix is sculpted en block from the base frame, then detached and slide up the body of the framework [8, 14]. Alternatively, his *expansile* technique and carving in one block can be used [14].

During the carving of the auricular framework, cartilage shavings and unusable cartilaginous fragments are collected, morcelized, and placed in a Vicryl® mesh (polyglactin, Ethicon, Somerville, NJ, USA) sleeve that is then used to reconstitute the costal margin [36]. Similar to the results reported by Nagata [25], histological analysis of this method of rib reconstitution demonstrated hyaline cartilage admixed with fibrous tissue. Moreover, this method validated that an intact perichondrial sleeve is not requisite for cartilage formation, as only the posterior perichondrium is preserved. The mesh is folded in half and sutured along the border to create a tube and the sleeve is measured to the same length of the donor defect with 1 cm added at either end to allow fixation to the lateral and medial borders of the defect. Intercostal nerve blocks (chirocaine, 2.5 mg/mL) are carried out for postoperative analgesia prior to inset of the mesh, and the cartilage block for the second stage is banked in a subcutaneous pocket along the inferior margin of the chest incision. No dressings are applied to the reconstructed ear(s) to enable constant surveillance of the skin envelope and underlying construct. Patients are admitted to hospital where the ear(s) is monitored and the vacutainer drains are changed every 4 h to maintain the skin maximally applied to the contours of the framework. Patients are placed on a course of intravenous antibiotics while the drains are in place. On postoperative day 4, the drains are removed, and the patient is discharged from hospital on oral antibiotics for 1 week. The junior author has patients fitted with a waterpolo cap for sleeping to avoid flattening of the helix and pressure necrosis of the skin envelope.

For hemi-facial microsomia, craniofacial deficiency is often associated with an insufficient skin envelope for framework coverage, as well as a low temporal hairline resulting in hair extending onto the skin that will drape the superior portion of the ear construct. Tissue expansion has been suggested to address the former, and temporoparietal flap harvest for framework cover is generally used to deal with the latter [10]. When tissue expansion is used, Firmin [37] reported that expansion should be limited to the temporal region (scalp) and should not include the actual skin intended for framework coverage. The expansion process creates a fibrous capsule beneath the expanded skin, which must be meticulously removed to maintain the required pliability of the cutaneous cover. Furthermore, in view of the subsequent contraction of the expanded skin, the cited benefit of expansion, namely a single stage reconstruction with formation of the posterior auricular sulcus, is unpredictable. Hypoplastic auricular skin is heralded by a darker skin tone compared to adjacent facial skin. A valuable adjunct to improve the quality of this hypoplastic cutaneous cover is fat grafting of the auricular region. To compensate for the hypoplasia of the mastoid, Firmin has suggested the addition of a cartilaginous segment beneath the inferior portion of the framework, extending from the anti-tragus to the lobule [32]. This piece augments the projection of the lobule and anti-tragus and impedes the descent of the framework into the mastoid hollow (projection piece III). Use of the temporoparietal fascial flap enables simultaneous coverage of the upper pole of the framework and formation of the superior retro-auricular sulcus. If a temporoparietal fascial flap is required for partial or complete coverage of the cartilaginous framework, it is harvested following dissection of a subcutaneous pocket through a 4 cm *chevron-type* incision placed at the apex of the temporal fossa, centered over the superficial temporal artery, in distinction to the vertical *zig-zig* incision described by Nagata and Firmin, which have been shown to result in a potentially unfavorable scar with alopecia. The fascial flap is then covered with a split-thickness skin graft harvested from the *contralateral* scalp.

The second stage is routinely performed 6 months following the first stage, with the exception of first-stage reconstruction necessitating temporoparietal fascial flap coverage of the construct, for which an interval of 12 months must elapse before framework elevation and sulcus formation [31] (Fig. 5.5a and b). Thc reconstructed ear is released through a peri-helical incision extending to fascia, and the framework is elevated to the level of the concha. In contradistinction to Nagata's technique for framework elevation, the authors have adopted Firmin's technique, where the framework is elevated denude of soft tissue attachments. The latter facilitates mobilization of the framework anteriorly to the concha, and the more extensive mobilization of the framework has the added advantage of enabling adjustments to the position of the reconstructed ear [27]. Projection of the ear construct is buttressed by placement of the cartilage block previously banked in the thoracic skin pocket in the first stage. The cartilage segment is carved to a height appropriate to achieve symmetric projection to the contalateral ear and shaped to mimic the curve of the overlying anti-helix, positioned to form the posterior conchal wall. Three to four wire sutures are placed along the anterior aspect of the anti-helix, passed through the base and cartilage block to fix the fragment into position. Although a temporoparietal fascial flap is commonly used for coverage of the framework and cartilage block, the authors, like Brent [22], prefer a random pattern anteriorly based mastoid fascial flap [38–40]. The flap is turned over to cover the cartilage block and posterior surface of the reconstructed ear [39]. This fascial flap provides reliable well-vascularized coverage of the ear without necessitating placement of potentially conspicuous scars and noticeable

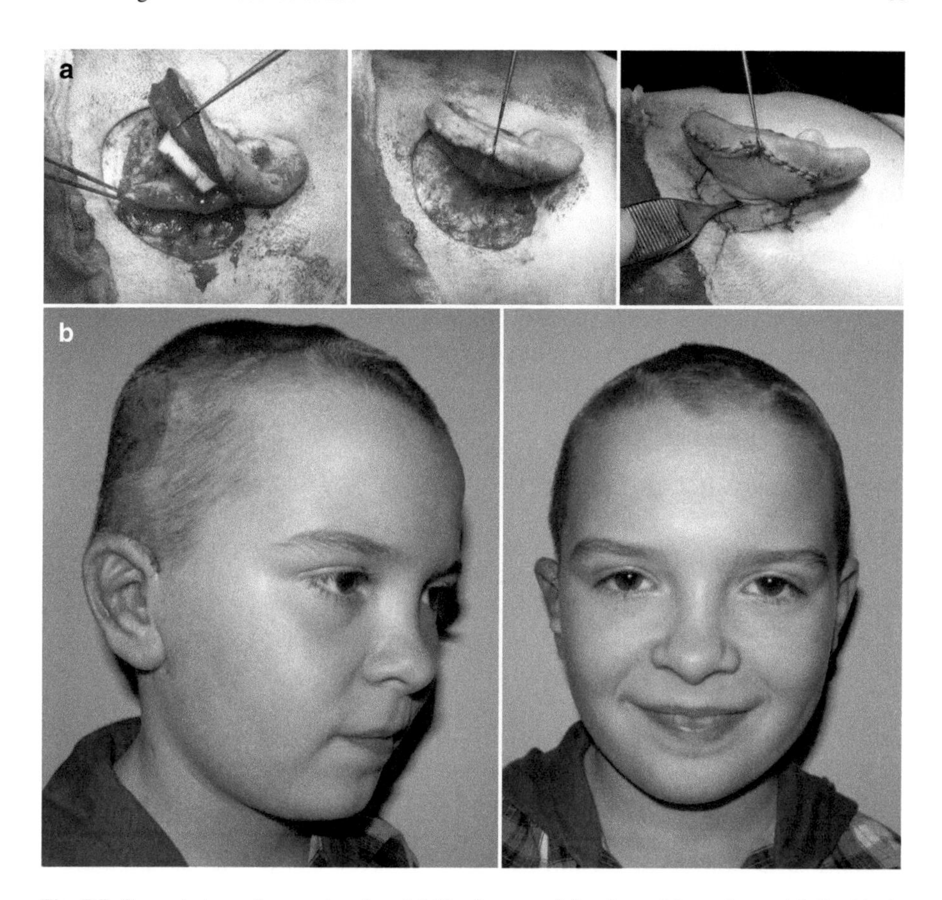

Fig. 5.5 Second stage of reconstruction. (**a**) The framework is released through a peri-helical incision extending to fascia and elevation of the ear construct is buttressed with a cartilage block. A random-pattern galeal fascial flap is used for the coverage of the framework and cartilage block. The retro-auricular skin is advanced toward the sulcus and the remaining areas surfaced with a split-thickness skin graft harvested from the scalp. (**b**) Early postoperative result achieved following completion of two-stage reconstruction in a patient with unilateral isolated microtia. (**a**, **b**: Used with permission of John Wiley and Sons from Cugno and Bulstrode [31])

scar alopecia in the scalp, preserving the temporoparietal fascia for any salvage procedure. Firmin has abandoned use of the mastoid fascial flap for the second stage stating the reliability of this random pattern flap is inconsistent and is associated with a higher rate of overlying graft failure, which along with greater filling of the retro-auricular sulcus with the pedicle of the flap, results in poorer depth of the sulcus (Firmin, personal communication). In our practice, we routinely use this fascial flap for the second stage and have not noted any difference in vascularity relative to the temporoparietal fascial flap. The retro-auricular skin is advanced toward the auriculocephalic sulcus and the posterior surface of the ear and, if required, the mastoid region is surfaced with a split-thickness skin graft. As described by Nagata and Firmin, we consistently use the *ipsilateral* scalp as a donor site for skin graft harvest in the second stage. If both the posterior surface of the ear and the mastoid area require coverage, two separate skin grafts are fixed to these areas, in an effort to minimize retraction of the sulcus. Following the second stage, patients are admitted overnight to complete a 24-h course of intravenous antibiotics, and then discharged on oral antibiotics for 7 days. The dressing remains in place until the first postoperative visit at 1 week. At 2 weeks, the auriculocephalic sulcus is fitted with an elastomer ear splint to counteract the contractile forces of the skin grafts in the retro-auricular sulcus in an effort to maintain the depth of the sulcus and projection of the ear.

In the last decade, reconstruction for cases of bilateral microtia has been executed simultaneously by the senior author, with each stage of this operative sequence performed in tandem [41]. For patients with bilateral microtia in whom adequate projection has been achieved following the first stage of reconstruction, the authors often do not perform the second stage of reconstruction. If the second stage is done for creation of the retro-auricular sulcus, and no further projection of the framework is required (i.e., no addition of a cartilage block), then the Brent technique can be used, as previously described.

The second stage presents an opportunity to carry out other refinements to the ear construct and/or additional reconstructive procedures to enhance facial form and/or symmetry [42]. This combined reconstructive approach has become the authors' routine practice, with complementary procedures including contralateral prominauris correction, ear piercing, fat transfer for soft tissue augmentation, as well genioplasty and malar augmentation to camouflage any associated bony deficiency. Ear piercing is often a principal motivation for auricular reconstruction in girls. In order to pierce the reconstructed ear, an incision is made along the border of the lobule, the cartilage within the lobe is partially excised, and the skin sutured. The point of piercing is identified, placed inferior to the reduced end of the costal cartilage framework (or at the level of the previously made perforation), and marked on the anterior surface of the lobule. A jelco needle is used to pierce the lobe, the needle retracted and a 4-0 nylon placed within the tubing and sutured to form a "hoop" earring. This fabricated earring is removed 3 weeks later and replaced with a true earring. Typical result achieved following completion of two-stage microtia reconstruction is shown in Fig. 5.6.

Complications

There are a number of complications associated with autologous auricular reconstruction, related to both donor site and the site of reconstruction. With regard to donor site, the most notable complication is chest wall depression or deformity [43, 44], often cited by proponents of synthetic reconstruction as a primary argument against costal cartilage harvest for framework fabrication. However, much of the contention surrounding attendant chest deformity stems from data gathered from the earlier decades of autologous reconstruction, where large amounts of cartilage were harvested in younger patients (below age 8 years) without any regard for

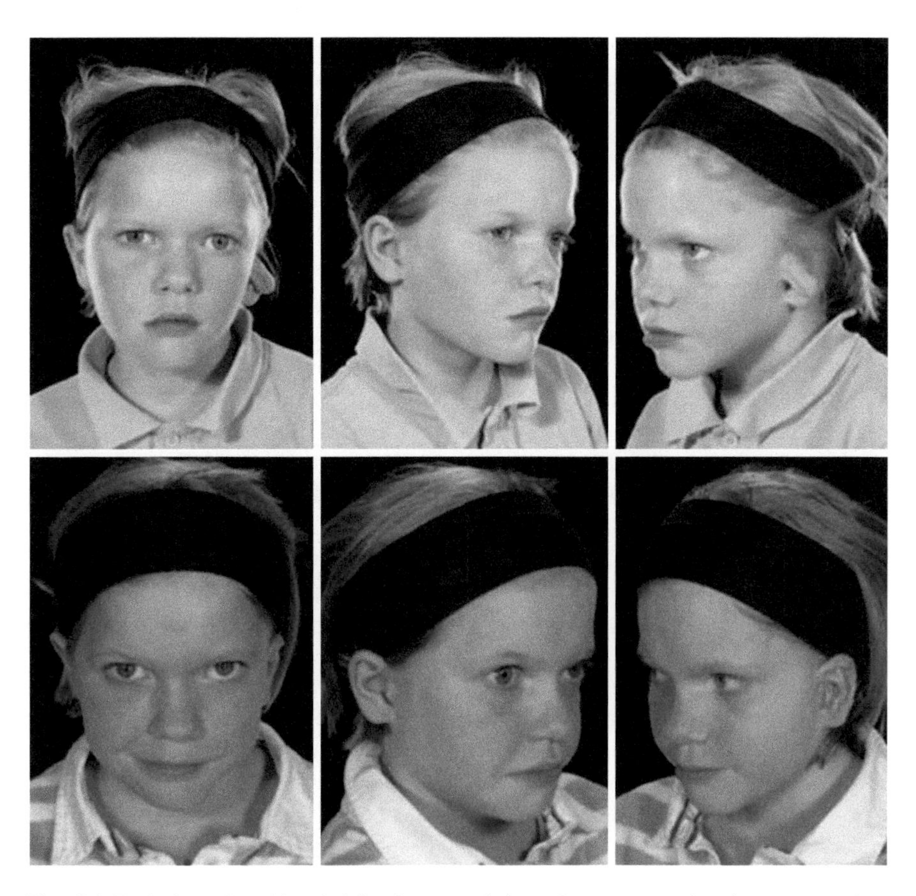

Fig. 5.6 Typical result achieved following completion of two-stage microtia reconstruction. (Used with permission of Elsevier from Cugno et al. [42])

preservation of the perichondrium [44, 45]. Furthermore, recent studies have demonstrated that there is a high prevalence of preoperative chest deformities among patients with microtia [46], which is not reflected in many longitudinal reports. Leaving the posterior or entire perichondrium in situ may potentially lessen chest wall morbidity by promoting cartilage regrowth at the donor site. In our practice, we have found that reconstitution of the costal margin as previously described, minimizes potential contour deformity, and Nagata maintains that preservation of the entire perichondrial envelope is integral to conserving maximum integrity of the chest wall. However, the benefit of the latter techniques remains to be definitively elucidated [47]. During rib harvest, one may inadvertently create a breach in the parietal pleura, resulting in pneumothorax. This is typically identified during the procedure and the pleural defect promptly repaired. Additional complications include hypertrophic scarring of the chest incision and postoperative respiratory problems, such as atelectasis. Most patients consider chest wall morbidity an acceptable compromise for a reconstructed ear [48].

At the level of the reconstructed ear, the most common complication is exposure of the cartilage framework. Draping the delicate auricular skin over the numerous convolutions of a rigid three-dimensional framework can result in vascular compromise to the overlying skin envelope, with consequent necrosis and cartilage exposure. The latter mandates early recognition and appropriate treatment as cartilage resorption and distortion to the final form of the ear construct may result. In general, small areas of cartilage exposure can usually be addressed conservatively with local wound care. However, larger areas of exposure require imminent surgical management with debridement and cutaneous or fascial flap coverage, depending on the location relative to the contours of the auricle and adjacent tissue mobility. In our experience, exposures greater than 10 mm^2 necessitate flap coverage. The mastoid and temporoparietal fascial flaps are most commonly used flaps in salvage operations following skin necrosis and exposure of the cartilage framework after reconstruction of microtia [49]. For harvest of a random mastoid fascial flap, a T incision is made adjacent to the defect, with the short limb of the incision placed along the periphery of the construct. The two resulting scalp flaps are elevated superficial to the superficial mastoid fascia. The dimensions of the fascial flap required for cover are outlined, the fascia incised, and the flap elevated superficial to the deep mastoid fascia. An anteriorly based fascial flap is turned over and inset over the denuded cartilage. The fascia is then covered with a split-thickness skin graft harvested from an adjacent area of scalp. A fascial turnover flap is commonly used for areas localized to the helix and anti-helix. For large concave surfaces, namely the concha, if sufficient viable surrounding skin is present, direct closure may be achieved by reliance on the *drawbridge effect*, which occurs when tissue lining a concave surface is mobilized anteriorly. However, use of this technique must be tempered with an understanding that unfavorable conchal effacement may result. Alternatively, a tunneled fascial turnover flap and skin graft can be used to satisfaction (Fig. 5.7a and b). In this case, following elevation of the cutaneous scalp flaps overlying the fascial flap, a tunnel is created beneath the cartilaginous framework from the periphery of the construct to the recipient site. The harvested fascial flap is then delivered into the wound and inset in place. In our experience, the extent of fascial flap harvest is 10 cm from the periphery of the framework and 4 cm in width, where the distal extremity of the flap is used for framework coverage. Others have described flap dimensions of 6 × 6 cm [49] and reported that the superficial mastoid fascial layer can be extended as far as 8–10 cm posteriorly and superiorly [50]. If the mastoid fascia was previously used to cover an area of exposure following the first stage of

Fig. 5.7 Local fascial flap coverage for cartilage exposure. (**a**) Patient with hemifacial microsomia who presented with right unilateral lobular microtia. Twenty-nine days following the first stage of reconstruction, she presented with total necrosis of skin overlying the concha. (**b**) Coverage of the area of exposed cartilage graft was restored with harvest of a random superficial mastoid fascial flap, which was tunneled beneath the cartilaginous ear construct to reach the distal extent of the defect. The fascial flap was then grafted with a split-thickness skin graft harvested from the scalp (skin graft donor site shown). (**a**, **b**: Used with permission of John Wiley and Sons from Cugno and Bulstrode [31])

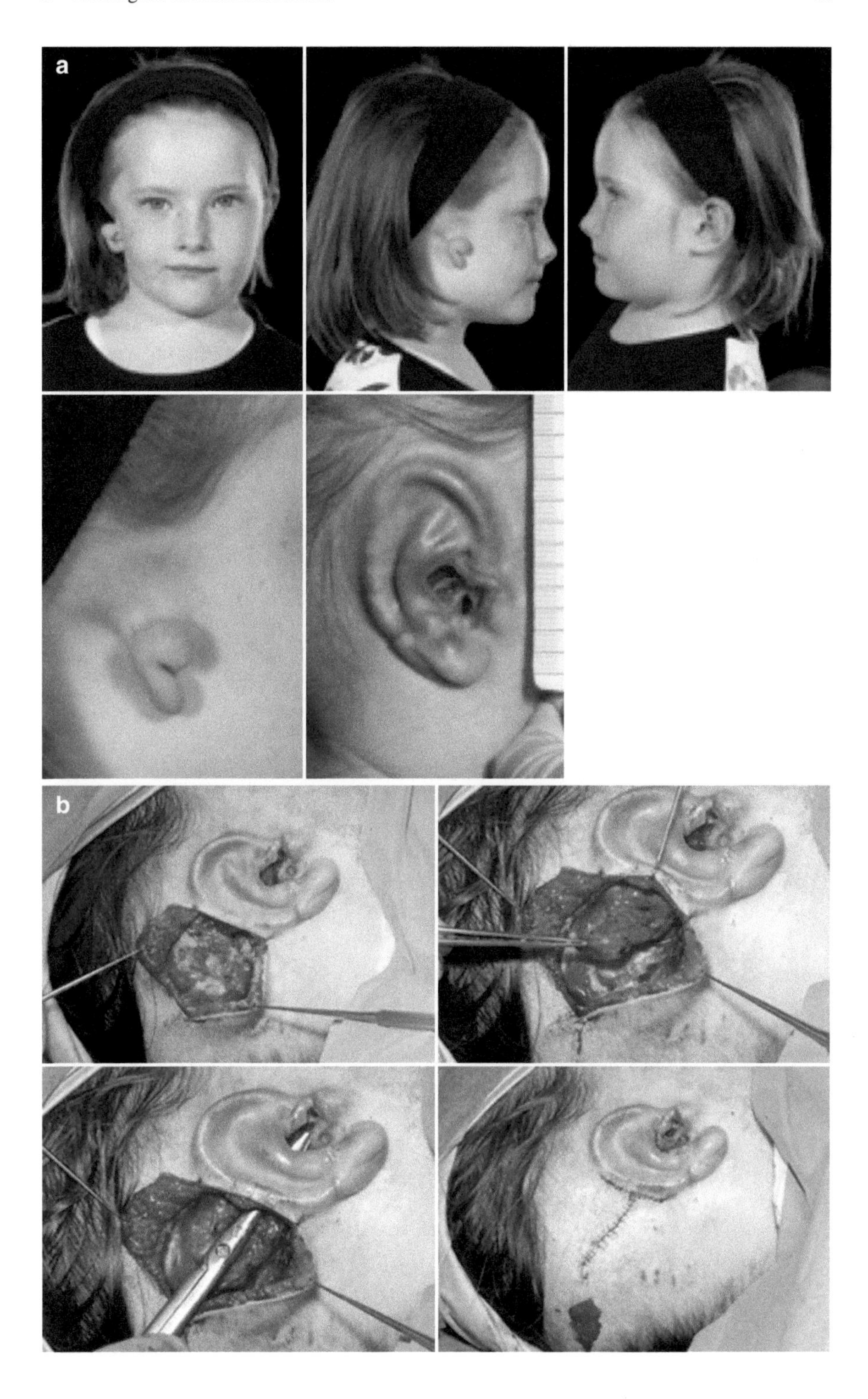
a
b

reconstruction, the fascial flap can still be utilized for the second stage. In this case, a tunnel is created between the previously elevated mastoid fascia and the framework to place the cartilage graft and the remaining fascia is raised for coverage of the adjacent areas of denuded cartilaginous framework.

The most devastating complication is infection. Although rare, infection is more commonly, if not almost exclusively, encountered following reconstruction of conchal-type microtia with presence of a true or vestigial external auditory canal. The presence of a remnant canal warrants preoperative cleaning and a course of prophylactic antibiotics for 5–7 days. Infection may also arise following cartilage exposure or prolonged neglect of any extruded material. Indeed, the wire sutures used to fix the pieces of the framework lie precariously under the thin auricular integument and bear great risk of frequent extrusion through the skin. If extrusion occurs, the wire should be removed promptly to prevent local infection and aesthetic compromise. The treatment of any suspected infection includes hospitalization of the patient for serial washouts of the skin pocket and a regimen of intravenous antibiotics. Despite efforts to control infection, cartilage resorption remains a certainty.

Additional complications include hematoma or seroma formation, cartilage framework resorption or fracture (most frequently, the helical rim), as well as fascial flap necrosis and associated skin graft loss (second stage).

Secondary Reconstruction

The main criticism of autologous reconstruction has remained the inconsistent and often unsatisfactory results obtained, with a construct that lacks definition and projection. However, this proposed disadvantage can be deterred by achieving proficiency in carving an ear framework prior to any reconstructive efforts. In cases where the reconstructed ear is deemed unsatisfactory, secondary reconstruction can be performed. Secondary reconstruction of a previously reconstructed ear is challenging and often disappointing [51]. While a new cartilaginous framework can be fashioned to satisfaction, a scarred inelastic skin envelope often results in a less than acceptable result, especially if secondary reconstruction is endeavored after the second stage has been performed. A fundamental principal in autologous ear reconstruction is to *only perform the second stage if a satisfactory result is achieved following the first stage of reconstruction*. If the result following the first stage is deemed unsatisfactory, it is preferable to sacrifice the reconstruction and begin anew. The approach to secondary ear reconstruction begins with an assessment of the retro-auricular skin. Despite previous dissection, the skin envelope following the first stage of reconstruction retains sufficient laxity and vascularity to be used for coverage of a new auricular framework. Secondary reconstruction following the second stage is a more challenging endeavor, where the skin is often unusable and alternative coverage options must be considered, namely, indirect tissue expansion and local fascial flaps. Indirect expansion is considered where sufficient skin is available to cover the framework but remains relatively inelastic. This process involves expansion of the hair-bearing scalp adjacent to the auricular area such that the expanded flap can be advanced and the non-hair bearing skin draped over the framework without tension. The rationale for indirect and direct expansion of the retro-auricular skin differs in that the former serves to decrease tension over the advanced non-hair-bearing skin, while the latter is performed to increase the amount of non-hair-bearing skin. Despite the popularity of the latter method in auricular reconstruction [50], it is seldom used in the authors' practice.

First introduced by Fox and Edgerton [52] as the *fan flap* and later popularized by Tegtmeier [53], the temporoparietal fascial flap has become an indispensable adjunct for reconstruction of the external ear [23, 54–56] and is often reserved for salvage of the unsatisfactory result when there is a paucity of well-vascularized skin available for complete or partial coverage or when previous scaring (including previous canuloplasty procedure) precludes skin use [55]. If the temporoparietal fascial flap has been used for the primary reconstruction, additional fascial flap options include mastoid fascia, deep temporal fascia, and other random-pattern turnover flaps (as described previously) [57]. Nagata has described using the innominate fascial flap for ear elevation in the second stage [55]. Free flaps, including the contralateral temporoparietal fascial flap, can also be considered.

Conclusion

The intricate contours of the external ear are attributed to delicate elastic cartilage covered with a thin layer of subcutaneous tissue and skin. Since the inception of costal cartilage use for microtia reconstruction, many modifications and refinements in technique have been developed over the last several decades, which have engendered an excellent replica of the complex three-dimensional structure of the external ear. However, autologous reconstruction remains a challenge necessitating an inherent artistic ability and is associated with a considerable learning curve. Despite advances in alternative methods of reconstruction, autologous cartilage remains the mainstay reconstructive option for microtia, particularly in the pediatric population, with proven durability and long-term success of the reconstructed ear that is at present unparalleled.

However, the optimal management of several aspects of autologous microtia reconstruction remains unresolved and debated by current leaders in the field of autologous ear reconstruction. Some authorities contend that the second stage of reconstruction should be reconsidered as creation of the auriculocephalic sulcus can result in a loss of framework definition. Further, optimal management of significant underlying bony deficit, as is common in cases of severe craniofacial microsomia, remains in dispute, as well as the optimal reconstructive sequence in these, and other, syndromic cases where auricular reconstruction is the only one in a series of procedures anticipated to address facial dysmorphism.

References

1. Gillies HD. Plastic surgery of the face, vol. 381. London: Hodder and Stoughton; 1920.
2. Tanzer RC. Total reconstruction of the external ear. Plast Reconstr Surg Transplant Bull. 1959;23(1):1–15.
3. Tanzer RC. An analysis of ear reconstruction. Plast Reconstr Surg. 1963;31:16–30.
4. Tanzer RC. Microtia—a long-term follow-up of 44 reconstructed auricles. Plast Reconstr Surg. 1978;61(2):161–6.
5. Tanzer RC. Total reconstruction of the auricle: a 10-year report. Plast Reconstr Surg. 1967;40(6):547–50.
6. Kirkham HL. The use of preserved cartilage in ear reconstruction. Ann Surg. 1940;111(5):896–902.
7. Tanzer RC. Total reconstruction of the auricle. The evolution of a plan of treatment. Plast Reconstr Surg. 1971;47(6):523–33.
8. Brent B. Ear reconstruction with an expansile framework of autogenous rib cartilage. Plast Reconstr Surg. 1974;53(6):619–28.
9. Brent B. The correction of mi-rotia with autogenous cartilage grafts: I. The classic deformity? Plast Reconstr Surg. 1980;66(1):1–12.
10. Brent B. The correction of microtia with autogenous cartilage grafts: II. Atypical and complex deformities. Plast Reconstr Surg. 1980;66(1):13–21.
11. Brent B. Auricular repair with autogenous rib cartilage grafts: two decades of experience with 600 cases. Plast Reconstr Surg. 1992;90(3):355–74; discussion 75–6.
12. Cronin TD, Greenberg RL, Brauer RO. Follow-up study of silastic frame for reconstruction of external ear. Plast Reconstr Surg. 1968;42(6):522–9.
13. Cronin TD. Use of a silastic frame for total and subtotal reconstruction of the external ear: preliminary report. Plast Reconstr Surg. 1966;37(5):399–405.
14. Brent B. Technical advances in ear reconstruction with autogenous rib cartilage grafts: personal experience with 1200 cases. Plast Reconstr Surg. 1999;104(2):319–34; discussion 35–8.
15. Nagata S, Burton B. Discussion. Modification of the stages in total reconstruction of the auricle, parts I to IV. Plast Reconstr Surg. 1994;93(2):267–8.
16. Nagata S. A new method of total reconstruction of the auricle for microtia. Plast Reconstr Surg. 1993;92(2):187–201.
17. Firmin F. Ear reconstruction in cases of typical microtia. Personal experience based on 352 microtic ear corrections. Scand J Plast Reconstr Surg Hand Surg. 1998;32(1):35–47.
18. Ishikura N, Kawakami S, Yoshida J, Shimada K. Vascular supply of the subcutaneous pedicle of Nagata's method in microtia reconstruction. Br J Plast Surg. 2004;57(8):780–4.
19. Nagata S. Modification of the stages in total reconstruction of the auricle: Part I. Grafting the three-dimensional costal cartilage framework for lobule-type microtia. Plast Reconstr Surg. 1994;93(2):221–30; discussion 67–8.
20. Nagata S. Modification of the stages in total reconstruction of the auricle: Part II. Grafting the three-dimensional costal cartilage framework for concha-type microtia. Plast Reconstr Surg. 1994;93(2):231–42; discussion 67–8.
21. Nagata S. Modification of the stages in total reconstruction of the auricle: Part III. Grafting the three-dimensional costal cartilage framework for small concha-type microtia. Plast Reconstr Surg. 1994;93(2):243–53; discussion 67–8.
22. Brent B. Microtia repair with rib cartilage grafts: a review of personal experience with 1000 cases. Clin Plast Surg. 2002;29(2):257–71, vii.
23. Nagata S. Modification of the stages in total reconstruction of the auricle: Part IV. Ear elevation for the constructed auricle. Plast Reconstr Surg. 1994;93(2):254–66; discussion 67–8.
24. Kawanabe Y, Nagata S. A new method of costal cartilage harvest for total auricular reconstruction: Part I. Avoidance and prevention of intraoperative and postoperative complications and problems. Plast Reconstr Surg. 2006;117(6):2011–8.

25. Kawanabe Y, Nagata S. A new method of costal cartilage harvest for total auricular reconstruction: Part II. Evaluation and analysis of the regenerated costal cartilage. Plast Reconstr Surg. 2007;119(1):308–15.
26. Chen ZC, Goh RC, Chen PK, Lo LJ, Wang SY, Nagata S. A new method for the second-stage auricular projection of the Nagata method: ultra-delicate split-thickness skin graft in continuity with full-thickness skin. Plast Reconstr Surg. 2009;124(5):1477–85.
27. Firmin F. State-of-the-art autogenous ear reconstruction in cases of microtia. Adv Otorhinolaryngol. 2010;68:25–52.
28. Firmin F. Auricular reconstruction in cases of microtia. Principles, methods and classification. Ann Chir Plast Esthet. 2001;46(5):447–66.
29. Firmin F, Marchac A. Auricular malformations. Ann Chir Plast Esthet. 2016;61(5):420–8.
30. Firmin F, Marchac A. A novel algorithm for autologous ear reconstruction. Semin Plast Surg. 2011;25(4):257–64.
31. Cugno S, Bulstrode N. Chapter 19. Congenital ear anomalies. In: Farhadieh R, Cugno S, Bulstrode N, editors. Plastic and reconstructive surgery: approaches and techniques. New York: Wiley Blackwell; 2015. p. 238.
32. Firmin F, Guichard S. Microtia in cases of oto-mandibular dysplasia. Ann Chir Plast Esthet. 2001;46(5):467–77.
33. Nagata S. Discussion. Balanced auricular reconstruction in dystopic microtia with the presence of the external auditory canal. Plast Reconstr Surg. 2002;109(5):1501–5.
34. Park C. Balanced auricular reconstruction in dystopic microtia with the presence of the external auditory canal. Plast Reconstr Surg. 2002;109(5):1489–500; discussion 501–5.
35. Gibson T, Davis WB. The distortion of autogenous cartilage grafts: its cause and prevention. Br J Plast Surg. 1958;10:257–74.
36. Fattah A, Sebire NJ, Bulstrode NW. Donor site reconstitution for ear reconstruction. J Plast Reconstr Aesthet Surg. 2010;63(9):1459–65.
37. Firmin F. Value of tissue expansion in total reconstruction of the external ear. Ann Chir Plast Esthet. 1996;41(5):495–502.
38. Park C. A single-stage two-flap method of total ear reconstruction. Plast Reconstr Surg. 1991;88(404):12.
39. Yoshimura K, Asato H, Nakatsuka T, Sugawara Y, Park S. Elevation of a constructed auricle using the anteriorly based mastoid fascial flap. Br J Plast Surg. 1999;52(7):530–3.
40. Wang Y, Zhuang X, Jiang H, Yang Q, Zhao Y, Han J, et al. The anatomy and application of the postauricular fascia flap in auricular reconstruction for congenital microtia. J Plast Reconstr Aesthet Surg. 2008;61(Suppl 1):S70–6.
41. Cugno S, Bulstrode N. Bilateral autologous microtia reconstruction: a simultaneous two-stage approach. Eur J Plast Surg. 2016;39(4):257–64.
42. Cugno S, Farhadieh RD, Bulstrode NW. Autologous microtia reconstruction combined with ancillary procedures: a comprehensive reconstructive approach. J Plast Reconstr Aesthet Surg. 2013;66(11):1487–93.
43. Ohara K, Nakamura K, Ohta E. Chest wall deformities and thoracic scoliosis after costal cartilage graft harvesting. Plast Reconstr Surg. 1997;99(4):1030–6.
44. Thomson HG, Kim TY, Ein SH. Residual problems in chest donor sites after microtia reconstruction: a long-term study. Plast Reconstr Surg. 1995;95(6):961–8.
45. Long X, Yu N, Huang J, Wang X. Complication rate of autologous cartilage microtia reconstruction: a systematic review. Plast Reconstr Surg Glob Open. 2013;1(7):e57.
46. Wu R, Jiang H, Chen W, Li Q, Zhao Y, Bi Y, et al. Three-dimensional chest computed tomography analysis of thoracic deformities in patients with microtia. J Plast Reconstr Aesthet Surg. 2015;68(4):498–504.
47. Wallace CG, Mao HY, Wang CJ, Chen YA, Chen PK, Chen ZC. Three-dimensional computed tomography reveals different donor-site deformities in adult and growing microtia patients despite total subperichondrial costal cartilage harvest and donor-site reconstruction. Plast Reconstr Surg. 2014;133(3):640–51.

48. Uppal RS, Sabbagh W, Chana J, Gault DT. Donor-site morbidity after autologous costal cartilage harvest in ear reconstruction and approaches to reducing donor-site contour deformity. Plast Reconstr Surg. 2008;121(6):1949–55.
49. Oyama A, Sasaki S, William M, Funayama E, Yamamoto Y. Salvage of cartilage framework exposure in microtia reconstruction using a mastoid fascial flap. J Plast Reconstr Aesthet Surg. 2008;61(Suppl 1):S110–3.
50. Park C. Subfascial expansion and expanded two-flap method for microtia reconstruction. Plast Reconstr Surg. 2000;106(7):1473–87.
51. Tanzer RC. Secondary reconstruction of microtia. Plast Reconstr Surg. 1969;43(4):345–50.
52. Fox JW, Edgerton MT. The fan flap: an adjunct to ear reconstruction. Plast Reconstr Surg. 1976;58(6):663–7.
53. Tegtmeier RE, Gooding RA. The use of a fascial flap in ear reconstruction. Plast Reconstr Surg. 1977;60(3):406–11.
54. Brent B, Byrd HS. Secondary ear reconstruction with cartilage grafts covered by axial, random, and free flaps of temporoparietal fascia. Plast Reconstr Surg. 1983;72(2):141–52.
55. Nagata S. Secondary reconstruction for unfavorable microtia results utilizing temporoparietal and innominate fascia flaps. Plast Reconstr Surg. 1994;94(2):254–65; discussion 66–7.
56. Edgerton MT. Discussion. Secondary reconstruction for unfavorable microtia results utilizing temporoparietal and innominate fascia flaps. Plast Reconstr Surg. 1994;94(2):266–7.
57. Hirase Y, Kojima T, Hirakawa M. Secondary ear reconstruction using deep temporal fascia after temporoparietal fascial reconstruction in microtia. Ann Plast Surg. 1990;25(1):53–7.

Chapter 6
Polyethylene Ear Reconstruction: A State-of-the-Art Surgical Technique

John F. Reinisch and Youssef Tahiri

Rationale

The purpose of outer ear reconstruction is the restoration of craniofacial balance by creating an aesthetically pleasing, symmetric, and long-lasting pinna. Ear reconstruction should be considered an aesthetic procedure, and its results should be held to the same critical standards as other cosmetic surgeries.

The traditional method of ear reconstruction has utilized an ear framework made from rib cartilage. Tanzer described this technique almost six decades ago [1]. Subsequent refinements of his procedure have reduced the number of needed surgical stages [2–5]. However, the amount of required harvested cartilage has increased, pushing back the age of reconstruction until 10 years of age or older.

Reconstruction at an older age, and its usual multiple stages, have made microtia reconstruction with autologous cartilage a more arduous physical and psychological endeavor for both children and their parents. If the final cosmetic result of the constructed ear is not ideal, the entire reconstructive journey can feel like *a long run for a short and disappointing slide*.

The use of an alloplastic framework covered by a thin temporoparietal fascia flap offers several advantages over the traditional method of cartilage reconstruction.

Electronic Supplementary Material The online version of this chapter (https://doi.org/10.1007/978-3-030-16387-7_6) contains supplementary material, which is available to authorized users.

J. F. Reinisch (✉)
Keck School of Medicine, University of Souther California, Los Angeles, CA, USA

Craniofacial and Pediatric Plastic Surgery, Cedars Sinai Medical Center, Los Angeles, CA, USA
e-mail: Jfr654@aol.com

Y. Tahiri (✉)
Plastic and Reconstructive Surgery, Cedars-Sinai Medical Center, Los Angeles, CA, USA
e-mail: Youssef.Tahiri@cshs.org

© Springer Nature Switzerland AG 2019

J. F. Reinisch, Y. Tahiri (eds.), *Modern Microtia Reconstruction*,
https://doi.org/10.1007/978-3-030-16387-7_6

Since ears reach 85% of adult size by 3.5 years [6], ear reconstruction can be performed at a younger age since the need for sufficient costal cartilage is not a factor. Other advantages of a fascia-covered alloplastic framework over the traditional rib cartilage technique include minimal patient discomfort, single outpatient procedure, and better ear definition and projection.

The main disadvantage of using an alloplastic framework is that it is not well tolerated under a thin skin flap, unlike rib cartilage constructs. Thus, the soft tissue coverage of an alloplastic ear needs to be different from a cartilage framework. To avoid exposure, it is critical that the alloplastic implant is completely enveloped by a thin fascia flap with its attached loose areolar layer [7]. Full-thickness skin grafts are then placed over the fascia.

Both cartilage and polyethylene frameworks are passive skeletons that provide shape and projection to the covering soft tissue. Cartilage has a low metabolic requirement because it has relatively few active cells within a large extra-cellular matrix. As a result, it survives nicely as a graft and is well tolerated beneath a thin skin flap. By contrast, when a porous polyethylene implant is placed beneath a thin skin flap, a significant rate of exposure of the implant is seen over time. A polyethylene implant should never be substituted for a cartilage framework when performing the traditional mastoid skin pocket soft tissue coverage.

While the harvest and assembly of the framework is the most challenging and time-consuming component of the rib ear reconstruction procedure, the most critical component of the alloplastic reconstruction is the soft tissue coverage of the framework. As long as a healthy fascia flap covers the implant without tension, an alloplastic reconstruction can be done with minimal complications. In addition, the ability to complete the procedure in a single, outpatient procedure before starting school is a very appealing feature of alloplastic ear reconstruction.

In this chapter, we describe the operative steps to reconstruct an outer ear using a porous high-density polyethylene (pHDPE) implant.

Indications and Contraindications

Candidates for pHDPE implant reconstruction include patients with congenital microtia, as well as patients with a traumatic loss of their ear or a prior unsatisfactory ear reconstruction. Patients must have either an intact superficial temporal artery (STA) supplying the superficial temporal-parietal fascia (STPF) or a patent occipital artery supplying the occipital parietal fascia (OCP). Free fascia flaps with a radial forearm fascia or a free contralateral TPF flap are possible in the rare case, in which no local arterial fascia flaps are available.

Conditions that would be relative contraindications for traditional rib reconstruction (low hair line, mastoid scaring, or a previous atresia repair) are not contraindications for pHDPE ear reconstruction, if the entire implant can be covered with well-vascularized fascia.

Surgical Technique

Anesthesia and Preparation

After satisfactory oral tracheal intubation, an intravenous line is started and intravenous antibiotics and steroids are given. A bladder catheter is placed and the patient is padded appropriately because of the expected length of the operative procedure.

The endotracheal tube is sutured to the upper central gingiva with a 2-0 silk mattress suture (Fig. 6.1). This is done to minimize the chance for tube displacement when turning the head during the procedure. The table is rotated 180°. The hair of the lower temporoparietal scalp is shaved, and the remaining hair is braided if needed. It is important that no paralytic agents are given during the procedure in order to assess nerve and muscle function.

For sterility, the eyes, nose, and mouth are covered with Tegaderms (3M, St-Paul, MN, USA) (Fig. 6.2a and b). These coverings further secure the endotracheal tube. The entire head is then prepped and draped, as well as the contralateral groin. If abdominal fat needs to be harvested for fat grafting of a hypoplastic, ipsilateral cheek, the abdomen is included with the groin draping. The patient's endotracheal tube and anesthetic tubing are then placed in a sterile camera drape to allow the anesthetic tubing to sit sterilely on top of the patient (Fig. 6.2a and b). This prevents the tubing from being caught beneath the drapes when rotating the head during the procedure. It also allows for the tubing to be moved as needed for fat graft harvest from the abdomen and full-thickness skin graft harvest from the groin.

Specific instruments needed for the procedure include the four lengths of straight and angled Colorado tip needles (Stryker, Kalamazoo, MI, USA) used for blended

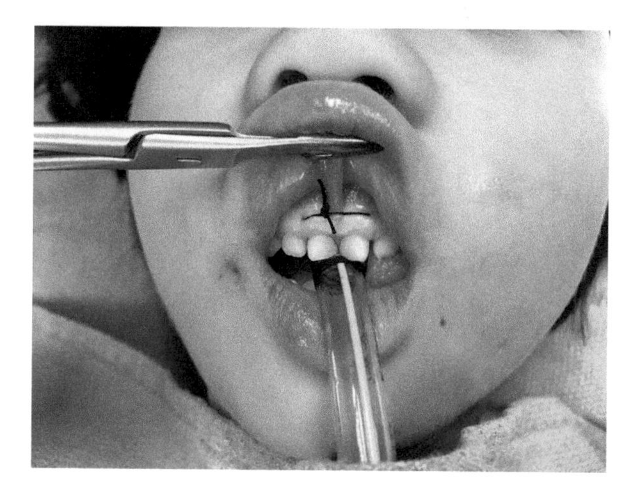

Fig. 6.1 The endotracheal tube is sutured to the upper central gingiva with a 2-0 silk suture

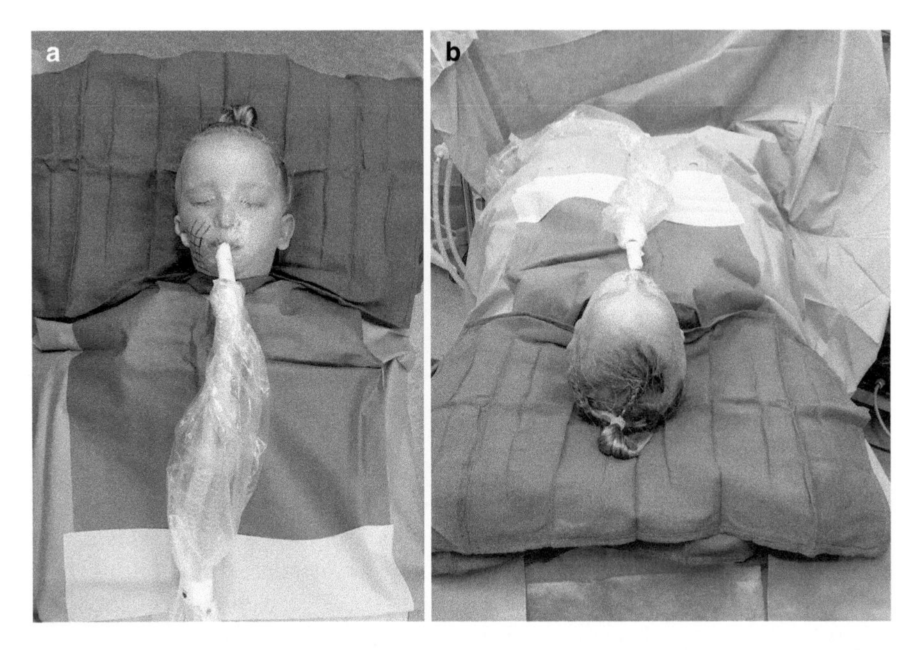

Fig. 6.2 (**a** and **b**) Eyes, nose, and mouth are covered with Tegaderms (3M, St-Paul, MN, USA). The patient's endotracheal tube and anesthetic tubing will be placed in a sterile camera drape to allow the anesthetic tubing to sit sterilely on top of the patient, allowing free movement of the head during the procedure, while decreasing the chance for inadvertent extubation

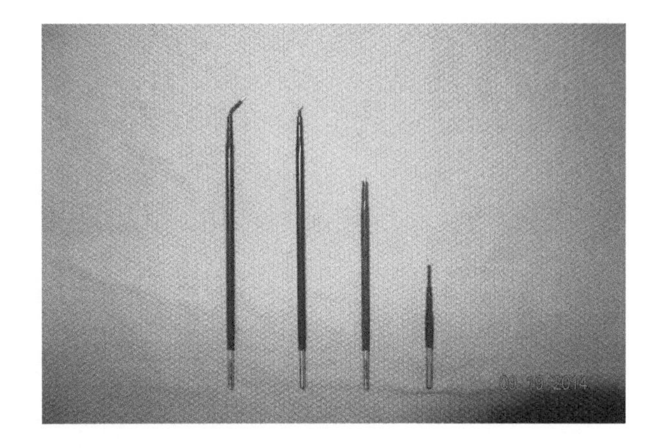

Fig. 6.3 Four lengths of straight and angled configurations of Colorado tip needle are used for blended cautery dissection during the harvest of the temporoparietal fascia flap

cautery dissection (Fig. 6.3), a Tessier retractor (Fig. 6.4), a #22 urethral sound (Fig. 6.5), two battery-operated high temperature cauteries, and an Edna clamp (Fig. 6.6), which is used during the assembly of the two components of the polyethylene framework.

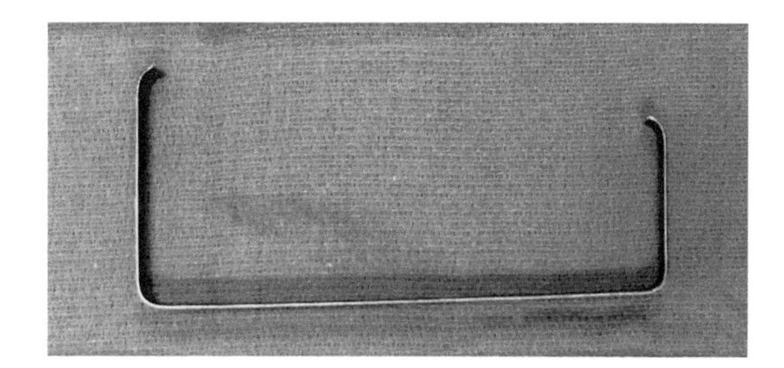

Fig. 6.4 Tessier retractor

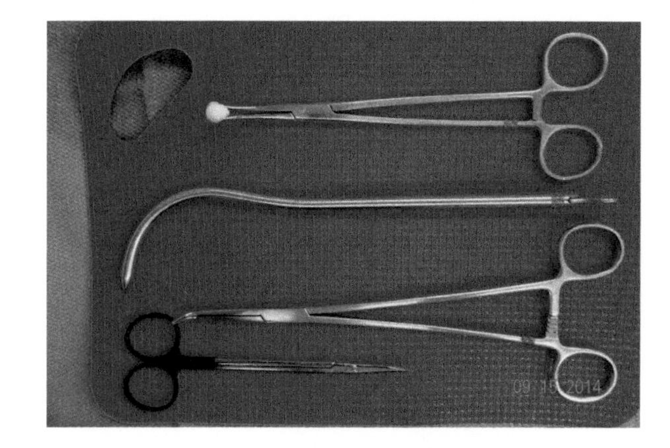

Fig. 6.5 Specific instruments used to raise the temporoparietal fascia flap include a #22 Urethral sound along with a peanut, curved scissors and a right angle clamp

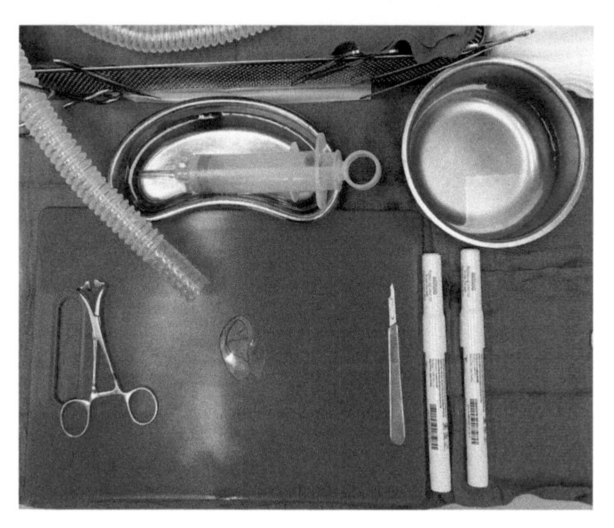

Fig. 6.6 Back table set up for carving of the implant

Markings and Vascular Considerations

The patient's normal ear is outlined on a template and transposed to the patient's affected side. The STA, along with the anterior and posterior branches, is identified by palpation, and marked. If palpation of the vessels is unsuccessful, a Doppler can be used to find the STA. The outline of the STPF flap is only marked after the prepping and draping (to avoid smearing of the ink during the prep). The anterior branch of the STA runs just posterior to the temporal branch of the facial nerve. Interestingly, the anterior branch of the STA turns and runs transversely in a posterior direction about 12 cm above the ear canal. If the transverse portion of this vessel is included in the STPF flap, it provides a healthy blood supply to the distal portion of the inferiorly based flap.

The size of the TPF has to be large enough to cover the entire implant without tension or tenting when shrink-wrapped onto the framework with suction. The width of the flap is approximately 10 cm, and the height is approximately 13 cm from the center of the ear. The flap must be long enough to include the transverse portion of the anterior branch. This transverse portion of the STA can also be used as a secondary landmark for the cephalic border of the flap, by dissecting 1 cm cephalic to the vessel. The anterior border of the flap is immediately anterior to the anterior branch of the STA (Fig. 6.7a and b).

In approximately 17% of cases, the STA has an origin posterior to the lobule and runs immediately beneath the small microtic cartilage remnant (Fig. 6.8). Since resection of the microtic cartilage is necessary to give a good conchal concavity and provide cartilage for the tragus, it is important to determine if this anomaly is present. The presence of this anomaly can be determined by palpation or by Doppler once the patient is anesthetized. When this variation is present, resection of the microtic cartilage must be done with extra care to avoid injury to the underlying artery.

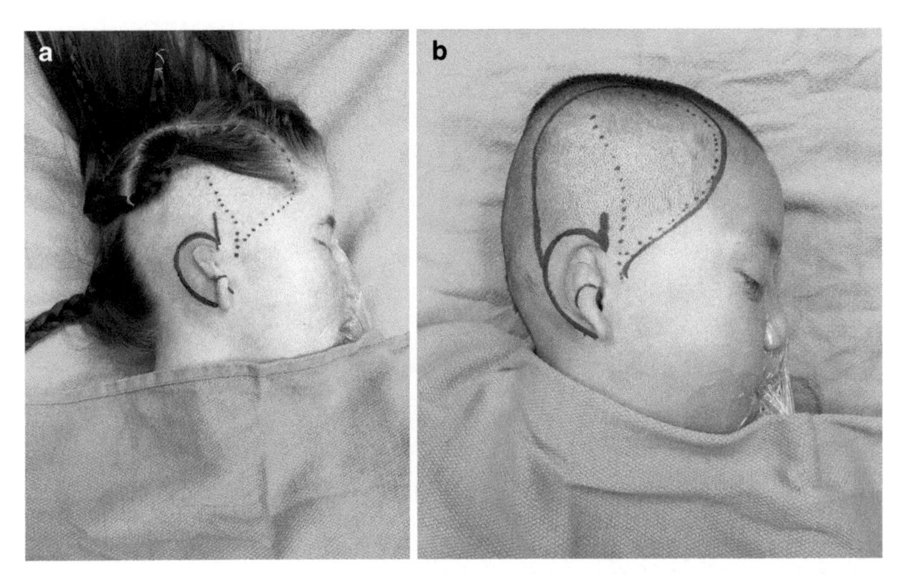

Fig. 6.7 (**a** and **b**) Preoperative markings demonstrating the superficial temporal artery with its anterior and posterior branches. The flap dimensions are approximately 10 cm in width by 13 cm in height from the canal (or the supposed position of the canal). The 13 cm height allows the inclusion in the flap of the transverse direction that the anterior branch of the superficial temporal artery takes at approximately the 12 cm mark

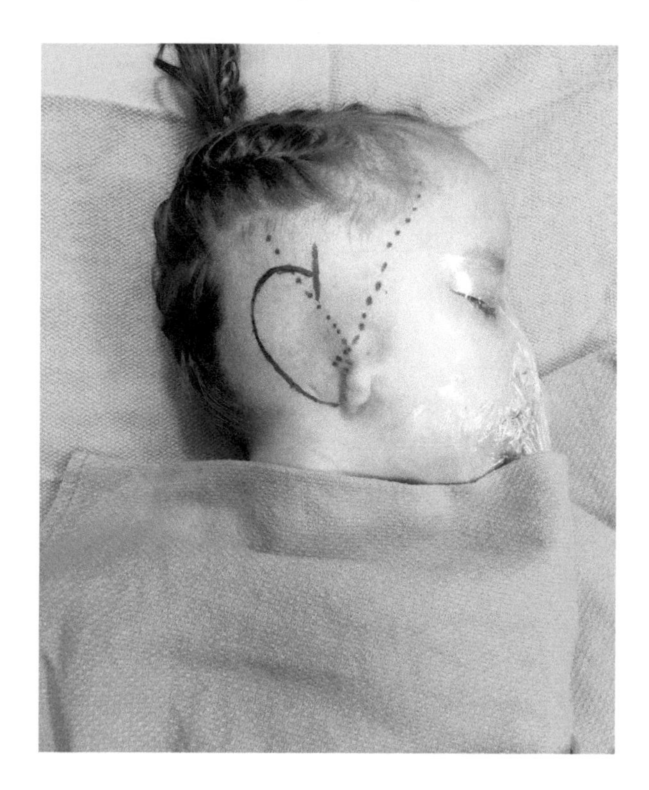

Fig. 6.8 In about 17% of cases, the STA has an origin posterior to the lobule and runs immediately beneath the small cartilage remnant

Finally, the lobule on the affected side is outlined for posterior transposition, and the remaining skin over the affected ear remnant and non-hair bearing mastoid area are outlined and infiltrated with a 0.5% lidocaine containing 1:200,000 epinephrine solution (Fig. 6.9).

Skin Graft Donor Sites

The contralateral medial thigh and groin are outlined for harvesting of a full-thickness skin graft (FTSG) to cover the postauricular surface of the reconstructed ear. The contralateral side is chosen as a donor site to allow simultaneous harvesting of the skin graft by an assistant while the principal surgeon harvests the TPF flap.

The lateral surface of the reconstructed ear is covered by the non-hair-bearing ipsilateral mastoid and ear remnant skin. While this skin can be defatted and used as an anteriorly based flap, it is most frequently divided from its anterior attachment and converted into a full-thickness skin graft (FTSG). Usually more skin is needed to cover the lateral surface of the reconstructed ear. One should avoid placing the thicker and usually darker groin skin on the lateral surface of the ear. In most patients, there is need for additional skin to cover that area. An adequately sized FTSG from the contralateral postauricular skin should be harvested and used to give a uniform color and texture to the more visible lateral surface of the new ear.

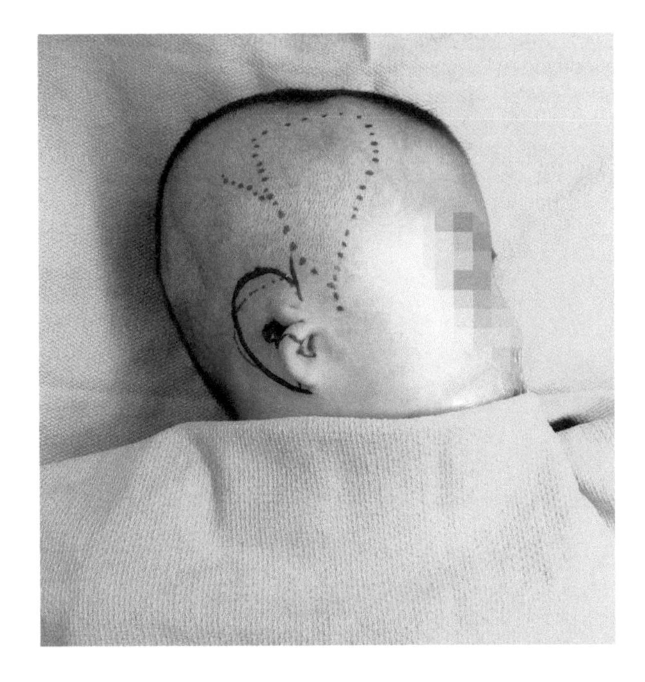

Fig. 6.9 Marking of the lobular remnant incision and inclusion

The donor sites are closed in layer after adequate undermining. The subcutaneous fascia is closed using 3-0 PDS and individual buried knots. The skin is then closed with interrupted 5-0 PDS sutures in buried individual subcuticular fashion. The two-layer closure is then sealed with Dermabond (Ethicon, Somerville, NJ, USA) to allow early bathing. A longitudinal Steri-Strip (3M, St-Paul, MN, USA) is applied for camouflage.

Initial Incisions

After vasoconstriction is obtained, the lobule of the affected ear is elevated as an inferiorly based flap for later posterior transposition and inset. The non-hair-bearing mastoid skin as well as the skin covering the microtic ear is then elevated as a thin anteriorly based flap. The microtic cartilage is removed carefully and saved as a potential cartilage graft for later tragal reconstruction. It is important to keep in mind that the ectopic cartilage is often larger than what it first appears to be. In patients without significant craniofacial microsomia, the area of cartilage resection leaves a concavity that becomes the depth of the future conchal bowl.

Harvesting of the Temporoparietal Fascia Flap (Video 6.1a and b)

Through the mastoid defect created by anterior reflection of the ear remnant and mastoid skin, the scalp is elevated from the surface of the superficial temporal fascia. The dissection is facilitated by using blended cautery (cutting at 20 and

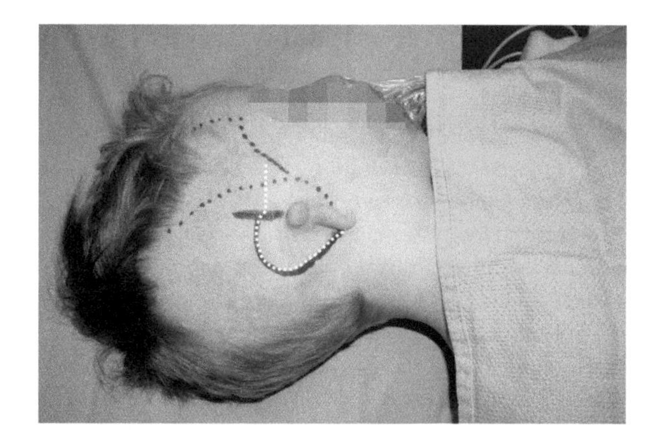

Fig. 6.10 Anterior transverse sideburn extension of the incision

coagulation at 15 and various lengths and configurations of fine tip cautery needles (Colorado needles, Stryker, Kalamazoo, MI, USA) as shown in Fig. 6.3. One should use the lowest effective electrocautery settings. The use of battery-operated headlamp helps the dissection. It is of great importance to first identify and preserve the anterior branch and main branch of the STA. An anterior transverse sideburn extension of the incision can be added if necessary to facilitate dissection (Fig. 6.10).

Once the scalp elevation is completed all the way to the outline of the flap, an incision through the superficial temporal and underlying subgaleal fascia is made down to the deep temporal fascia immediately anterior to the anterior branch of the superficial temporal artery. If the anterior branch of the STA is not easily seen, the anterior incision through the STPF flap can be delayed, and the head can be turned to harvest an FTSG from the opposite postauricular ear and mastoid skin. If the anterior branch has narrowed because of spasm, stopping the TPF dissection makes the vessel easier to visualize. Turning the head at this point also keeps the neck from being in one position too long during the procedure.

An incision where the posterior border of the flap is marked is then made through the superficial temporal fascia and carried down to the subgaleal space, right above the periosteum. Through the upper portion of this posterior incision, the upper scalp (cephalic to the scalp elevation) is dissected bluntly in the subgaleal space using a #22 urethral sound. The #22 urethral sound can be tunneled beneath the STPF and be used to strip the scalp and fascia from the periosteum 3–4 cm beyond the proposed 13 cm upper border of the flap. This blunt elevation of the scalp and fascia facilitates the eventual division of the distal cephalic border of the TPF flap from the under surface of the scalp. Furthermore, this elevation helps to ensure the inclusion of the transverse portion of the anterior branch of the STA in the distal flap. The superficial temporal fascia is then converted into an inferiorly based flap along with its subgaleal layer, by dividing these two layers from the undersurface of the scalp superiorly with a long, angled Colorado tip needle (Stryker, Kalamazoo, MI, USA). Using this technique, the STPF flap can be elevated and divided without a cephalic scalp incision. The superficial temporal fascia and its underlying subgaleal layer are then bluntly dissected from the periosteum superiorly and the deep temporal fascia inferiorly. The inferiorly based superficial temporal fascia is then transposed inferiorly through the mastoid defect. The base of the TPF flap should start several centimeters below the future site of the helical rim to allow for a good sulcus between the head and the reconstructed ear. It is important to include the thin subgaleal areolar fascia with the STPF flap. This loose areolar layer lies external to the STPF when it is transposed inferiorly and becomes the outer surface of the TPF flap upon which the skin is placed. This layer allows the healed skin graft to move over the STPF, which becomes adherent to the porous implant.

Once the temporal fascia flap is elevated, it can be returned to its original location under the scalp to keep it warm and allow any vasospasm to resolve. Time is then spent carving the implant; this will be discussed in the next section.

Once carving of the implant is done, attention is then turned back to the patient's STPF flap, which is brought out from beneath the scalp and transilluminated. The STA and its bifurcation into its two main branches are identified. Good pulsations are usually seen. Any distal bleeding is cauterized. The flap can be lengthened by incising the anterior border of the flap back to the STA inferior to its anterior branch. With prolonged vascular spasm, it can be challenging to visualize the vessels. In this situation, the flap can be replaced beneath the scalp and the head wrapped in sterile plastic bag for 15–30 min to warm the flap and allow the vascular spasm to subside.

Postoperative caudal descent of the implant is a possible complication of this procedure. To prevent implant migration, a 1 cm wide, inferiorly based, vertically oriented flap of deep temporal fascia (DTPF) can be raised from the temporalis muscle to suspend the implant. This narrow flap must be tunneled through the base of STPF flap using two very fine tip pediatric hemostats. The STPF flap should be transilluminated when making the tunnel to avoid injuring its vascular pedicle. The DTPF leash is then wrapped around the anterior portion of the inferior crus of the ear implant and sutured to itself to prevent future lowering of the implant.

Of note, if the elevation of the scalp and harvest of the underlying STPF flap through the mastoid defect seems difficult, a superior transverse scalp incision can be made. The incision should be placed perpendicular to the hair growth about 10–11 cm above the position of the absent canal (Fig. 6.11). The length of this counter incision can vary, based on surgeon's comfort to continue the flap dissection. Through this upper incision, one can dissect caudally to meet the inferior dissection from the mastoid. The scalp can then be dissected cephalically to reach the distal extent of the outlined flap. Although the scalp incision allows easier division of the upper portion of the STPF flap, it leaves a horizontal scalp scar. If the scalp incision is placed too high, and therefore runs parallel to the growth of the hair, the scar will be noticeable. This incision should be placed more caudally on the scalp where the hair growth would run perpendicular to a transverse scar, making the incision difficult to see. With more experience and confidence with harvesting of the STPF flap, the transverse incision can be abandoned.

Carving of the Implant (Video 6.2)

The two-piece implant can be assembled on the back table, while the assistant surgeon is harvesting the contralateral postauricular FTSG. The implant consists of two parts: a base and a helical rim. They are both soaked and impregnated in a

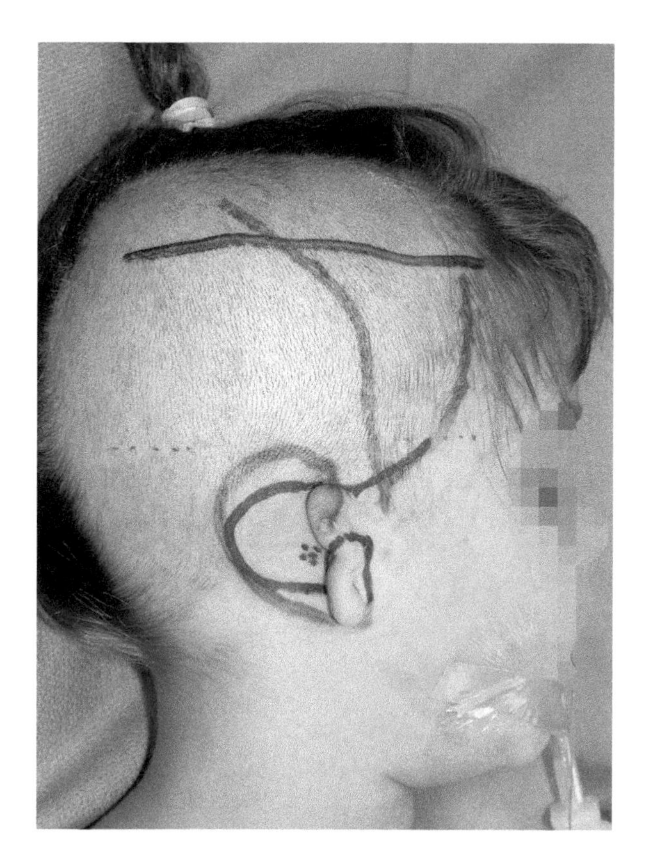

Fig. 6.11 Scalp counter incision that can be used to help during the flap harvest. The length of this counter incision can vary based on surgeon comfort to continue the flap dissection

bacitracin antibiotic solution. The thicker base can also be placed in a 60 cc syringe filled with the antibiotic solution. With a finger over the end of the syringe, negative pressure is then applied in order to remove air from the interstices of the porous implant and to fill the implant with the antibiotic solution; this cannot be done once the implant is fully constructed since it will not fit in the syringe.

The base component is carved by removing the tragal component. Some of the lower portion of the base may be removed so that the vertical height of the base with the rim attached plus the lobule will equal the vertical height of the patient's normal contralateral ear. If the child is between 3.0 and 4.5 years of age, the reconstructed ear is made approximately 6 to 2 mm longer, respectively. The helical rim is attached to the base, using remnants of polyethylene material from the removed helical root or tragal extension to fuse the two components of the implant together. The two pieces are melted together with a battery-operated, high temperature ophthalmic cautery (Argent Surgical Systems, Jacksonville, FL, USA). The helical root is removed to make room for a larger conchal bowl. A portion of the removed helical rim is used as a strut between the superior crus and the lateral helical rim to add additional strength to the lateral helical rim of the implant. The medial surface of the implant can be reduced to match the projection of the patient's contralateral ear. Once the construct is finalized, it is then left soaking in the antibiotic solution.

External Auditory Canal or Faux-Canal Formation

Microtia is accompanied by congenital absence or stenosis of the external auditory canal with variable middle ear anomalies, which causes a significant conductive hearing loss [8–11]. Children with unilateral microtia seem to develop normally. Parents usually do not notice a significant difference between their young children and their siblings without microtia. This is the reason why unilateral hearing loss has been undertreated by many otolaryngologists and usually ignored by plastic surgeons treating microtia [12].

However, when children with microtia are older, and communication becomes more sophisticated, hearing issues become more obvious. Sound localization and hearing comprehension especially in noisy environments become more difficult [13, 14].

Patients with microtia tend to turn their unaffected ear in the direction of sound, because the head itself casts a sound shadow, which reduces comprehension in the unturned normal ear.

Once a child is 2.5 years of age, a computed tomography (CT) scan of the temporal bones can allow an otologist to determine if an atresia patient is a possible candidate for a canalplasty. The otologist needs to view the actual scan rather than the radiologist's report. The Jahrsdorfer 10-point grading scale is commonly used to predict surgical candidacy depending on key features seen on the CT scan [15].

The treatment of hearing loss by an otologist should be coordinated with the surgeon responsible for the outer ear surgery. Traditionally, atresia repair is done after the costal cartilage ear reconstruction, since almost all otologists perform the ear canal reconstructions through a posterior mastoid skin incision to access the temporal bone. This approach compromises the blood supply of the mastoid skin that is used to cover the cartilage framework. However, prior atresia repair does not jeopardize the success of ear reconstruction using an implant covered by a vascularized fascia flap. With an alloplastic reconstruction, atresia repair is best done before or at the same time as the ear reconstruction because the canal helps with positioning of the reconstructed pinna. Also, early atresia repair potentially improves hearing at a critical period of early brain development [16].

If the patient is not a candidate for atresia repair and a functional canal, a faux-canal can be created at the time of microtia reconstruction.

The faux-canal is reconstructed by resecting the entire microtic cartilage remnant with additional soft tissue down to the mastoid periosteum to increase the depth of the auricular concavity. The tragus is later made by medially transposing an anteriorly based mastoid flap, which contains a cartilage graft for support (Fig. 6.12).

Implant Insetting and Coverage

Following canal or faux-canal creation and once hemostasis is obtained, the custom-made implant is positioned in its appropriate location, and suspended using the 1 cm deep temporal fascia leash. One suction drain is then placed beneath the implant and

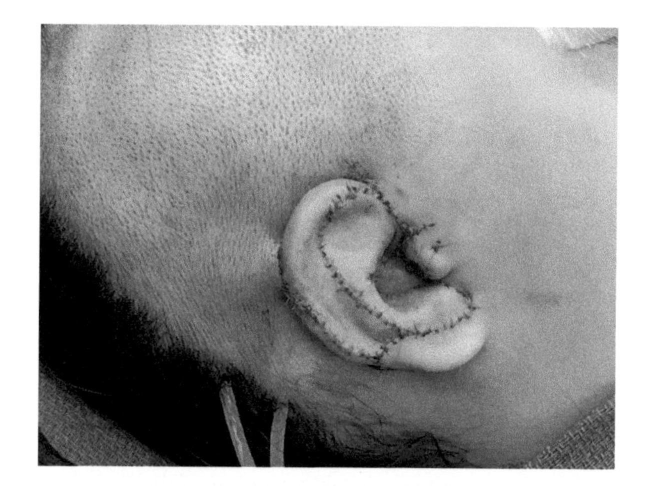

Fig. 6.12 Pseudo canal reconstruction using a combination of anteriorly based local flaps and full-thickness skin grafts

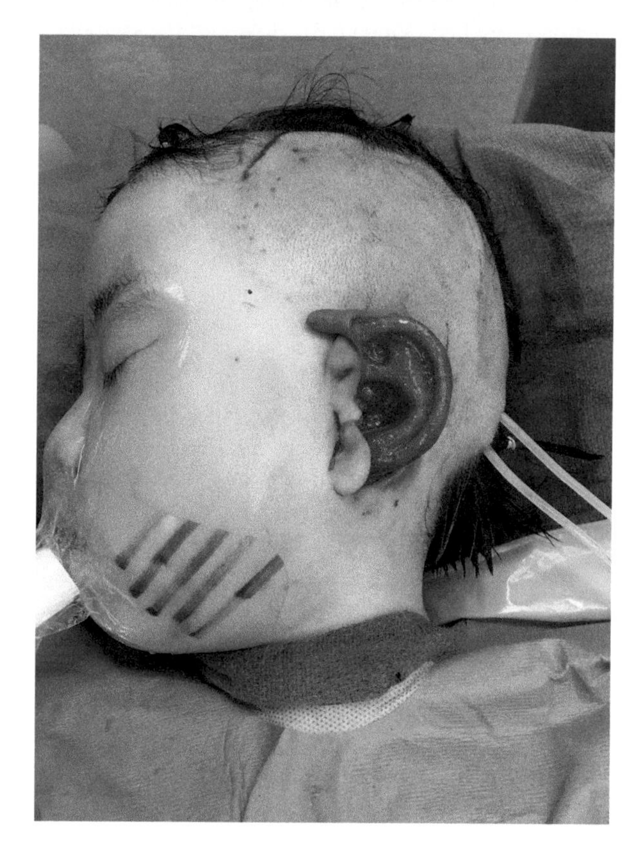

Fig. 6.13 Once the implant is covered completely, suction applied good contouring of the fascia over the implant was noted

another one under the scalp (where the flap was harvested). Both drains exit through the parietal scalp approximately 4 cm behind the reconstructed ear. The drains are not sutured, as they will be removed after the ear mold and dressing are placed.

The ear implant is then wrapped completely with the superficial temporal fascia flap. Suction is applied to shrink-wrap the fascia over the implant (Fig. 6.13).

The postauricular surface of the fascia-covered implant is then covered with the full-thickness skin graft obtained from the patient's medial thigh and groin. The skin is sutured in place to the mastoid skin with 5-0 chromic catgut sutures. The lobule is filleted longitudinally and defatted distally before being inset along the lower pole of the ear. This is also done with 5-0 chromic catgut sutures. The anterior surface of the ear is covered using the anteriorly based ear remnant and mastoid skin. This skin can be defatted and used as a flap, but is usually converted to a full-thickness skin graft. In most cases, there will not be sufficient ipsilateral skin to completely cover the entire lateral surface of the ear. In patients with unilateral microtia, the previously harvested contralateral postauricular skin can be added to cover the entire lateral reconstructed ear with skin of similar color, thickness, and texture. Suturing is done anteriorly with 6-0 chromic catgut sutures and posteriorly with 5-0 chromic catgut sutures. Each stitch is placed as a simple individual suture rather than as a running closure.

We observe a nice shrink-wrapping of the STPF flap over the implant once the suction is applied (Video 6.3). However, the skin placed over the STPF flap often does not contour as well to the implant initially, due to the presence of air between the skin and underlying STPF. This can be resolved by placing multiple, closely spaced sutures along the suture lines of the ear, obtaining an airtight closure. If the skin does not contour to the implant, additional sutures should be placed until all air can be expressed and the skin maintains its concavities over the scapha, triangular fossa, and conchal bowl (Fig. 6.14 and Video 6.4).

Tragal Reconstruction

To reconstruct the tragus, an appropriately sized piece of cartilage from the resected cartilage remnant is selected and inserted into a preauricular pocket. This pocket is created by medial transposition of an anteriorly based horizontally oriented flap of skin. Once positioned correctly, the cartilage is initially kept in place using a 25-gauge needle inserted through and through the cartilage transcutaneously. Definitive fixation is done using a 5-0 or 6-0 chromic gut mattress suture transcutaneously (Fig. 6.15a and b).

Dressings and Postoperative Care

The ear is then covered with bacitracin ointment. A calcium alginate dressing (Kaltostat, Convatec, Inc., Skillman, NJ, USA) is placed into the conchal bowl and along the postauricular sulcus. If the patient is prone to scarring and keloid formation (depending on ethnic background and skin Fitzpatrick type), a steroid ointment can be mixed with the bacitracin and applied to the ear prior to dressing application. A custom-made silicone ear splint (Azoft, Detax, Ettlingen, Germany) is then

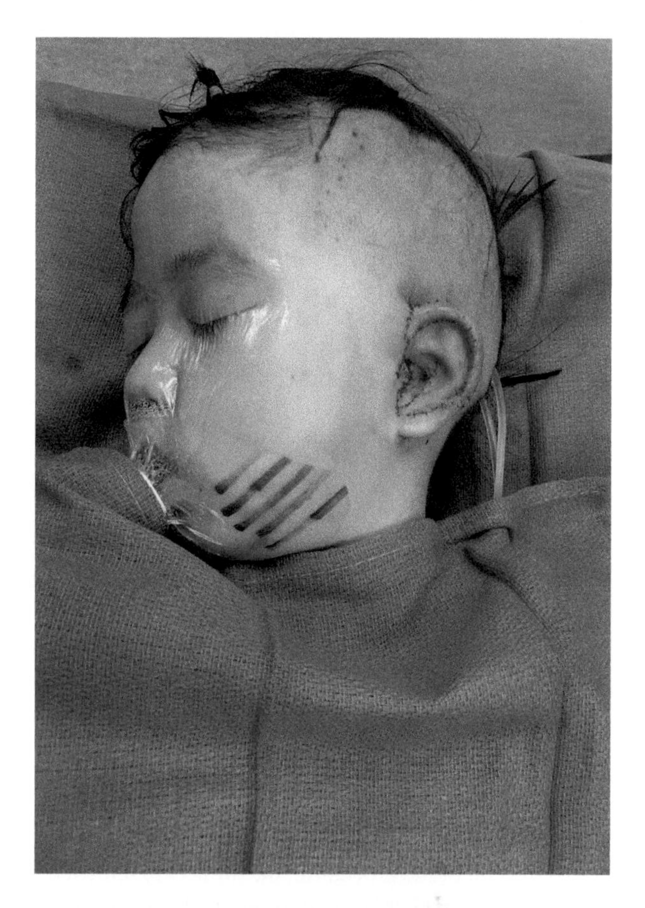

Fig. 6.14 Appearance of the ear following application of full-thickness skin grafts

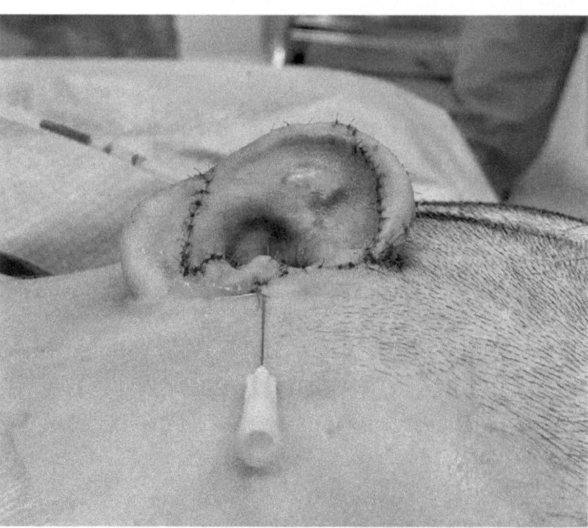

Fig. 6.15 Once positioned properly, the cartilaginous graft is maintained temporarily using a 25-gauge needle. It is then secured permanently using a 5-0 or 6-0 chromic suture mattressed through the skin and cartilage

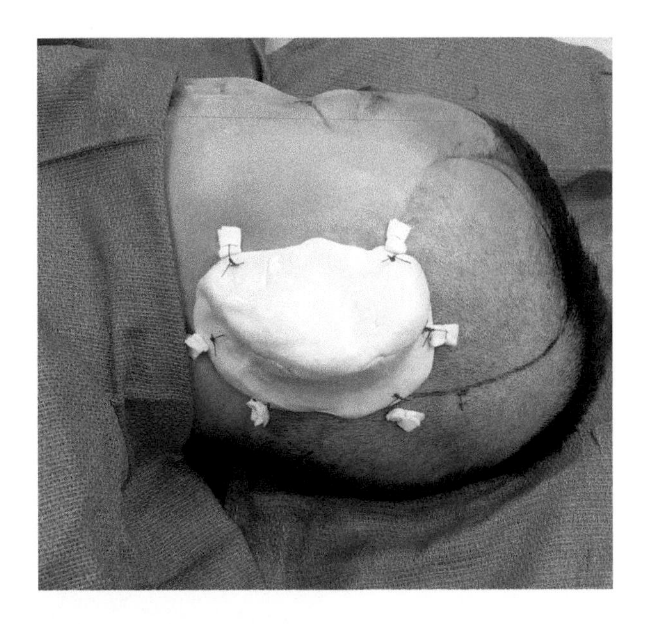

Fig. 6.16 A custom-made silicone ear splint is then fabricated and applied to the ear. It is contoured to the ear and allowed to become firm before being sutured to the surrounding scalp and cheek with horizontal mattress sutures of 2-0 Prolene® (Ethicon, Somerville, NJ, USA) tied over silicone pledgets

fabricated, applied, and contoured to the ear. Once the material becomes firm, the silicone is sutured to the surrounding scalp and cheek with horizontal mattress sutures of 2-0 Prolene® (Ethicon, Somerville, NJ, USA) tied over cottonoid pledgets (Fig. 6.16).

Plain 0.25% Marcaine® (Hospira, Lake Forest, IL, USA) is then infiltrated into the scalp drain, around the ear, and at the level of the skin graft donor sites. This allows for decreasing or eliminating any immediate postoperative discomfort.

At the end of the procedure, the drains are removed and the head is wrapped with an absorptive head dressing in order to absorb the drainage from the drain sites. The dressing is covered with a decorative head cap (Fig. 6.17). The Foley catheter is removed and the gingival suture placed to prevent movement of the endotracheal tube is released. Once extubated, the patient is taken to the recovery room. After 1–2 h spent in the recovery room, the patient is sent home with a prescription of cephalexin for 7 days. Children less than 6 years of age require little or no analgesia on the first postoperative day. Older children and adults may require some oral pain medication for a day or two.

The first postoperative appointment occurs at postoperative day #2 or #3. The absorptive dressing is removed during this appointment. If fluid is noticed beneath the scalp at that time, it can be easily drained percutaneously with a butterfly needle. The silicone ear splint is left in place for a total of 2 weeks postoperatively (Fig. 6.18). During that period, the head should be kept dry, and the patient should not sleep on the side of surgery to avoid pressure on the reconstructed ear.

For young children, parents should sleep with the child to make sure they do not inadvertently turn and sleep on the operated side.

At 2 weeks postoperatively, the silicone ear mold is removed and the ear and head are washed with shampoo in the office. Parents are shown how to wash it gently

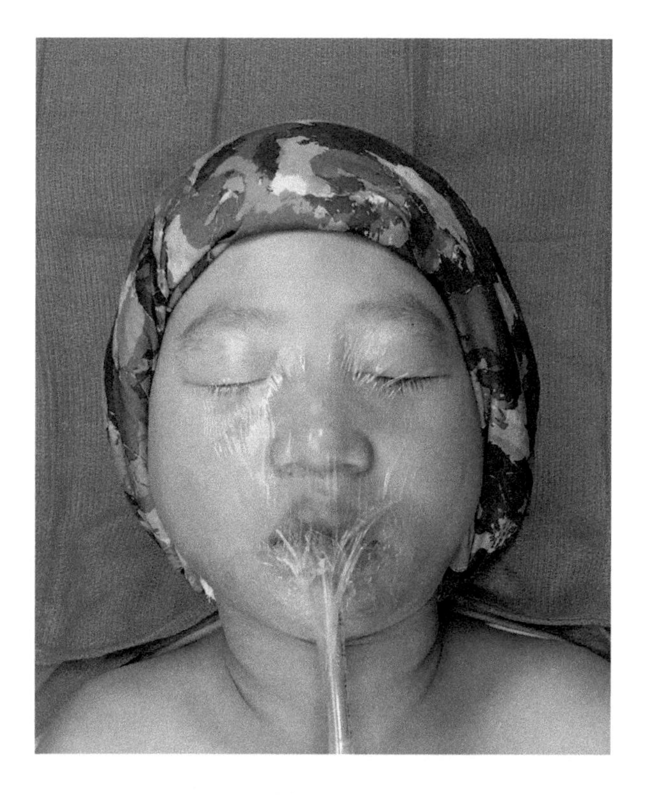

Fig. 6.17 Once the dressing is done, a decorative head cap is applied

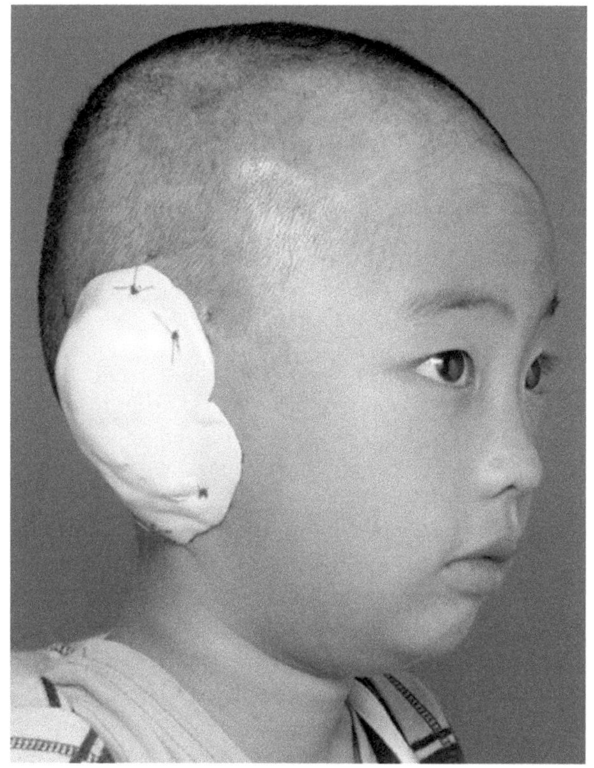

Fig. 6.18 On the first postoperative visit (usually on the second or third 2–3 day after surgery), the absorptive dressing is removed at that time and the silicone ear splint is left in place for a total of 2 weeks postoperatively

with their fingers on a daily fashion. A new silicone ear mold is made for the patient to use at night for the following 4 months. A light coating of ointment is applied on the ear before applying the ear mold for the next week.

The third postoperative visit occurs after 3 weeks. Washing can now be done with a gauze pad to encourage removal of the dissolving chromic sutures. Parents are taught how to make the silicone ear mold, which will be worn every night for the following 4 months (parents are provided with the silicone mold packets). This helps to protect the ear, but more importantly, it helps to maintain the projection of the ear.

Bilateral Ear Reconstruction

The overall similar procedure is performed for bilateral ear reconstruction. However, a few differences are important to note.

Since matching a contralateral ear is not an issue here, and since the amount of FTSG that can be harvested is limited, one can aim to reconstruct slightly smaller ears in a staged fashion.

Moreover, the contralateral postauricular skin is not available in patients with bilateral microtia. Therefore, other donor sites with reasonable color match are needed for coverage of the lateral surface of the ear. Possible donor sites include a split-thickness skin graft from the scalp (make sure to remove all the hairs/hair follicles), or an FTSG from the upper inner arm or clavicular areas (author's preferred method).

Additionally, since the two ears are reconstructed in staged fashion, when reconstructing the second ear, it is important to warn the family that definition of the first ear may be lost for the first 1–2 weeks postoperatively. This is due to swelling caused by positioning the patient on that side of the head while performing the contralateral ear reconstruction.

Fat Grafting

If a patient presents with cheek/malar asymmetry and hypoplasia on the affected side, fat grafting is offered in addition to ear reconstruction. The subcutaneous tissue of the central abdomen is infiltrated with a dilute Marcaine solution made by adding 10 mL of 0.25% Marcaine containing 1:200,000 part epinephrine with 30 mL of normal saline.

Liposuction is performed using a stab incision in the inferior portion of the umbilicus to allow pretunneling and harvesting of fat. The collected fat is then centrifuged at 3000 revolutions per minute for 3 min.

The fat, separated from the infiltration fluid, is then loaded into 1 mL syringes attached to 18-gauge blunt-tipped cannulae (Fig. 6.19). Through the existing ear incision, fat is injected into the area of the malar hypoplasia for improved contour (Fig. 6.20).

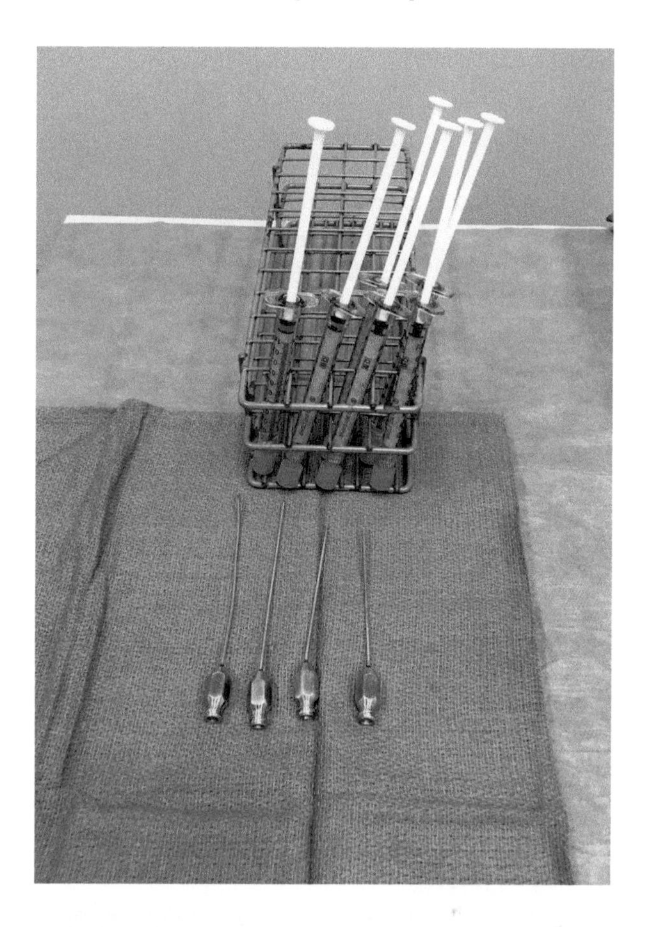

Fig. 6.19 Processed fat is loaded into 1 mL syringes attached to 18-gauge blunt-tipped cannulae

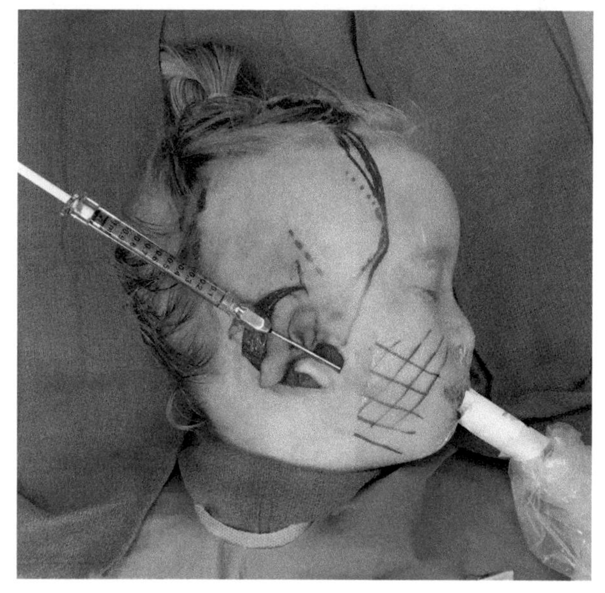

Fig. 6.20 Through the existing ear incision, fat is injected into the area of the malar and mandibular hypoplasia for improved contour

Conclusion

Ear reconstruction in young children with a porous high-density polyethylene implant is preferred by the authors because the necessary fascial flap coverage is thinner and easier to harvest than in older patients. Additionally, the surgery can be done at a young age, in a single outpatient procedure with minimal discomfort or psychological trauma. In our experience, excellent results are obtained. Video 6.5 demonstrates some of our long-term results and highlights the ear mobility obtained.

References

1. Tanzer R. Total reconstruction of the external ear. Plast Reconstr Surg Transplant Bull. 1959;23(1):1–15.
2. Brent B. The correction of microtia with autgenous cartilage grafts: 1. The classic deformity? Plast Reconstr Surg. 1980;66(1):1–12.
3. Nagata S, Fukuda O. A new reconstruction for the lobule type microtia. Jpn J Plast Reconstr Surg. 1987;7:689.
4. Firmin F. Ear reconstruction in cases of typical microtia: personal experience based on 352 microtic ear corrections. Scand J Plast Reconstr Surg Hand Surg. 1998;32(1):35–47.
5. Ksrai L, Snyder-Warwick A, Fisher D. Single-stage autolog ous ear reconstruction for microtia. Plast Reconstr Surg. 2014;133(3):652–62.
6. Adamson J, Horton C, Crawford H. The growth pattern of the external ear. Plast Reconstr Surg. 1965;36(4):466–70.
7. Tolhurst D, Carstens M, Greco R, et al. The surgical anatomy of the scalp. Plast Reconstr Surg. 1991;87(4):603–12; discussion 613–14.
8. Klockars T, Rautio J. Embryology and epidemiology of microtia. Facial Plast Surg. 2009;25(3):145–8.
9. Reed R, Hubbard M, Kesser BW. Is there a right ear advantage in congenital aural atresia? Otol Neurotol. 2016;37(10):1577–82.
10. Kesser BW, Krook K, Gray LC. Impact of unilateral conductive hearing loss due to aural atresia on academic performance in children. Laryngoscope. 2013;123(9):2270–5.
11. Jensen DR, Grames LM, Lieu JEC. Effects of aural atresia on speech development and learning. JAMA Otolaryngol Head Neck Surg. 2013;139(8):797–802.
12. Kuppler K, Lewis M, Evans AK. A review of unilateral hearing loss and academic performance: is it time to reassess traditional dogmata? Int J Pediatr Otorhinolaryngol. 2013;77(5):617–22.
13. Lieu JEC. Speech-language and educational consequences of unilateral hearing loss in children. Arch Otolaryngol Head Neck Surg. 2004;130(5):524–30.
14. Lieu JEC, Tye-Murray N, Fu Q. Longitudinal study of children with unilateral hearing loss. Laryngoscope. 2012;122(9):2088–95.
15. Jahrsdoerfer RA, Yeakley JW, Aguilar EA, Cole RR, Gray LC. Grading system for the selection of patients with congenital aural atresia. Am J Otol. 1992;13:6–12.
16. Roberson JBJ, Reinisch J, Colen TY, Lewin S. Atresia repair before microtia reconstruction: comparison of early with standard surgical timing. Otol Neurotol. 2009;30(6):771–6.

Chapter 7
Complications and Management of Alloplastic Ear Reconstruction

John F. Reinisch and Youssef Tahiri

Introduction

Auricular reconstruction is a challenging procedure. Because microtia is relatively uncommon and has a significant learning curve, complications, especially as one gains experience, are inevitable. While a good surgeon learns to treat complications, an excellent surgeon has learned to avoid them.

As mentioned in the previous chapter, the authors prefer to use a porous high-density polyethylene framework (pHDPE) for ear reconstruction. The authors feel that ear reconstruction with an alloplastic framework allows a more holistic approach to microtia as it better addresses the cosmetic, functional, and psychological issues associated with microtia.

One of the most important differences between a cartilage and a pHDPE ear reconstruction is the soft tissue coverage of the framework. The composition of the framework is less important as the internal construct merely acts as a passive skeleton to shape its overlying soft tissue. While a cartilage framework is well tolerated in a thin, skin pocket, pHDPE frequently becomes exposed if placed under a thin skin flap. Thus, the soft tissue coverage of an alloplastic ear needs to be different than that of a cartilage framework. To avoid exposure, it is essential that the

---

Electronic Supplementary Material The online version of this chapter (https://doi.org/10.1007/978-3-030-16387-7_7) contains supplementary material, which is available to authorized users.

J. F. Reinisch (✉)
Keck School of Medicine, University of Souther California, Los Angeles, CA, USA

Craniofacial and Pediatric Plastic Surgery, Cedars Sinai Medical Center,
Los Angeles, CA, USA
e-mail: Jfr654@aol.com

Y. Tahiri (✉)
Plastic and Reconstructive Surgery, Cedars-Sinai Medical Center, Los Angeles, CA, USA
e-mail: Youssef.Tahiri@cshs.org

© Springer Nature Switzerland AG 2019

J. F. Reinisch, Y. Tahiri (eds.), *Modern Microtia Reconstruction*,
https://doi.org/10.1007/978-3-030-16387-7_7

alloplastic framework be completely enveloped by a thin fascia flap which becomes adherent to the porous implant [1].

Over the years, the senior author has modified and refined his technique to reduce complications and improve the aesthetic and functional outcomes of ear reconstruction.

This chapter will highlight the potential complications associated with alloplastic ear reconstruction. The management of complication and how to prevent them will be discussed.

Intraoperative Complications and Management

The most common intraoperative complications are injury to the superficial temporal artery, failure to raise a flap with sufficient size to cover the entire implant, damage to the temporal branch of the facial nerve, and injury to scalp hair follicles.

As mentioned previously, a polyethylene framework requires a different type of soft tissue coverage to avoid exposures. The covering fascia must be well vascularized, must include it underlying loose areolar layer, and must be large enough to envelope the entire implant without tension (Video 7.1).

Vascular Injury

It is important to identify and preserve the vascular pedicle of the STP fascia while dissecting the fascial flap. The STP artery divides into an anterior and posterior branch. The anterior branch of the STA runs just posterior to the temporal branch of the facial nerve. It turns posteriorly and runs transversely approximate 12 cm above the locations of the missing or stenotic ear canal (Fig. 7.1). It is important to include the transverse portion of the artery in the distal flap as it forms an arcade linking the blood supply from the anterior and main branches. If the anterior branch of the superficial temporal artery is injured or is too close to the frontal branch of the facial nerve, the STPF flap will survive on its main branch. If the main branch is injured, the fascia will survive on an intact anterior branch especially if the distal, transverse component is maintained within the distal flap. However, if the STA is injured proximal to its bifurcation, a microvascular repair of the artery is necessary. If not possible, an occipital flap should then be used.

It should be noted that approximately 18% of microtia patients have an abnormal posterior origin of the STA. In these patients, the origin of the STA is behind the earlobe. The vessel courses in an anterior direction immediately beneath the microtic cartilage remnant to take its normal position in the upper preauricular area. This anomaly can be suspected preoperatively as these patients often have a slight anterior tilt to the lobule and a small cartilage remnant (Fig. 7.2). Digital pressure over the posterior cheek does not obliterate the pulse in the STA in the temporal area as it would in patients with the normal course of the vessel. It is important to identify this abnormality because the artery can be injured either when resecting the microtic cartilage remnant or when removing soft tissue more inferiorly to make a faux-canal.

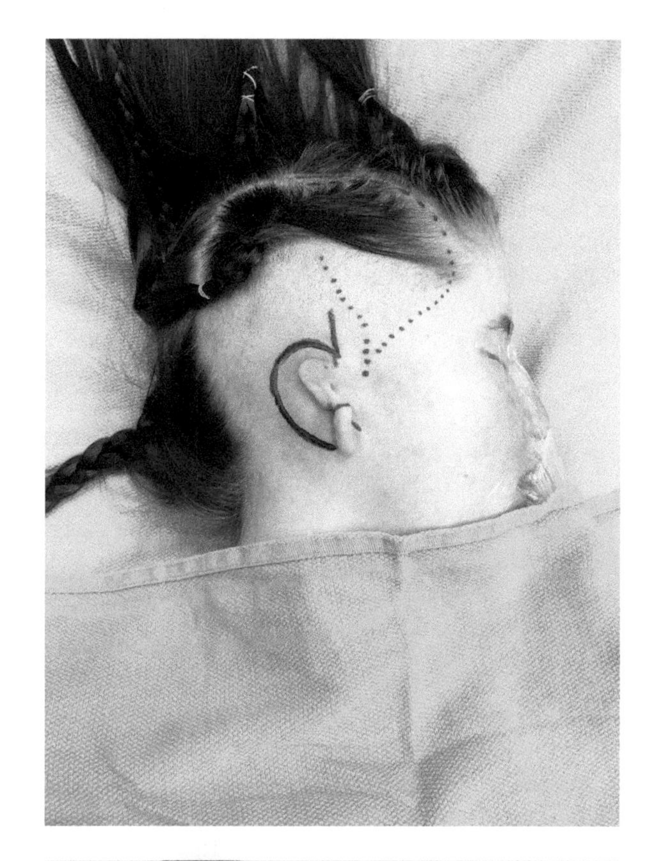

Fig. 7.1 Preoperative markings demonstrating the superficial temporal artery with its anterior and posterior branches. The flap dimensions are approximately 10 cm in width by 13 cm in height from the canal (or the supposed position of the canal). The 13-cm height allows the inclusion in the flap of the transverse direction that the anterior branch of the superficial temporal artery takes at approximately the 12-cm mark

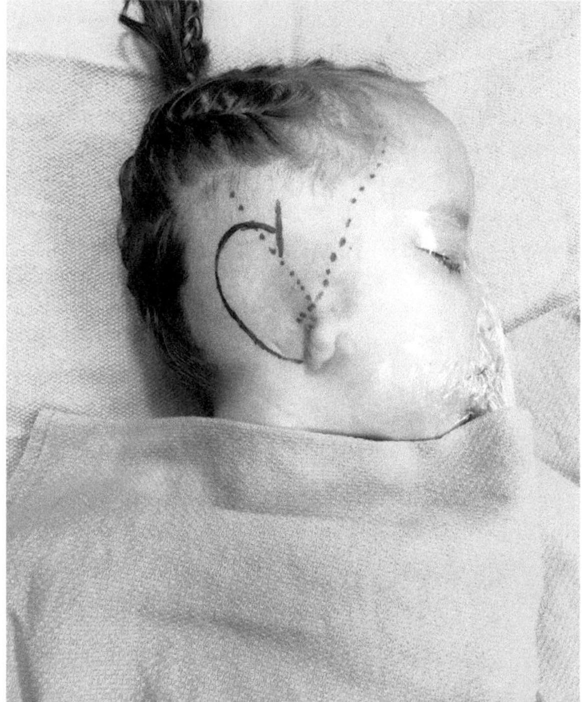

Fig. 7.2 In about 18% of cases, the STA has an origin posterior to the lobule and runs immediately beneath the small cartilage remnant

Once the STPF flap is elevated, one ideally will see good pulsations within the flap and will need to cauterize bleeding at its distal edge. If the flap dissection and elevation cause arterial spasm, replacing the flap beneath the scalp and wrapping the head for 15 min to warm the flap will usually restore pulsations within the flap and allow one to cauterize bleeding points. On rare occasions, the arterial spasm persists and is not relieved by warming the flap. If the pedicle is intact and no major arterial bleeding was encountered during elevation, the surgery can be completed with the expectation that the spasm will improve and the flap will survive. One should not rely on the color of the flap to assess viability, as an ischemic flap often looks pink for quite some time.

Insufficient Flap Size

The STPF needs to be large enough to envelope the entire implant without tension (Video 7.1). Raising a flap with insufficient vertical length can leave the inferior portion of the implant covered only by the lobule without an intervening fascia layer. This situation will increase the chance for a later inferior exposure. Placing tension on the flap also increases the risk of exposure by jeopardizing the viability of the flap over the helical rim of the implant. Even if the flap survives, the tension prevents the flap from completely conforming to the contour of the implant and gives a less defined reconstructed ear.

When harvesting the STPF flap without a scalp incision, one can maximize the vertical length of the STPF flap by stripping the scalp from the periosteum beyond its outlined (13 cm) cephalic boarder. This maneuver allows one to divide the galea and its underlying loose areolar tissue more cephalically by dividing the distal flap from inside out above the cephalic extent of the subcutaneous dissection. If a transverse incision is used to give better access to the distal flap, one should make the transverse scalp incision perpendicular to the hair growth. One will then need to dissect the scalp in a cephalic direction before dividing the distal flap. A higher scalp incision that runs parallel to the hair growth will leave a noticeable scar.

A slightly short flap can be lengthened by improving its anterior pivot point by dissection anterior to the STA proximal to the division into its anterior and main branches. This dissection is facilitated by transilluminating the flap and visualizing the vessels. Another method of improving the coverage of an inadequate flap is by reducing the projection of the implant by reducing its medial surface.

Temporal Nerve Branch Injury

Injury to the frontal branch of the facial nerve is uncommon, but can occur during flap elevation. This usually happens when dissecting the TPF flap and including the anterior branch of the superficial temporal artery. In some patients, the anterior branch of the STA can be quite anterior and very close to the frontal branch. The nerve can be identified and preserved using a nerve simulator. With an assistant watching for frontalis and orbicularis stimulation while separating the scalp from the STPF along the course of the anterior branch of the STA, one can determine if the flap can be divided immediately anterior to the anterior branch. It is common to see some muscle stimulation. In the rare case of strong muscle stimulation during anterior scalp elevation, the anterior branch can be divided inferiorly and not included in the flap to preserve frontalis function.

The anesthesiologist should not give a paralytic agent during the procedure in order to be able to assess nerve proximity during flap dissection. Anterior division of the flap can be done easier in patients who have a preoperative frontalis paralysis.

If a patient with no preoperative palsy presents with a frontal branch palsy postoperatively, it could be either a neuropraxia or a complete intraoperative injury of the frontal branch of the facial nerve (Fig. 7.3). In the majority of the cases, if a meticulous technique was used, it is a neuropraxia and the patient would observe a progressive return of function within the first 6–9 months postoperatively. If a non-reversible injury frontal branch injury is observed, symmetry can be achieved by using/injecting a neuromodulator on the contralateral side.

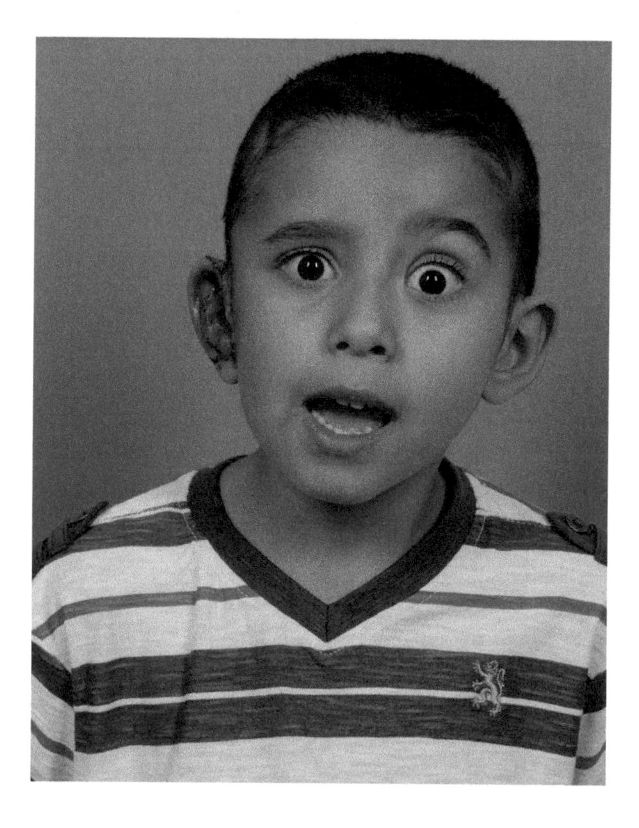

Fig. 7.3 5-year-old patient who presents with a right frontal nerve palsy 2 weeks following right ear reconstruction

Others

Other intraoperative complications include an insufficient amount of full-thickness skin harvested and harvesting hair-bearing skin. Thus, it is important to accurately estimate how much skin graft will be needed. Ideally, using non-hear-bearing skin grafts is recommended. The anterior surface of the reconstructed ear is covered with local skin as well as contralateral postauricular skin grafts, while the posterior surface of the ear is covered with groin skin graft. In the instances where no contralateral postauricular skin is available (bilateral microtia, Treacher Collins syndrome), a full-thickness skin graft (FTSG) from the inner upper arm or a split-thickness skin graft from the scalp (while making sure to remove all hair/hair follicles) can be used.

Finally, implant malposition during insetting of the pHDPE implant and hair follicle injury during the scalp dissection and the TPF flap harvest can occur in the intraoperative period. The former can be prevented by adequate preoperative planning and marking, while the latter can be prevented by meticulous dissection of the scalp at a plane right below the hair follicles and above the fascial layer.

Early Postoperative Complications and Management

We define early postoperative complications as those that occur within the first 2 months following porous polyethylene ear reconstruction. Early complications include infection, scalp hematoma or seroma, skin graft necrosis, implant exposure, pain and stiffness related to positioning, and scalp alopecia.

Infection

Without an exposure, infection is a rare complication. When it occurs, it happens early in the postoperative period. While infection can cause swelling and erythema (Fig. 7.4a and b), most infections are subtle and result in drainage without cellulitis or significant swelling. Antibiotics may temporarily reduce drainage, but are unlikely to resolve an infection involving the implant. Removal of the implant, debridement of the surrounding granulation tissue in the pocket with a curette, irrigation with an antibiotic solution, and replacement with a new implant are usually successful. The infected implant can be placed in alcohol, rinsed in saline, and used as a model to size the new implant. The sterile implant is placed in the debrided pocket over a suction drain (Fig. 7.5a–d). A preoperative or intraoperative culture should be taken to confirm the appropriate antibiotic selection. Suction is applied once the access incision is closed and a silicone ear splint is applied and sutured in place. The drain can then be removed.

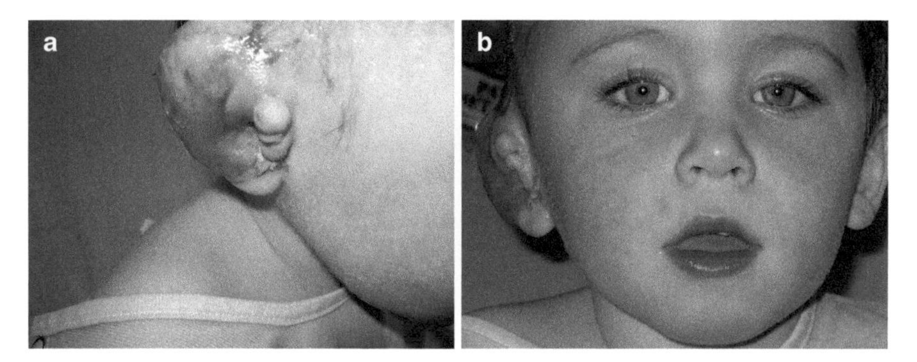

Fig. 7.4 (**a** and **b**) 5-year-old boy with a deep purulent staphylococcus infection. Notice the significant swelling, redness, and loss of definition

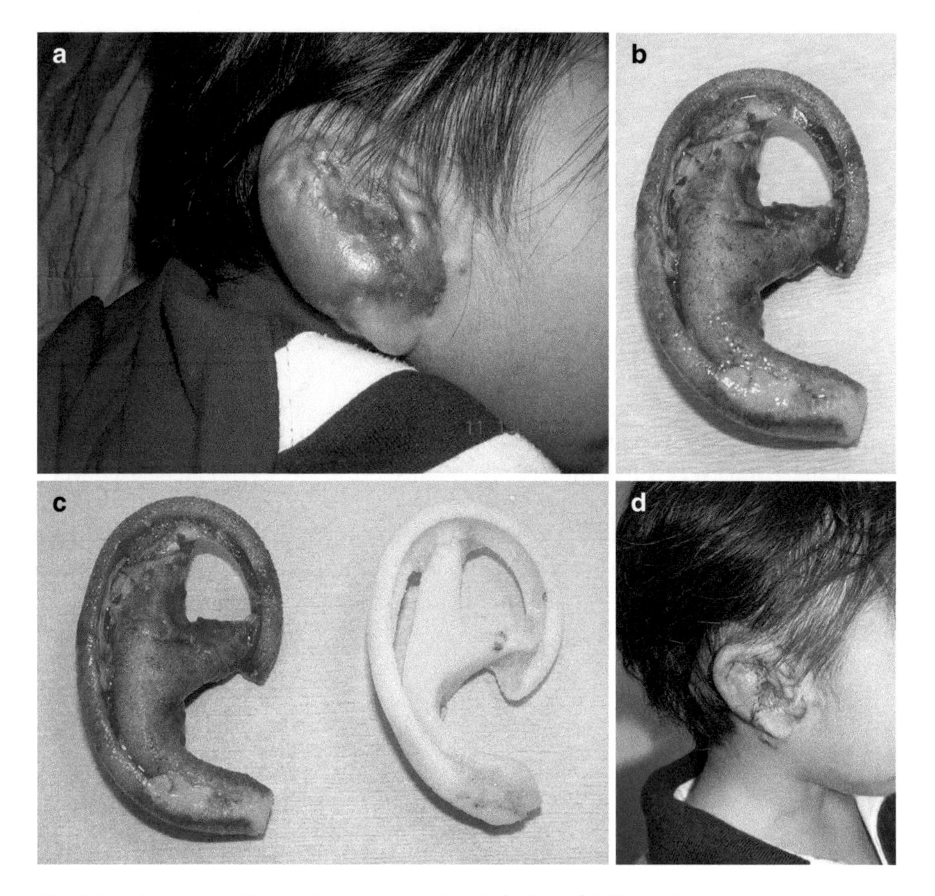

Fig. 7.5 (**a**) 4-year-old boy with a deep purulent infection. (**b**) Through an anti-helical incision, the old implant is removed, and the pocket is debrided with a curette and irrigated thoroughly. (**c**) Once removed, the old implant is submerged in alcohol and is used as model for the carving of the new implant. (**d**) Photograph of the ear at 2 weeks postoperatively

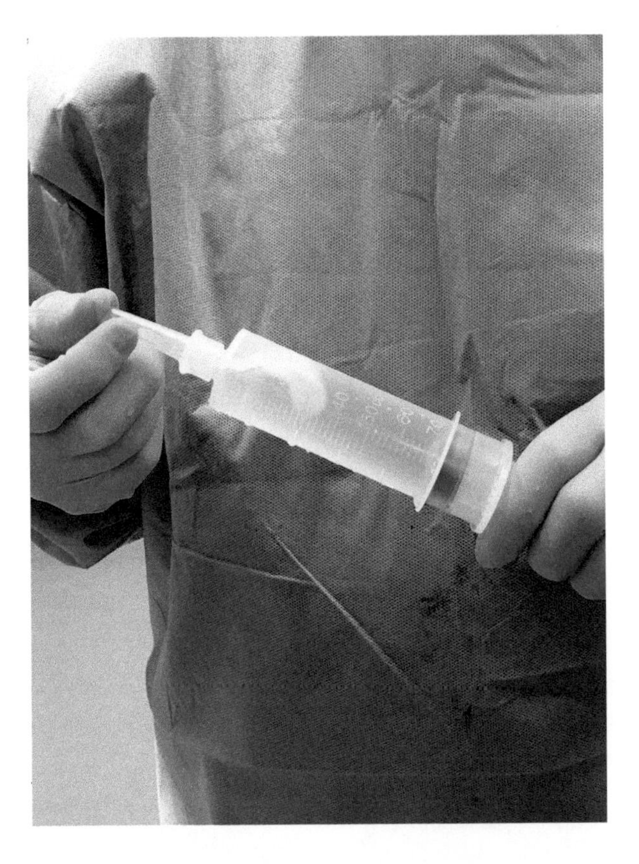

Fig. 7.6 By placing the implant in a syringe filled with an antibacterial solution, one can replace the air in the porous framework with the antibiotics by creating negative pressure

By adhering to a strict sterile protocol during surgery, one can make infections a rare occurrence. Intravenous antibiotics should be started at the beginning of anesthesia and given every 4-h during the procedures. Fresh gloves should be used when assembling the framework. Moreover, by placing the implant in a syringe filled with an antibacterial solution, one can replaces the air in the porous framework with the antibiotics by creating negative pressure (Fig. 7.6). Oral antibiotics should be given for a week postoperatively until the suture line under the silicone mold have sealed. We had two infections in a relatively short period when the postoperative antibiotic selection did not cover skin flora.

Hematoma or Seroma

A scalp hematoma or seroma can form postoperatively in the dead space created by the fascia flap harvest. Hematomas are very unusual and can be eliminated by a second hemostasis check before final closure.

Seromas are more common and harder to prevent. Occasionally at the first follow-up visit, on the first or second postoperative day, a patient will present with a small collection beneath the lower scalp flap donor site. Seromas are usually accompanied by periorbital swelling. Small seromas will resolve, but larger collections can be drained with minimal discomfort using a small butterfly needle through the temporarily insensate scalp.

Skin Graft Loss

Necrosis of the skin over the ear usually is secondary to necrosis of the underlying STPF. Bleeding between the STPF and the overlying skin grafts is rare following meticulous hemostasis and the application of a closely fitting initial silicone mold. If a small hematoma does occur in this location, the skin over the hematoma will not survive (Fig. 7.7). If the area is small and the fascia covering the implant is healthy, one can debride the necrotic skin graft and apply a wet to dry gauze dressing twice a day with the expectation that the area will contract and heal quickly. In the rare instance of a large area of skin loss, application of additional skin will allow more rapid healing and prevent significant contracture and loss of ear definition.

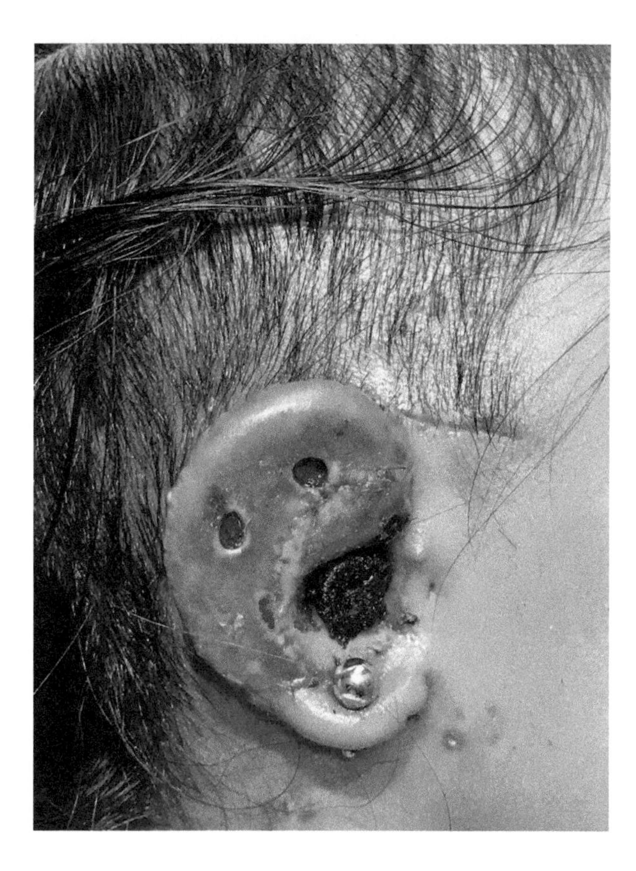

Fig. 7.7 A hematoma under the skin graft can cause skin graft failure and loss

Implant Exposure

Exposure of the alloplastic framework is almost always an early postoperative complication. It is caused by vascular compromise of the enveloping fascia flap either from direct vascular injury during harvest of the flap or from postoperative pressure from the dressing (e.g., from sleeping on the fresh ear). Recognition of an impending exposure, especially when small, can be missed. The covering skin that was placed on the fascia enveloping the implant should be viable at 2 weeks when the silicone ear splint is first removed and the ear and scalp are washed. One can notice a small impeding exposure by the appearance of a demarcated area of nonviable skin. If the skin adjacent to the questionable area is pink and healthy, it should be assumed that the presence of the necrotic area means that the underlying fascia is nonviable and that an exposure of the implant will occur with time. It is important to recognize this complication early. If there is uncertainty about the tissue's viability, an operating time can be scheduled for the following week, and the tissue given another week to declare itself. Needle puncture of the dermis should result in some bleeding. If the area of concern is relatively small (>2.5 cm^2), one can salvage the ear reconstruction by debriding the nonviable tissue over the implant, irrigating the implant with an antibiotic solution using an angiocath to push the irrigation fluid into the interstices of the implant, and then covering the defect with an adjacent fascia flap and skin graft before the implant becomes contaminated. With an impeding exposure, and even an early exposure of only 1–2 weeks in the absence of obvious infection or granulation tissue, the original implant can be maintained and not replaced (Fig. 7.8a–f).

The design of the fascia flap needed to cover a freshly exposed implant depends on the location of the exposure. The two most common areas for early exposure are either the upper helical rim or inferior pole of the implant. If the superior portion of the helix is about to be exposed or is acutely exposed, transposition of an inferiorly based, deep temporoparietal fascia (DTPF) flap harvested through a new temporal or parietal zigzag scalp incision can be used for coverage (Fig. 7.9a–d). One must elevate a flap significantly larger than the defect so that the fascia not only can cover the exposed implant without tension but can also be tucked well under the surrounding viable tissue.

In the case of an exposure of the lower portion of the implant, the necrotic soft tissue is removed, and an anteriorly based postauricular fascia flap can be transposed anteriorly like a book page to cover the debrided defect. The fascia needs to be large enough to cover the exposure area as well as 5–6 mm of the implant under the surrounding healthy tissue. The fascia-covered defect is then covered with a full-thickness skin graft (Fig. 7.10a–i).

A more anterior defect can be covered by the anterior transposition of a long vertically oriented, inferiorly based postauricular flap. The lobule can be elevated to allow the transposition of the flap and then be reattached. Again, it is important to design a flap that is wider and longer to allow tensionless closure that allows the transposed tissue to underlap the tissue surrounding the defect.

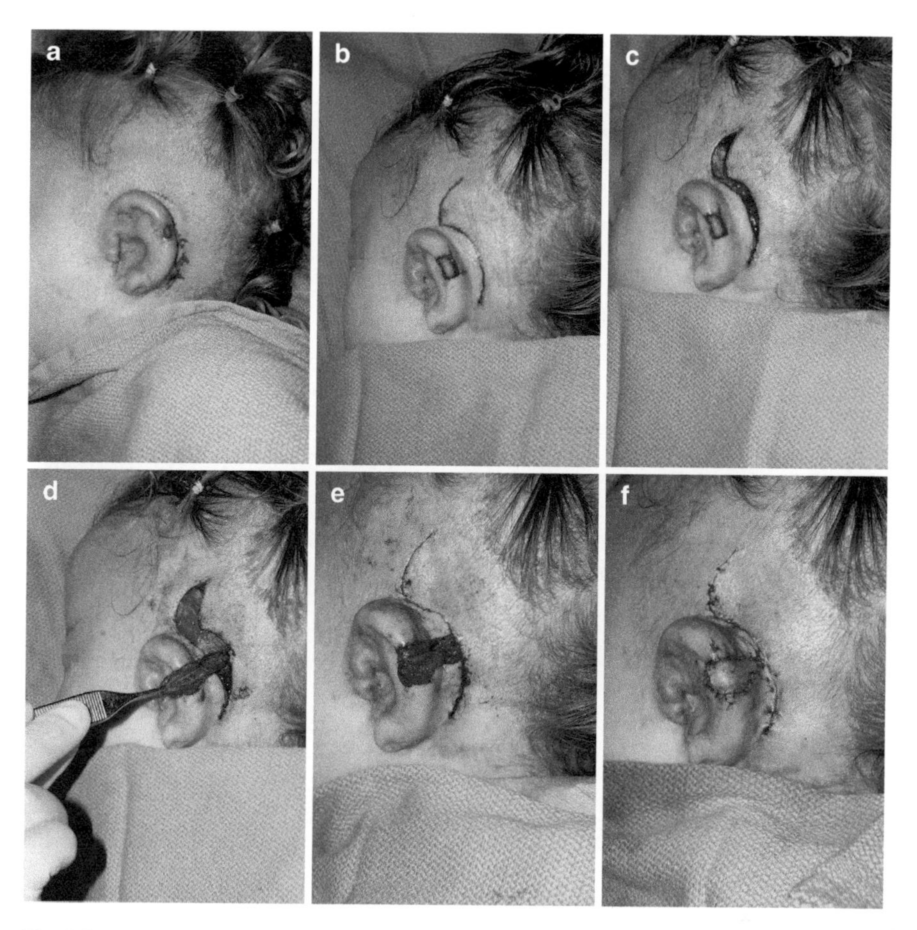

Fig. 7.8 (**a**) 4-year-old boy with early exposure at the level of the helix. (**b**) He was taken to the operating room for debridement and irrigation. (**c–e**) An inferiorly based local flap is used for coverage. (**f**) A FTSG is used for skin coverage

If the implant has been exposed for more than 3 weeks or shows drainage or granulation tissue, one must assume that the implant is contaminated. Salvage of the ear reconstruction is possible if the implant is removed and the pocket debrided and irrigated with antibiotic solution. The old implant should not be reused; do not autoclave the old implant since it will melt. It should be placed in alcohol for 10 min washed with saline to remove all traces of the alcohol and then used as a template to help assemble a framework of similar size. The new implant is placed in the freshly debrided and irrigated pocket. The area of exposure is covered with a local fascia flap and full-thickness skin graft. A suction drain is used to shrink-wrap the soft tissue to the new implant, and a silicone splint is applied around the ear. The splint is sutured in place and the drain removed. If the implant is removed and not replaced, the soft tissue harvested to cover the implant will contract, making it impossible to

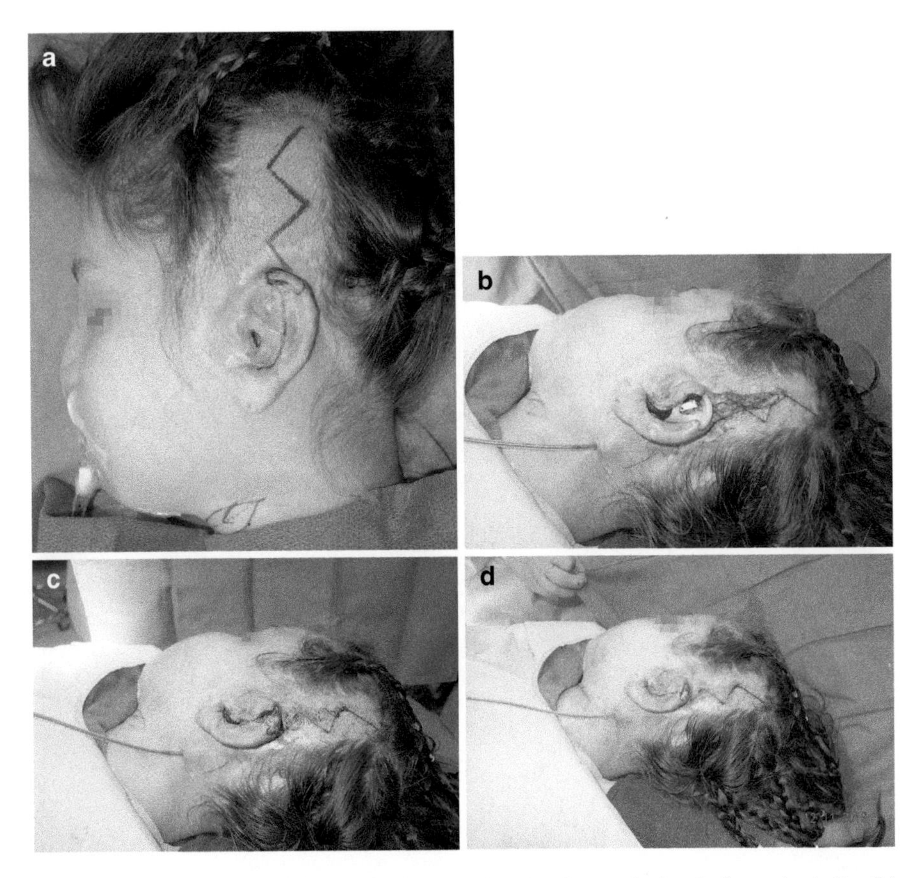

Fig. 7.9 (**a**) 5-year-old girl with early exposure of the implant at the level of superior helix. (**b**) A partial zigzag coronal-type incision is designed and used to access and raise a deep temporal fascial flap that will be used to cover the irrigated implant. (**c** and **d**) The flap is used to cover the exposed implant and is used tucked in as an "inlay" below the original flap all around the exposed area

use the same pocket for later insertion of a new framework, and thus needing a new reconstruction with a different fascia flap, if available.

If there is a large area of soft tissue necrosis, a local fascia flap will be insufficient to salvage the reconstruction. In this case the implant should be removed, and the soft tissue debrided and closed loosely. Future reconstruction of the ear is possible using a different fascia flap such as anterior transposition of a large occipital artery fascia flap or a free flap.

While successful salvage of an ear reconstruction with an impending or early small exposure is possible, prevention of exposure should be the kept in the surgeons' mind throughout the initial surgery. Success requires the meticulous dissection of a sufficiently large TPF flap to cover the entire implant without tension. Maintaining the structural integrity and vascularity of the flap during harvest is critical. The application of a custom-fitted silicone ear splint as described in the

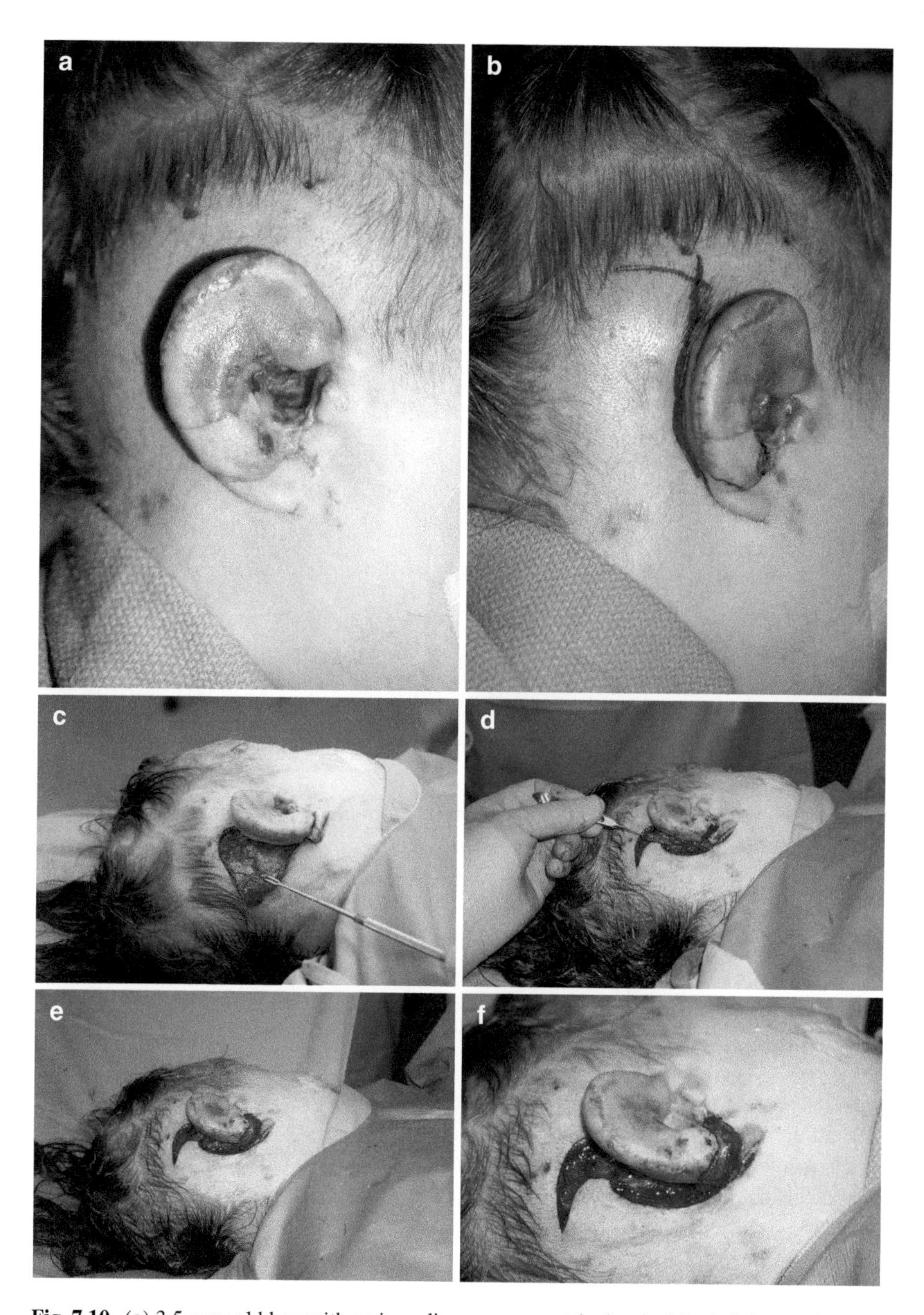

Fig. 7.10 (**a**) 3.5-year-old boy with an impeding exposure at the level of the inferior medial portion of the conchal bowl. (**b**) He was taken to the operating room for debridement and irrigation. (**c–f**) A local inferiorly based fascial flap is raised in the postauricular region and tunneled to the exposed area. The tunnel can be created by releasing the lobule, insetting the flap. (**g**) Once the flap is insetted, the lobule is reattached, and a full-thickness skin graft is applied in the area where the exposure was. (**h** and **i**) PA and lateral photograph demonstrating adequate healing of the ear

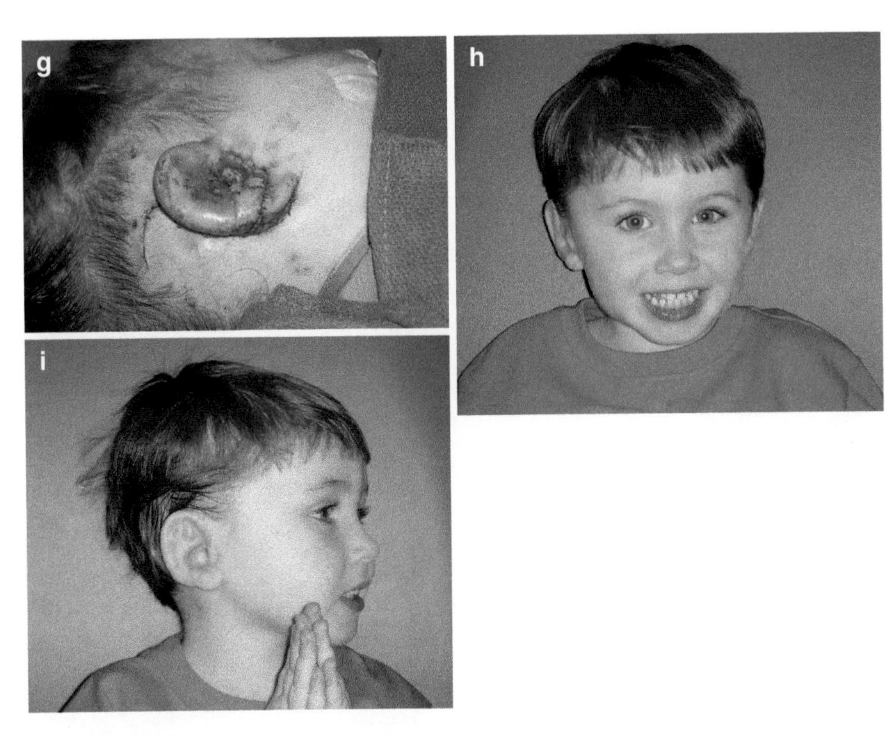

Fig. 7.10 (continued)

previous chapter is helpful for gentle compression and protection in the immediate postoperative period. Finally, the need to sleep with young children in order to avoid pressure on the ear during the first 2–3 weeks after reconstruction must be impressed on parents.

Complications Due to Patient Positioning

Because ear reconstruction is a long procedure, the position of the anesthetized patient during surgery can lead to several non-ear complications.

Prolonged neck stiffness and limited range of motion is occasionally seen after ear reconstruction. It can last for 3–6 weeks and can be distressing for both patients and their family. Heat and massage can be tried, but in the authors' experience, are ineffective in restoring cervical range of motion. The condition resolves eventually, and family reassurance is necessary. We know of child who had limited cervical motion postoperatively. She was referred to physical therapy and placed in cervical traction. The traction device applied pressure to the newly reconstructed ear and caused a large area of necrosis and subsequent implant exposure.

Avoidance of postoperative cervical issues requires an awareness of neck position during surgery. Dissection of the STPF flap in children is facilitated by extending the neck by placing a foam or silicone pad beneath the patient's shoulders. One must not over extend the neck. The head is also rotated to the side during dissection of the STPF flap. One can reduce the amount of neck rotation by tilting the operating room table. Limiting the time the head is in one position is also important. This happens automatically when one needs to harvest skin from the opposite normal ear. Remembering to move the neck from the side at intervals during surgery is important, especially in bilateral cases where the patient has no available opposite postauricular skin. This is also the case in patients with a large microtic ear remnant. These patients usually have enough skin from the ipsilateral remnant and mastoid area to cover the entire lateral surface of the reconstructed ear so one does not need to turn the head to harvest additional color matched skin from the contralateral ear.

With long operative procedures, one needs to be aware of the potential for soft tissue pressure ischemia. Pain, prolonged skin erythema, and hair loss are seen as the result of prolonged constant soft tissue pressure. Adult patients are at greater risk for skin pressure complications than are children. This is probably related to their greater weight and the fact that ear reconstruction in adults usually requires more time. One can prevent these complications by moving the patient and changing the side tilt and longitudinal inclination of the operating room table to redistribute pressure areas.

Severe postoperative elbow pain can be seen in adult patients when their elbows are kept in an extended position during ear reconstruction. This complication is not seen in children. It occurs when adult arms are placed along the body and held in place with the draw sheet. The elbows of adult patients should be kept slightly flexed during surgery and ideally be given some range of motion during the procedure.

Scalp Alopecia

Hair loss can occur over the area of the STPF flap dissection in some patients. It is not common and, fortunately, is transient and resolves without treatment within 3–4 months (Fig. 7.11a–c). The alopecia seems to occur in children rather than adults and therefore may be related to scalp thickness.

To prevent postoperative scalp alopecia, it seems logical to elevate the scalp from the surface of the STPF with the lowest effective blended cautery setting. It may help to keep the dissection on the surface of the STPF flap to leave as much subcutaneous tissue between the dissection plain and the hair follicles as possible.

Late Postoperative Complications

Late postoperative complications are seen 2 months or longer after the porous polyethylene ear reconstruction. These complications include implant fracture, loss of ear projection, pigment changes, and implant descent.

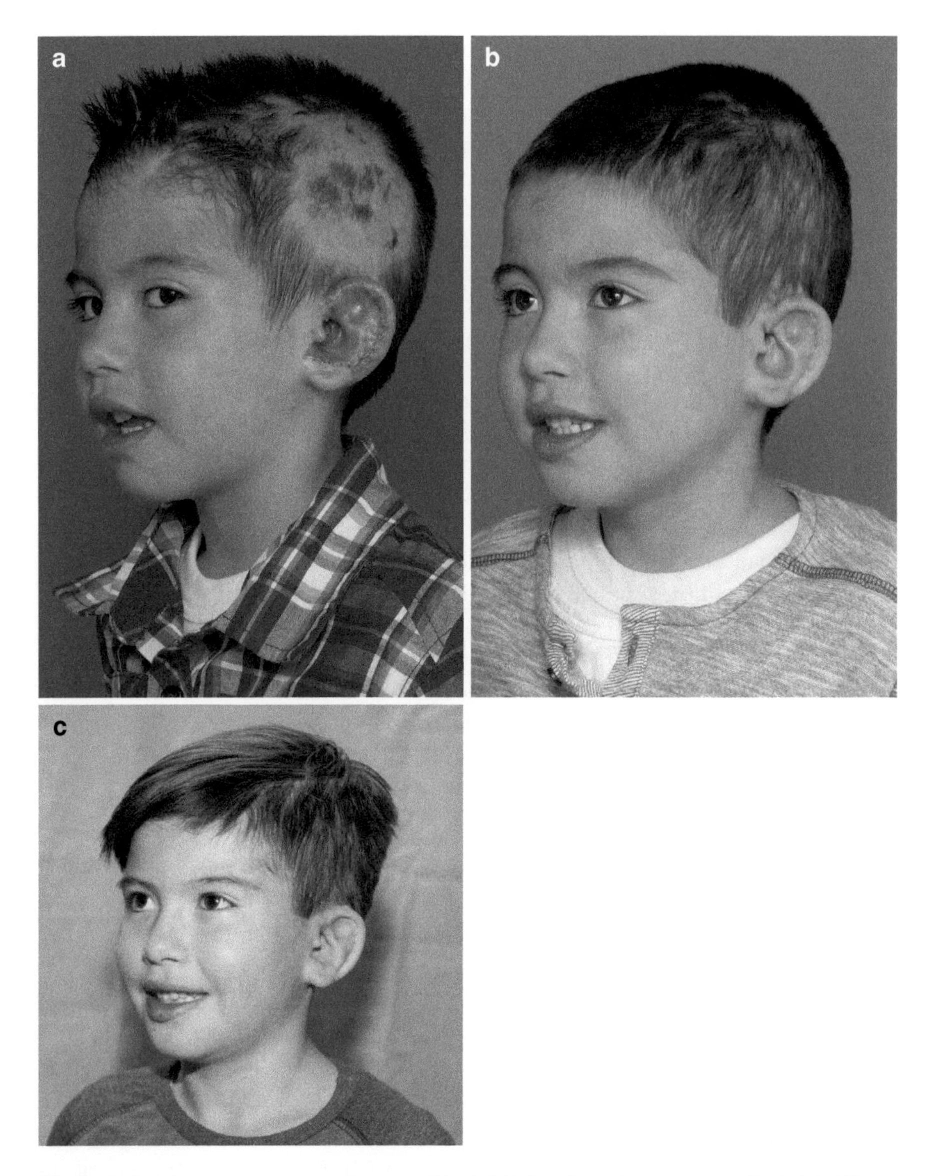

Fig. 7.11 Hair loss can occur over the area of the STPF flap dissection in some patients (**a**). It is not common and, fortunately, is transient and resolves without treatment within 3–4 months (**b** and **c**)

Implant Fracture

While an implant fracture theoretically can occur within the immediate postoperative period, it has always been seen as a late complication, often years after the alloplastic ear reconstruction. Almost all the fractures seen have occurred in young patients rather than adults. Since the porous implant allows soft tissue ingrowth, fractures can be subtle since the soft tissue supports the implant and keeps it from collapsing. An implant fracture can sometimes present with a loss of shape and definition (Fig. 7.12a and b). Many parents are unaware of the presence of a fracture until pointed out by the surgeon. A fractured implant rarely causes an exposure by disrupting its covering soft tissue.

Two types of fractures are seen. The first is a medial subluxation of the helical rim, which occurs with fracture of the distal superior crus upon which the rim should rest. This fracture can be subtle, but the reconstructed ear shows some loss of the original helical prominence. The superior helical rim, which should be more lateral than the antihelix, lies in the same plane after it dislocated medially. This type of fracture is caused either by surgical thinning of the medial aspect of the superior crus or insufficient overlap and support of the crus behind the helical rim.

Fracture of the helical rim is the second and more obvious type of fracture. It results in discontinuity of the smooth curve of the helical rim and is more easily identified (Fig. 7.13a and b). On rare occasions, a small exposure occurs from penetration of the sharp edge of the fractured rim (Fig. 7.14a–c).

Before 1996 when the current helix component of the framework was designed, rim fractures were frequent and eventually occurred in most patients done early in the authors' series. The use of dedicated helical rim portion has lowered the rate of fractures of this component of the implant to 4% in the first 10 years following ear reconstruction. We started doing ear reconstructions in patients with prior atresia repairs in 2005 and began the combined atresia repair and ear reconstructions (CAM) in early 2008. In 2011, it became apparent that the patients that had prior or simultaneous canal reconstructions had a higher rate of implant fractures. The framework in these patients is made less mobile by the tethering canalplasty and, therefore, absorbs more of the force of an impact than implants without canals. In 2011, we changed the method used to coapt the two components of the framework by maintaining the thickness of the superior crus and adding a strut to support the lateral helical rim. These two modifications have made a dramatic difference in implant disruption. In the nearly 600 patients since 2012, even with a higher percentage of atresia repairs, we have seen only one fracture.

Treatment of a fractured implant without an exposure is not urgent and can be done electively even years later (Fig. 7.12a and b). A lateral incision over the antihelical portion of the implant facilitates elevation of both an anterior-based soft tissue flap and a posterior-based flap. Separation of the ingrown soft tissue from the implant is done with a combination of blended cautery and an elevator. Freeing the caudal end of the implant first and then working in a cephalic direction gives the best chance to remove the implant intact so that it can be used as a template for a new implant of similar size. The helical rim will be imbedded in the posteriorly based flap and needs to be separated from the flap carefully so as not to injure the viability of the posterior flap. The removed implant should be used to make a new implant of similar size. The new implant is inserted into the pocket over a drain. An air tight, two-layer closure allows suction to pull the soft tissue around the new implant. Once a silicone splint is mixed, contoured to the ear, and becomes firm, it is sutured to the surrounding scalp and cheek and the drain is removed.

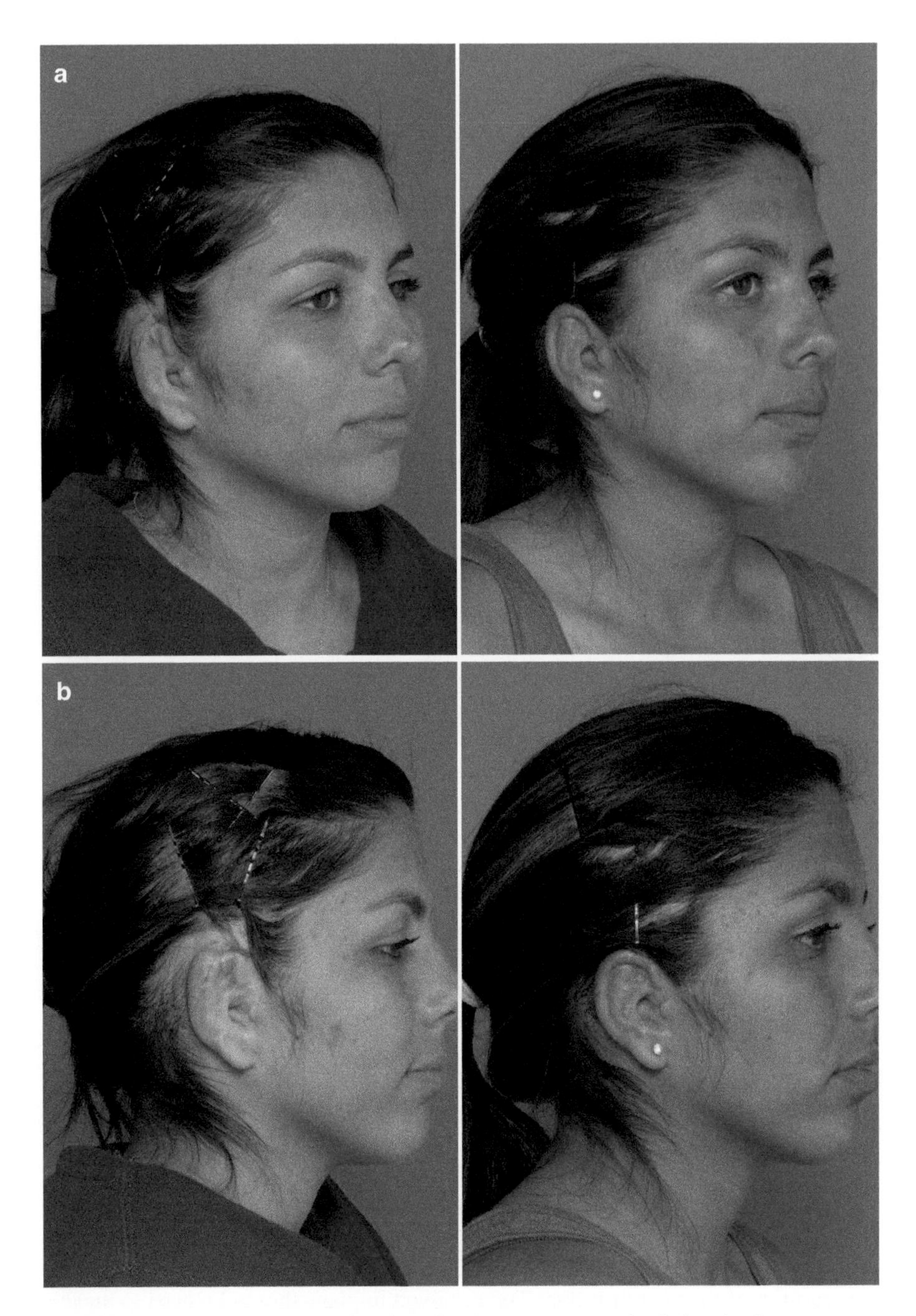

Fig. 7.12 This patient had a right microtia and underwent porous polyethylene implant ear reconstruction at 4 years of age. At 15 years of age, she had an implant fracture. She then underwent implant exchange at 19 years old age. (**a**) ¾ view photographs of the pre- and post-op ear after implant replacement. (**b**) Lateral view photographs of the pre- and post-op ear after implant replacement

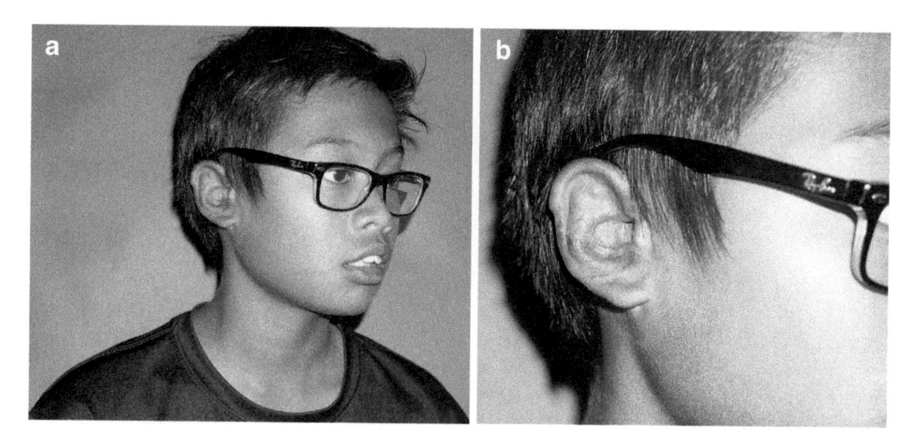

Fig. 7.13 (**a** and **b**) A fracture of the helical rim can result in discontinuity of the smooth curve of the helical rim

Late Implant Exposure

Late implant exposures in the absence of an implant fracture are surprisingly rare in our series. In contrast to an impeding or early exposure, a late exposure is likely to have been present for some time. In a patient with a late, and likely chronic exposure, the implant has to be removed. To keep the soft tissue from shrinking, a new implant needs to be placed, and a new local fascia flap and FTSG are used to cover the previously exposed area. Figure 7.15a–m illustrates a 9-year-old boy with a chronic exposure at the level of the superior rim. The patient presented late and needed an implant exchange and deep temporal fascia flap closure.

Late Infections

Late infections in the absence of an exposure are extremely rare. The ingrowth of vascularized tissue protects an establish implant against late infections. We have never recommended prophylactic antibiotics prior to dental procedures. If a late infection occurs, one should suspect an infection from an underlying cholesteatoma. This tumor must be removed completely before another ear reconstruction is attempted. In this unfortunate setting, an occipital flap (Fig. 7.16) is harvested to perform the secondary ear reconstruction at some point well after the infection has resolved. Even when parents are not considering an atresia repair, a temporal bone CT scan prior to primary ear reconstruction should always be obtained to rule out the possibility of a later complication from an unrecognized cholesteatoma.

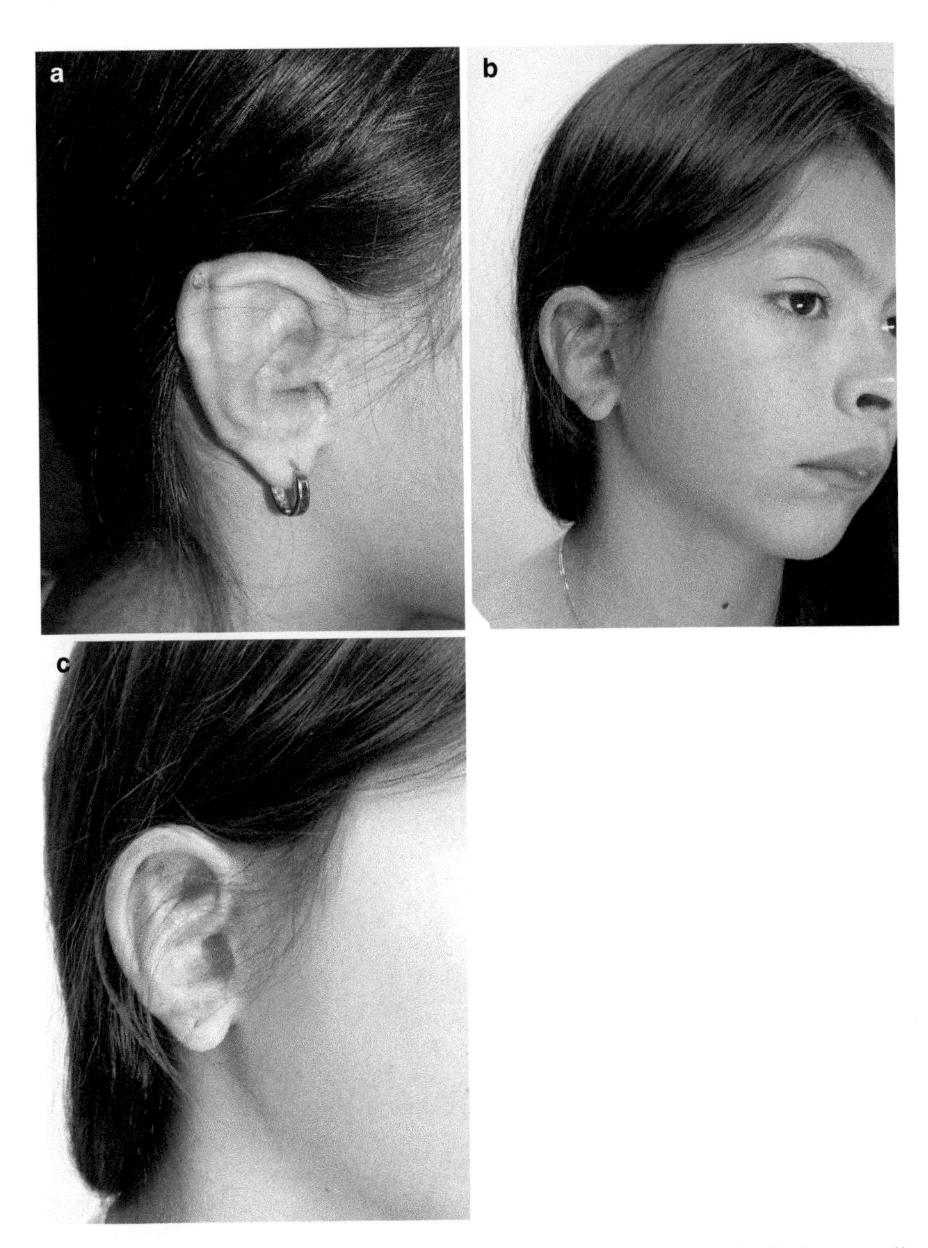

Fig. 7.14 (**a**) 12-year-old female presents with a late right ear implant fracture that leads to a small exposure at the level of the superior portion of the helix. Through an anti-helical incision, the implant was removed and replaced, and the previous area of exposure was covered with local deep temporal parietal fascia flap and a FTSG. (**b**) One can appreciate adequate healing 1 year postoperatively. (**c**) Close-up of the healed ear

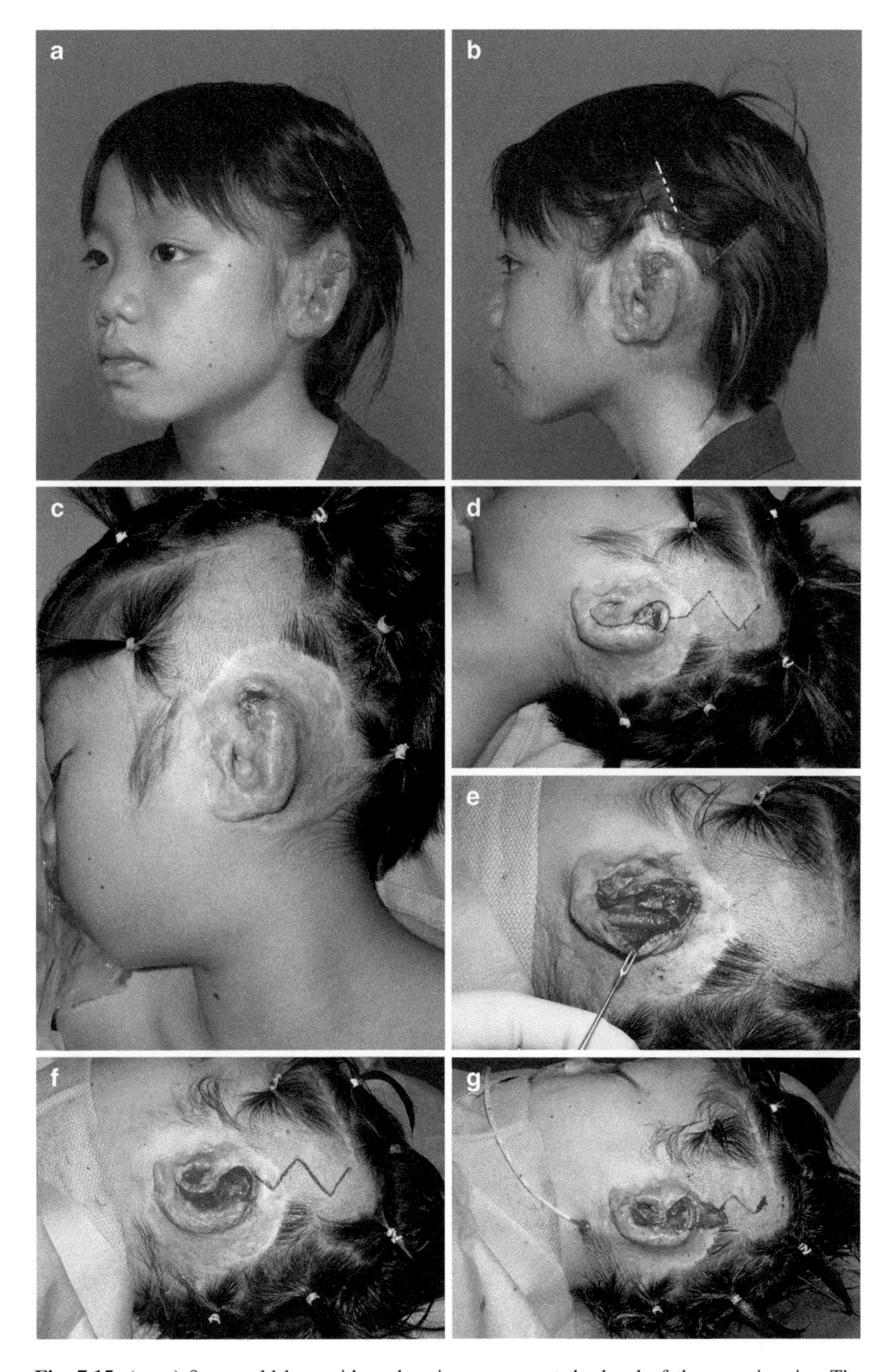

Fig. 7.15 (**a–m**) 9-year-old boy with a chronic exposure at the level of the superior rim. The patient presented late and needed an implant exchange and deep temporal fascia flap closure

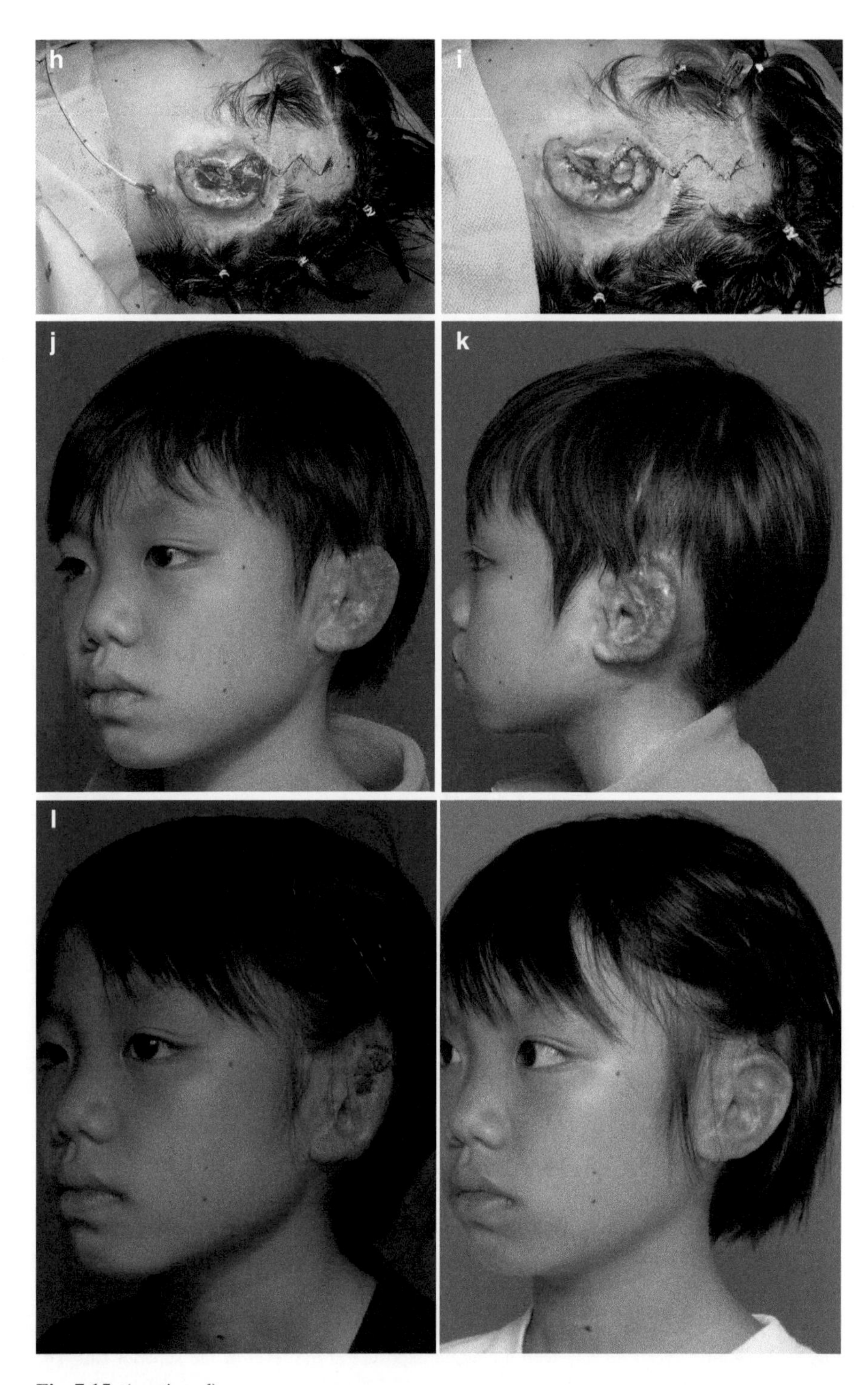

Fig. 7.15 (continued)

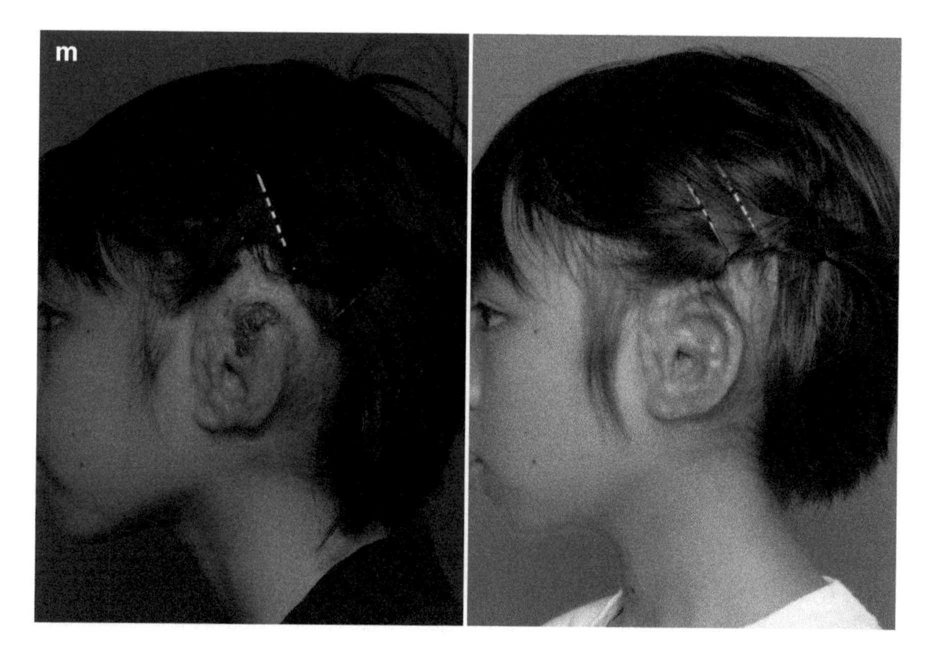

Fig. 7.15 (continued)

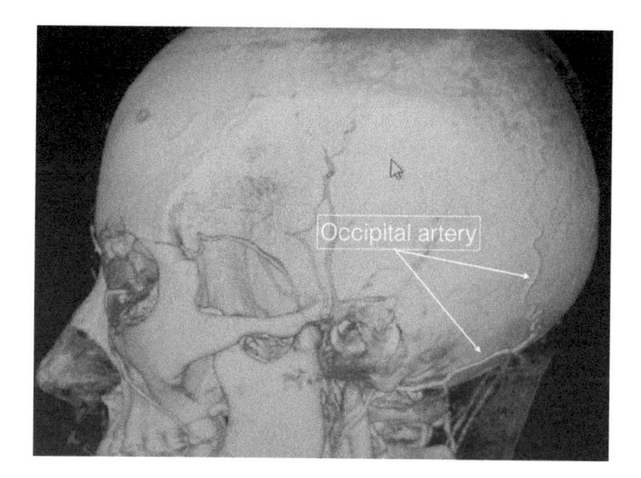

Fig. 7.16 3D CT scan demonstrating the course of the occipital artery. In salvage cases, when a temporoparietal fascia flap has already been used, an occipital fascia flap based on the occipital artery is used to cover the alloplast

Implant Descent

Descent of the reconstructed ear over time has been noticed. In patients without an atresia repair, descent of the implant is an aesthetic issue. When it occurs in a patient with an ear canal, the lower implant can cause partial or complete obstruction of the external auditory canal. The loss of canal aeration can lead to chronic canal moisture and infection. With complete obstruction, it can decrease hearing. As we described in the previous chapter, to prevent implant descent, we use a suspension "leash" of deep temporal fascia to suspend the framework. This leash is a vertically oriented flap1cm wide and an "as long as possible" long inferiorly based deep temporoparietal fascia flap that is raised and passed through a safe tunnel at the base of the flap and is used to wrap around an arm of the implant and sutured back to the deep temporal fascia. This prevents future lowering of the implant.

Others

Blunt trauma to the reconstructed ear can occur over time. Most of the time, like for any soft tissue trauma, swelling and bruising can occur; however, it is self-limiting, and the definition gets better with time. If a trauma is associated with a laceration, the wound should be irrigated and closed in layer, as for any laceration. The main goal of the ear reconstruction is to help the patient feel better about his appearance and resume a "normal" life. We do not have any activity restrictions in the long term. If a trauma occurs, it will be dealt with accordingly. We aim to address the cosmetic, the functional, and the psychological issues associated with microtia and not apply long-term restrictions.

Moreover, since the reconstructed ear is less sensate and the hearing is not completely normal (even with an atresia repair), the ear is more susceptible to more prolonged insect bites. Observation and reassurance while the swelling improves is the treatment of choice.

Keloid and hypertrophic scars at the donor sites can occur in the long term. We chose to close our donor site with deep dermal inverted PDS sutures that take a long time to dissolve and provide an extended closure support.

One rare late complication seen sometimes in male teenagers who had an ear reconstruction in infancy is slight loss of ear definition and skin thickening. It is unclear if these skin changes and thickening are related to puberty.

Conclusion

As with any surgical procedure, complications can occur following an alloplastic ear reconstruction. Those complications have various degrees of severity and can be treated by following the guidelines we provide here. Most importantly, by adhering to a very meticulous technique, one can reduce the risks of complications quite significantly.

Reference

1. Reinisch J. Ear reconstruction in young children. Facial Plast Surg. 2015;31(6):600–3.

Chapter 8
Other Techniques for Microtia Management

Sabrina Cugno and Neil Bulstrode

Camouflage

There are many patients with microtia who never seek consultation for reconstruction, either having accepted the deformity or having resorted to camouflage to obscure the malformed vestigial remnant. As described in detail in Chap. 5, it is often necessary to accept a compromise in the location of the auricle in the antero-posterior (horizontal) plane; however, placement in the vertical plane must be precisely determined as disparity in the position of the two ears would be noted on frontal view. In like manner, when the inferior portion of the microtic auricle resembles the contralateral normal (or malformed) side in morphology and location, the superior portion can be concealed with hair resulting in a remarkable camouflage of the underlying deformity (Fig. 8.1a–c).

Prosthesis

For children, a prosthesis is, at present, considered a salvage option following failed secondary reconstruction where costal cartilage or soft tissue coverage remains insufficient for consideration of additional autogenous or alloplastic reconstructive

S. Cugno (✉)
Department of Plastic and Reconstructive Surgery, Montreal Children's Hospital, Shriners Hospital for Children, CHU Sainte-Justine, Montreal, QC, Canada
e-mail: microtia@drcugno.com

N. Bulstrode
Department of Plastic and Reconstructive Surgery, Great Ormond Street Hospital, London, UK
e-mail: neilbulstrode@doctors.org.uk

© Springer Nature Switzerland AG 2019
J. F. Reinisch, Y. Tahiri (eds.), *Modern Microtia Reconstruction*,
https://doi.org/10.1007/978-3-030-16387-7_8

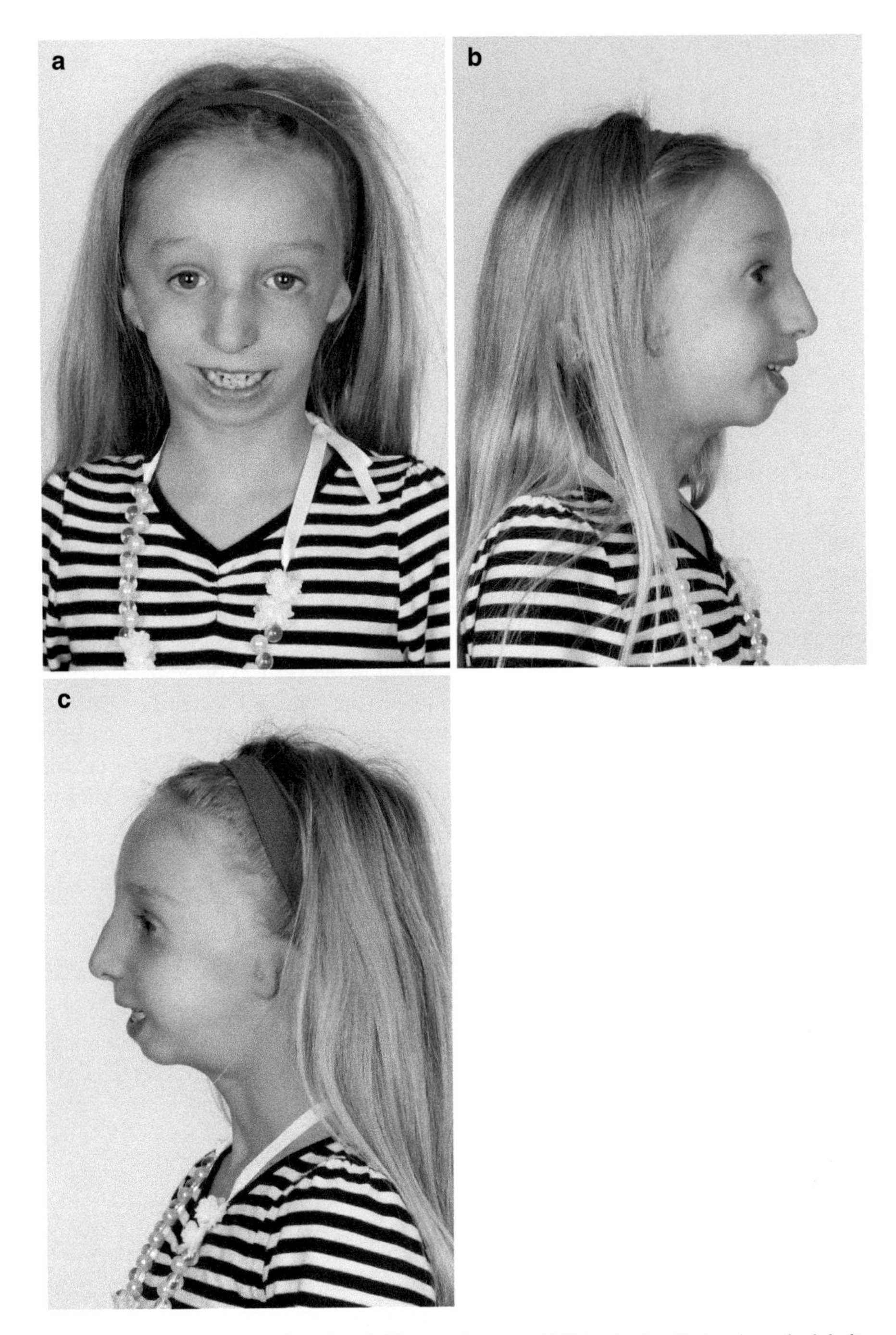

Fig. 8.1 (**a–c**) Patient with Treacher Collins syndrome and bilateral microtia in whom the lobules were symmetric in size and located at the same height on frontal view. This patient achieved excellent camouflage of her malformed ears by placing her hair over the superior portion of the remnant vestiges

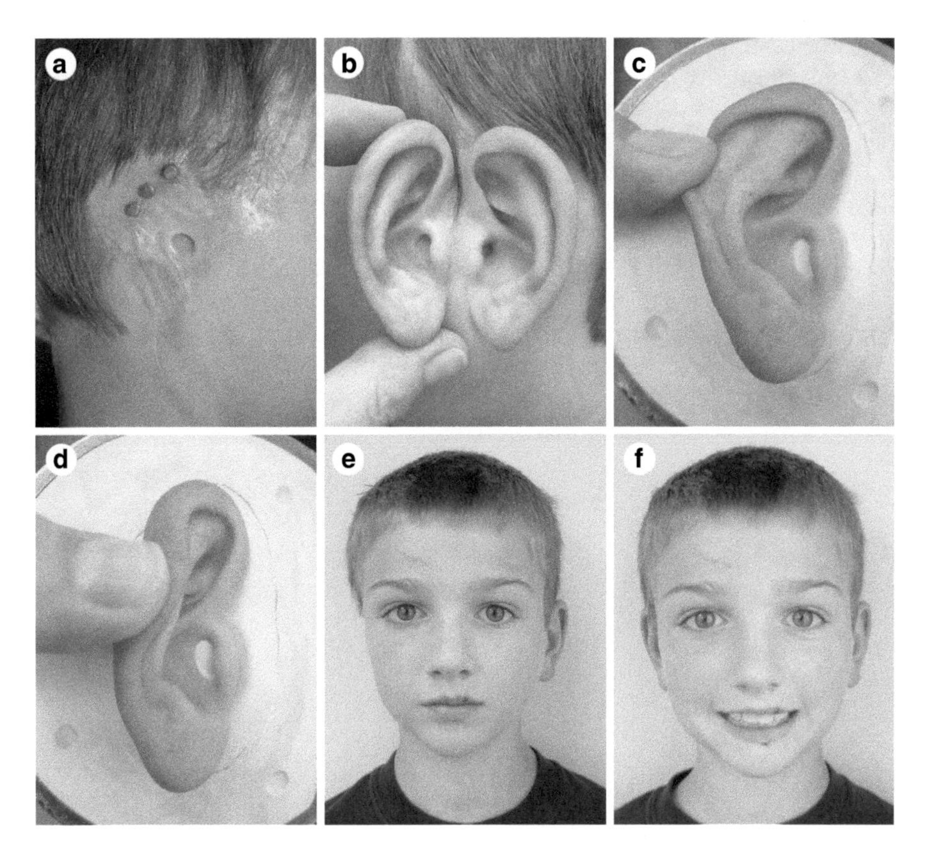

Fig. 8.2 Pediatric patient fitted with an osseointegrated prosthetic ear (**a**, **e**, **f**). Comparison of the prosthesis to the contralateral normal ear demonstrates the remarkable replication of the ear that can be achieved (color and resistance to typical displacement forces) (**b**–**d**). (Used with permission of Elsevier from Gion [5])

efforts. The use of prosthesis in primary reconstruction remains an area of contention in pediatric patients, particularly in cases of microtia. Aside from failed autologous reconstruction, potential indications for prosthesis may include severe soft tissue and/or skeletal hypoplasia and a considerably low hairline [1, 2] (Fig. 8.2a–f). However, in the adult population, prosthetic reconstruction is often considered in lieu of other more complex reconstructive endeavors for either congenital or acquired auricular restoration.

Early methods for retention of the prosthesis, including adhesives, have been largely supplanted by the advent of osseointegration, first described by Branemark and colleagues [3]. The surgical technique for osseointegration generally involves two stages [4]. In the first stage, the titanium screw implants are placed into the temporal bone through an incision posterior to the external auditory meatus, if present. Following a period of osseointegration, approximately 3–6 months, the second stage is performed, wherein the implants are revealed and the abutments are loaded onto the implants. The silicone prosthesis is then fitted onto the abutments.

In the case of failed autologous reconstruction, the tragus should be preserved or augmented with a piece of the excised framework as it serves to hide the anterior edge of the prosthesis, imparting a more natural appearance. Likewise, preservation of a well-positioned lobule imparts a more esthetic margin, preserving continuity between the ear and cheek [5]. Alternatively, enhancement of the unsatisfactorily reconstructed ear with an overlying prosthetic surface or *sleeve* can serve to improve the final esthetic result. In this situation, the autogenous construct functions as a retention device for the prosthetic ear, reducing or eliminating reliance on adhesive [5]. In like manner, the prosthesis can be integrated with the vestigial tissue of the microtic ear. This can be beneficial in situations where osseointegration is being considered, such that the possibility for reconstruction is not precluded (Fig. 8.3a–c).

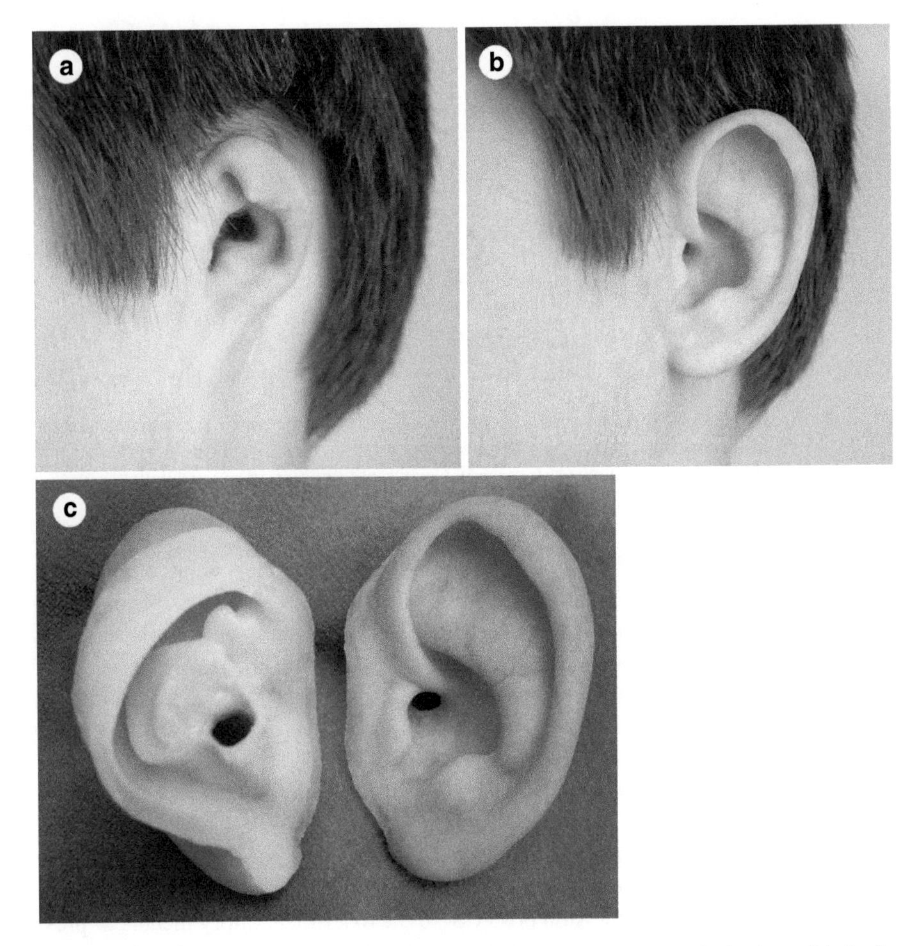

Fig. 8.3 Patient with untreated left microtia (**a**) and with an overlying prosthetic *sleeve* (**b**). As the microtic ear serves as a retention device, the possibility for later reconstruction is not precluded. Sleeve prosthesis and duplicate shown (**c**). (Used with permission of Elsevier from Gion [5])

Osseointegrated prosthetic reconstruction is associated with a low morbidity and is readily performed on an outpatient basis. The primary complications associated with osseointegrated auricular prostheses are cutaneous reactions [6] and failure of the implant to integrate into the bone. In the pediatric population specifically, appositional growth of the temporal bone may necessitate revision surgery [7]. However, as adolescence is attained, the appositional growth of bone is retarded, and, thus, revisions are fewer [8]. Despite the fact that the osseointegrated prosthesis is not permanently positioned, requires daily maintenance, and must generally be changed every 2–5 years, patients are mostly satisfied with the results [9–12]. Indeed, a superior esthetic product with remarkable anatomic exactness can be achieved with osseointegrated implantation. Moreover, a principal advantage rendered by prosthetic reconstruction is *symmetry*.

Pre-lamination/Prefabrication

Pre-lamination has been used for auricular reconstruction when regional options for secondary reconstruction have been expended. Under these circumstances, the framework is implanted beneath a cutaneous cover within the vascular territory of a recognized axial flap, thereby fashioning a composite flap. In the first stage, the framework is fabricated as described in previous chapters and buried beneath the flap with the alignment of the construct reflective of the projected orientation of the flap once inset into the area of the future reconstructed ear. Three to 6 months later, the second stage is performed, where the composite flap is transferred to the auricular region for microsurgical anastomosis. The radial forearm flap remains the most commonly utilized axial flap for the purposes of auricular reconstruction [13–15]. Following transfer of the flap to the auricular region, the radial artery and vein are typically anastomosed to the ipsilateral facial vessels, as the superficial temporal artery and associated vein have generally been previously sacrificed. The primary criticism of this reconstructive method is the lack of definition of the auricle given the thick skin of the forearm relative to that of the mastoid region. In an effort to circumvent this problem, tissue expansion has been utilized to create a thin skin envelope such that the details of the convolutions of the underlying framework can be appreciated [16]. Moreover, expansion provides extended coverage for the posterior surface of the ear. Harvest of the radial forearm flap with the antebrachial cutaneous nerve (for later anastomosis to the great auricular nerve) may address the problem of anesthesia frequently reported by patients. The latter reconstructive undertaking remains a salvage procedure when the retro-auricular skin is scarred and inelastic, local fascial flap options have been extinguished, and transfer of a free fascial flap is considered a lesser option. Disadvantages of this technique include multiple stages to reach completion, prolonged reconstructive time relative to alternative options, extended hospital stay, and necessity for microsurgical techniques.

The concept of framework prefabrication was initially conceived by Young [17] and Peer [18] as early as the 1940s. Diced fragments of autologous costal cartilage were placed in a fenestrated Vitallium mold shaped in an ear, which was then banked in the patient's abdominal wall to instigate connective tissue ingrowth. Several months later, the mold was retrieved, and the framework extracted. Despite initial enthusiasm for this technique, the results were inconsistent with deformation and effacement of the resultant framework [19]. In recent years, there has been considerable interest in generating a prefabricated cartilaginous ear framework from autogenous chondrocytes to circumvent the need for cartilage harvest and fabrication of a detailed construct as previously outlined in Chap. 5. While modern tissue engineering techniques have impelled extensive efforts to culture chondrocytes and produce cartilage matrix in the laboratory, these endeavors have thus far failed to generate a firm three-dimensional framework and do not simulate the environment in which reconstruction is accomplished; namely, placement of an auricular framework beneath a constrictive two-dimensional skin envelope. Future endeavors in prefabrication of auricular frameworks will also have to account for the variation in morphology and size of the auricle in order to mirror its contralateral counterpart.

Conclusion

Although primary reconstructive efforts should be centered on the use of costal cartilage or porous polyethylene for framework fabrication, when reconstruction has failed, salvage options must be considered. Placement of hair over the malformed vestigial remnant or unsatisfactory reconstructive result is often used by patients to camouflage the deformation. Otherwise, osseointegrated prosthetic reconstruction remains a suitable option. More complex endeavors such as prelamination of a composite auricular flap with subsequent microsurgical transfer are generally considered as a last resort, while tissue-engineered frameworks will perhaps in the future circumvent the need for cartilage harvest for framework fabrication or the use of alloplastic materials for the ear construct.

References

1. Wilkes GH, Wolfaardt JF. Osseointegrated alloplastic versus autogenous ear reconstruction: criteria for treatment selection. Plast Reconstr Surg. 1994;93(5):967–79.
2. Thorne CH, Brecht LE, Bradley JP, Levine JP, Hammerschlag P, Longaker MT. Auricular reconstruction: indications for autogenous and prosthetic techniques. Plast Reconstr Surg. 2001;107(5):1241–52.
3. Branemark R, Branemark PI, Rydevik B, Myers RR. Osseointegration in skeletal reconstruction and rehabilitation: a review. J Rehabil Res Dev. 2001;38(2):175–81.
4. Tjellstrom A. Osseointegrated implants for replacement of absent or defective ears. Clin Plast Surg. 1990;17(2):355–66.
5. Gion GG. Surgical versus prosthetic reconstruction of microtia: the case for prosthetic reconstruction. J Oral Maxillofac Surg. 2006;64(11):1639–54.

6. Holgers KM, Tjellstrom A, Bjursten LM, Erlandsson BE. Soft tissue reactions around percutaneous implants: a clinical study of soft tissue conditions around skin-penetrating titanium implants for bone-anchored hearing aids. Am J Otol. 1988;9(1):56–9.
7. Granstrom G, Bergstrom K, Odersjo M, Tjellstrom A. Osseointegrated implants in children: experience from our first 100 patients. Otolaryngol Head Neck Surg. 2001;125(1):85–92.
8. Korus LJ, Wong JN, Wilkes GH. Long-term follow-up of osseointegrated auricular reconstruction. Plast Reconstr Surg. 2011;127(2):630–6.
9. Hamming KK, Lund TW, Lander TA, Sidman JD. Complications and satisfaction with pediatric osseointegrated external ear prostheses. Laryngoscope. 2009;119(7):1270–3.
10. Westin T, Tjellstrom A, Hammerlid E, Bergstrom K, Rangert B. Long-term study of quality and safety of osseointegration for the retention of auricular prostheses. Otolaryngol Head Neck Surg. 1999;121(1):133–43.
11. Han K, Son D. Osseointegrated alloplastic ear reconstruction with the implant-carrying plate system in children. Plast Reconstr Surg. 2002;109(2):496–503; discussion 4–5.
12. Wright RF, Zemnick C, Wazen JJ, Asher E. Osseointegrated implants and auricular defects: a case series study. J Prosthodont. 2008;17(6):468–75.
13. Sucur D, Ninkovic M, Markovic S, Babovic S. Reconstruction of an avulsed ear by constructing a composite free flap. Br J Plast Surg. 1991;44(2):153–4.
14. Akin S. Burned ear reconstruction using a prefabricated free radial forearm flap. J Reconstr Microsurg. 2001;17(4):233–6.
15. Zhou G, Teng L, Chang HM, Jing WM, Xu J, Li SK, et al. Free prepared composite forearm flap transfer for ear reconstruction: three case reports. Microsurgery. 1994;15(9):660–2.
16. Chiang YC. Combined tissue expansion and prelamination of forearm flap in major ear reconstruction. Plast Reconstr Surg. 2006;117(4):1292–5.
17. Young F. Cast and precast cartilage grafts: their use in the restoration of facial contour. Surgery. 1944;15:735.
18. Peer LA. Reconstruction of the auricle with diced cartilage grafts in a Vitallium ear mold. Plast Reconstr Surg. 1948;3:653.
19. Brent B. Technical advances in ear reconstruction with autogenous rib cartilage grafts: personal experience with 1200 cases. Plast Reconstr Surg. 1999;104(2):319–34; discussion 35–8.

Chapter 9
Management of Conductive Hearing Loss Associated with Aural Atresia and Microtia

Craig Miller, Randall A. Bly, and Kathleen C. Y. Sie

Introduction

Craniofacial microsomia (CFM) refers to a variable pattern and spectrum of facial hypoplasia secondary to malformation of structures derived from the first and second branchial arches. Characteristic clinical features include but are not limited to microtia, external auditory canal (EAC) atresia, hearing loss, preauricular tags, mandibular hypoplasia, maxillary hypoplasia, macrostomia, facial nerve palsy, and epibulbar dermoid [1]. Severity can range from subtle facial asymmetry with a small preauricular skin tag adjacent to an otherwise normal-appearing ear, microtia or anotia with atresia of the ear canal, microphthalmia, and airway compromise due to severe mandibular hypoplasia [2]. The term *craniofacial microsomia* is the currently favored term of the condition previously described as *hemifacial microsomia*, owing to the high frequency of bilateral involvement. Individuals with features of CFM have been classified under a number of different diagnoses in addition to hemifacial macrosomia. CFM for this chapter includes the following conditions:

C. Miller
Department of Otolaryngology – Head and Neck Surgery, University of Washington School of Medicine, Seattle, WA, USA

R. A. Bly
Pediatric Otolaryngology, Seattle Children's Hospital, Department of Otolaryngology-Head and Neck Surgery, University of Washington School of Medicine, Seattle, WA, USA

K. C. Y. Sie (✉)
Pediatric Otolaryngology, Childhood Communication Center, Seattle Childrens Hospital, Department of Otolaryngology – Head and Neck Surgery, University of Washington School of Medicine, Seattle, WA, USA
e-mail: Kathleen.sie@seattlechildrens.org

© Springer Nature Switzerland AG 2019

J. F. Reinisch, Y. Tahiri (eds.), *Modern Microtia Reconstruction*,
https://doi.org/10.1007/978-3-030-16387-7_9

oculo-auriculo-vertebral syndrome, Goldenhar syndrome, first and second branchial arch syndrome, otomandibular dysostosis, facio-auriculo-vertebral syndrome, and lateral facial dysplasia.

Multiple classification schemes have been used to describe the degree of microtia. Marx described a four-stage classification system for the classes of microtia. In grade 1, the ear is small or abnormal, but all landmarks are identifiable, and the auricular superstructure is present. In grade II, some of the landmarks are identifiable. Grade III ears have very small external auricle components without definitive presence of superstructure; often only a skin tag is present. Grade IV signifies anotia. Other classification systems have been used to summarize the craniofacial anomalies associated with microtia. Mulliken proposed OMENS, a classification system for CFM that examines variables of orbital, mandibular, auricular, neural and soft tissue phenotypes [3]. Roberson's recently described classification scheme is known as HEAR MAPS [4]. This system uses multiple staging systems and incorporates hearing status and assessment of aural atresia with the aim of improving communication among a team of multidisciplinary providers [4].

The reported incidence of CFM varies from 1 in 3500 to 1 in 26,000 live births [1]. Varying prevalence has been reported, mainly due to discrepancies in characterization of malformations, such as congenital ear tags and mild unilateral mandibular hypoplasia. The lack of standard diagnostic criteria likely leads to underestimation of the true prevalence of the condition.

The etiology of CFM is not known. The condition is likely multifactorial with contributing factors ranging from abnormal genes with various epigenetic and intrinsic modifiers to extrinsic insults including teratogens and vascular events. The diverse influences and phenotypic heterogeneity of this condition make genetic and family counseling challenging; however, the empirically stated recurrence rate of CFM within a family is ~2–3%.

Hearing loss associated with CFM has been well described in individuals with microtia and EAC atresia. Patients with microtia and malformed ears are typically diagnosed at birth and should undergo audiological testing. Hearing loss in these patients is typically conductive in nature due to external ear abnormalities, aural atresia, and Eustachian tube dysfunction. Sensorineural hearing loss is less common but may also be present in individuals with CFM due to inner ear anomalies seen in these patients. In this chapter we will describe congenital aural atresia (CAA) and current options for management of conductive hearing loss associated with aural atresia and microtia.

Congenital Aural Atresia

Patients with microtia and malformed ears are typically diagnosed at birth. In cases of unilateral microtia, although the contralateral ear appears normal, detailed measurements reveal a smaller than average size compared to a normal control group [5]. Ears should be carefully examined for the presence of an ear canal. In patients with a patent ear canal, standard newborn screening should be performed in the first few days of life. Affected patients should also undergo diagnostic assessment of audiological function.

Congenital aural atresia (CAA) refers to the failure of normal development of the EAC that is often associated with anomalies of the tympanic membrane (TM), ossicles, and middle ear space. This typically results in a dysmorphic middle ear and ossicular chain anomalies leading to conductive hearing loss. Aural atresia has a prevalence of 1 in 10,000 to 20,000 live births [6]. Congenital aural atresia has been associated with other congenital anomalies that must be excluded, including hydrocephalus, posterior cranial hypoplasia, hemifacial microsomia, cleft palate, and genitourinary abnormalities. Early hearing evaluation is essential and will be discussed in a later section.

Embryology of Aural Atresia

The embryologic development of the external ear begins early in gestation, and the external ear itself becomes identifiable by 6 weeks of gestation (see Chap. 1). Inner ear and internal auditory canal embryogenesis develops separately and is beyond the scope of this chapter.

Ossicles

The ossicles are mesenchymal derivatives from the first and second branchial arch and begin to develop around 5 weeks of gestation. The portions of the ossicles occupying the epitympanic recess (head of the malleus and body and short process of the incus) derive from the first arch, also known as Meckel's cartilage. The portions of the ossicular chain occupying the mesotympanum (long process of the malleus, long process of the incus, and stapes suprastructure) derive from the second arch, also known as Reichert's cartilage. At 6 weeks of gestation, the malleus and incus are a single mass. Separation occurs at 8 weeks.

Stapes development begins at 4–5 weeks of gestation from the blastema [7]. Cranial nerve VII divides the blastema into the stapes; the future stapedial tendon, known as the interhayle; and the future pyramidal eminence, known as the laterohayle. The tympanic portion of the stapes footplate develops along with the middle ear from Reichert's cartilage, while the vestibular portion of the footplate is derived from the otic capsule. These are independent embryologic processes and the two portions eventually fuse.

By 15 weeks of gestation, the ossicles are full sized, but ossification is not complete until 25 weeks of gestation. During this period of ossification, the tympanic cavity expands, pneumatizes, and eventually suspends the bones. By 32 weeks of gestation, the ossicles are fully ossified, and the conductive mechanism is mature. The middle ear cavity continues to increase in size into childhood.

Hypoplasia of the first and second branchial arches underlies the ossicular malformations seen in aural atresia. Ossicular anomalies are widely variable and include malleus-incus fusion, absent manubrium, and partial or total absence of ossicles. Qin and colleagues demonstrated that ossicular anomalies are more severe in patients with canal atresia than those with EAC stenosis [8]. Fusion or hypoplasia of the malleus and incus typically leads to maximal conductive hearing loss (50–60 dbHL). In cases of malleus and incus underdevelopment, ossicular chain reconstruction is often a surgical option to improve hearing.

Tympanic Membrane (TM)

During the 5th week of gestation, the first branchial groove and pouch approximate, initiating the development of the TM. The most medial cells of the meatal plug form the outer layer of the TM. The middle layer of the TM derives from mesenchyme, which develops between the endoderm lining the tympanic cavity and the surface ectoderm. This mesenchymal layer differentiates into the collagen fibers that give the TM its elasticity. The medial surface of the TM is derived from the endoderm of the first branchial pouch. As the TM develops, it thins while expanding its surface area. By 28 weeks of gestation, the surface area of the membrane is similar to that of an adult.

External Auditory Canal (EAC)

The EAC is derived from the ectoderm that makes up the dorsal end of the 1st branchial groove. During the initial stage of EAC development, this ectoderm thickens and grows medially toward the tympanic cavity, resulting in the formation of a meatal plug or plate. The inner cells of this plug degenerate to form the ear canal. The distal end of the EAC remains closed as it elongates. It does not reopen until 24–35 weeks of gestation.

Failure of canalization results in EAC malformations including atresia of the membranous and/or bony EAC. If canalization is not complete, the process can result in a stenotic cartilaginous canal laterally with a more normal caliber of the osseous canal and TM medially. This may predispose individuals to cholesteatoma formation within the EAC. Cole described the increased risk of cholesteatoma formation in stenotic canals with diameters of 2 mm or less [9]. Incomplete canalization can manifest clinically as an atretic (aplastic) or hypoplastic (stenotic) EAC. Some patients may have a patent cartilaginous and bony canal with a bony atretic plate at the level of the tympanic membrane.

Facial Nerve

Facial nerve development begins at 3 weeks of gestation from the facio-acoustic primordium and is intimately related to the structures of the middle ear, external ear, parotid gland, and facial muscles [10, 11]. The facial nerve separates from the acoustic nerve at 5–6 weeks of gestation, and neural connections are completely established by the 16th week. The geniculate ganglion, nervus intermedius, and greater superficial petrosal nerve appear at this time. The chorda tympani nerve enters the mandibular arch and terminates near a branch of the mandibular nerve that will develop into the lingual nerve.

The facial canal continues to develop after the 16th week when neural connections are established. Ossification continues and is complete by the end of the first year of life.

At birth, the facial nerve lies approximately in the same position as that of an adult, with the exception of the exposed superficial stylomastoid foramen. The mastoid tip continues to develop postnatally to provide more protection to the nerve at this point.

Congenital aural atresia is frequently accompanied by hypoplasia of the temporal bone. The incidence of associated facial nerve canal deformity is as high as 75% [12]. The two most common anomalies of the facial nerve encountered in patients with congenital malformations of the middle ear or atresia of the EAC are displacement of the nerve and lack of a bony cover [13]. These two conditions place the nerve at risk of injury during atresia surgery. Studies show a strong correlation between more severe atresia or stenosis with abnormalities of the tympanic segment, mastoid segment, and angle of the second genu of the facial nerve canal [12]. The facial nerve may pass lateral to the middle ear making it vulnerable to injury during atresia surgery. These patients may have dehiscence of the bony canal in the middle ear. Manipulation or transposition of the facial nerve in these situations is possible but may lead to injury and resultant paresis and is rarely performed [14]. In other situations, the facial nerve may cover the oval window stapes, either completely or partially. In atresiaplasty, this may preclude surgical access to the oval window and increase the risk of potential injury to the stapes and/or facial erve. Knowledge of these variants in addition to preoperative imaging is essential prior to surgical correction.

Associated Middle Ear Anomalies

Anomalies of the middle ear can lead to malformation of the tympanic cavity, as well as the ossicles. Varying degrees of middle ear involvement can lead to change in the size or configuration of the tympanic cavity, as well as the number, size, and configuration of the ossicles. The oval window and, in rare cases, the round window may be affected as well.

Persistent stapedial artery is a rare anatomic variant that can be identified on CT imaging in patients with aural atresia. The characteristic CT finding is absence of the foramen spinosum and soft tissue in the area of the oval window shown in Fig. 9.1. The stapedial artery is the embryologic source of the middle meningeal artery that develops during the fetal period. The stapedial artery normally regresses during the 10th week of fetal development [7, 15]. Overall prevalence of persistent stapedial artery is estimated at 0.48% using data from a histopathologic study of 1045 temporal bones [16]. When present, the vessel courses through the floor of the

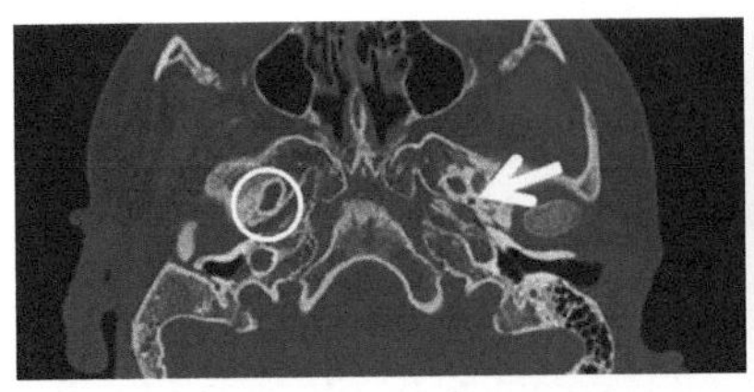
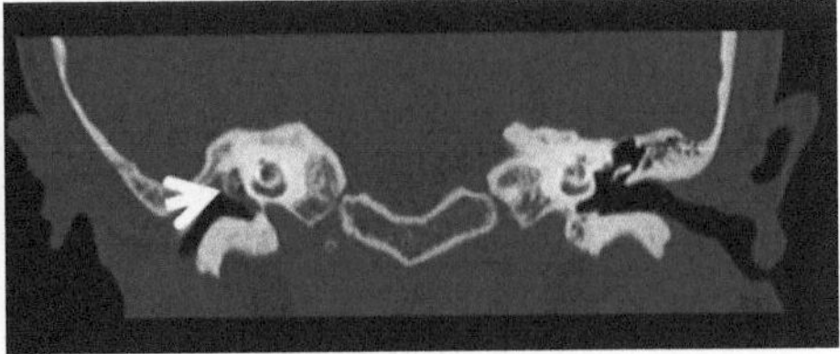

Fig. 9.1 Left panel shows axial high resolution CT scan of patient with persistent stapedial artery. The normal appearance of the foramen spinosum is shown by the arrow. The foramen spinosum and the nearby foramen ovale form the "high heel sign." The absence of the foramen spinosum is denoted in the circle. The right panel shows a coronal image from the same patient with soft tissue in the area of the oval window representing the aberrant stapedial artery (arrow)

middle ear, superiorly through the obturator foramen of the stapes and through the fallopian canal into the middle cranial fossa where it continues as the middle meningeal artery. Clinically, the persistent stapedial artery can cause pulsatile tinnitus and conductive hearing loss by limiting stapes mobility. If encountered intraoperatively, the surgeon may consider cauterization of the vessel though there is a risk of associated facial palsy. Recent studies have suggested that the risk of hemiplegia following stapedial nerve coagulation is minimal [15].

Surrounding Structures (Tegmen and Temporomandibular Joint)

In cases of EAC atresia or stenosis, surrounding structures tend to migrate toward the area normally occupied by the EAC. This leads to a cranial and dorsal displacement of the temporomandibular joint (TMJ) [8]. Consequently, the distance between the vertical portion of the mastoid facial nerve and TMJ is often shortened. The distance from the vertical facial nerve and the bony posterior wall of the TMJ is a safe surgical margin for canaloplasty. This space is larger in patients with EAC stenosis than in those with aural atresia, affording a larger operating space in patients with EAC stenosis than complete atresia.

The tegmen defines the superior margin in surgery for the atretic ear. In cases of EAC stenosis or atresia, the tegmen mastoideum may be inferiorly displaced, leading to a low-lying middle cranial fossa and therefore limiting access to the epitympanum and middle ear. This may significantly complicate atresiaplasty or preclude it as an option. Recent studies have not found significant differences in tegmen location or displacement in the stenotic ear versus the atretic ear [8]. This finding underlies the importance of evaluation of relative tegmen positioning prior to surgical intervention.

Clinical Assessment

An audiologist and otolaryngologist should evaluate patients with CAA in the first few months of life to perform diagnostic hearing assessment and discuss early intervention and amplification options. A thorough history and physical should be performed with special focus on the anomalous ear, the contralateral ear, and other possible associated anomalies. A prenatal history should also be obtained with attention to potential teratogen exposure.

It is helpful to counsel families about the timing of diagnostic testing and therapeutic options. These infants will require audiological testing at regular intervals. Based upon the diagnostic audiological testing, amplification options will be discussed. The otolaryngologist works with the audiologist and primary care provider to monitor the child's speech and language development and discuss the role of early intervention.

High-resolution CT scanning of the temporal bones is typically deferred until the child is 3–5 years of age. Obtaining the imaging at this age allows for mastoid growth, eliminates of the need for sedation to obtain the scan, and affords adequate time to screen for congenital cholesteatoma. The management of microtia reconstruction should be coordinated with the management of the hearing loss.

Hearing Assessment

Early Hearing loss Diagnosis and Intervention (EHDI) is a federal mandate with the goals of screening all newborns by 1 month of age, diagnosis of hearing loss by 3 months of age, and enrollment in early intervention by 6 months of age. Craniofacial anomalies are one of the Joint Commission on Infant Hearing (JCIH) risk factors for congenital hearing loss. Infants with microtia should have diagnostic hearing assessment in addition to hearing screening. An audiologist should perform diagnostic brainstem auditory evoked response (BAER) within the first 3 months of life. BAER is an electrophysiological test that can typically be performed without sedation in infants to obtain ear-specific frequency-specific information about hearing status. BAER can also provide information about the nature of the hearing loss, specifically whether it is conductive, sensorineural, or mixed in nature. In most cases of CAA, bone conduction thresholds are normal, highlighting the separate and distinct embryology associated with inner ear development. Conductive hearing loss in CAA is usually maximal at 60 dB due to the absence of the EAC, as well as ossicular fixation.

At about 6 months of age, infants are generally able to cooperate with behavioral testing. The type of testing recommended is based upon the child's developmental status. Visual reinforced audiometry (VRA) testing should be performed between 6 and 12 months of age. An audiologist must perform VRA in a sound-treated booth. VRA can be performed in the sound field or with insert earphones. VRA relies on operant conditioning and can result in ear-specific and frequency-specific responses, especially as the patient approaches 12 months of age.

Conditioned play audiometry (CPA) becomes the preferred testing modality in children 2–5 years of age. Its accuracy is excellent with ear-specific bone and air conduction thresholds reliably reported at multiple frequencies. Conventional audiometry is typically used in patients 5 years or older.

The audiologist chooses the behavioral audiometric testing based on the developmental, not the chronological, age of the child. Thus, the audiological evaluation of children with developmental, cognitive, and/or physical disabilities must be tailored to the patient's developmental status.

Radiographic Assessment

Imaging is typically delayed until the patient is greater than 3 years old. Although information at a younger age can be useful, we prefer to wait until closer to the age of a potential operation in most cases. High-resolution helical CT scan of the temporal bones, in both axial and coronal planes, is the recommended imaging modality to evaluate the surgical candidacy for atresiaplasty. Cone beam CT scans provide excellent resolution with lower radiation exposure than standard CT scans. If the EAC is stenotic and cannot be examined clinically due to narrow caliber, imaging at a younger age may be necessary to rule out canal cholesteatoma [17]. The risk of congenital cholesteatoma in patients with complete aural atresia is not well studied and only reported in a handful of case reports [17, 18]. Nevertheless, the theoretical possibility and reported series makes thorough review of imaging with attention to possible aberrant soft tissue essential.

The radiographic findings will determine the patient's potential candidacy for atresiaplasty. Numerous classification systems have been described. Stapes fixation can occur in isolation and result from bony plates or from aplasia or dysplasia of the annular ligament [19]. Altman proposed a system that differentiates combined malformations of the EAC and middle ear [20]. This classification scheme highlights the important observation that the severity of the EAC malformation is mirrored by similar severity in middle ear anomalies. This three-degree system can be applied to describe isolated middle ear deformities as necessary. Jahrsdoerfer established a ten-point grading system for candidacy for surgery in patients with congenital aural atresia (Table 9.1) [21]. In order to improve multidisciplinary and longitudinal care of patients with microtia and aural atresia, the HEAR MAPS classification system was developed and validated [4]. This system is used to help create a comprehensive plan tailored to patients with congenital aural atresia with or without other associate craniofacial anomalies.

The Jahrsdoerfer scale is based on radiographic and physical exam findings of nine structures resulting in a score ranging from 1 to 10. Each characteristic in the grading system is awarded one point except for the stapes suprastructure that is assigned two points. The following features are awarded one point when they are present: open oval window, well-pneumatized middle ear, favorable facial nerve position, favorable incus/malleus, incudostapedial joint, mastoid pneumatization, round window patency, and normal auricle. When the stapes suprastructure is present, albeit anomalous, it is awarded a single point. A score of less than 7 indicates poor surgical candidacy, whereas a score of 7 or greater indicates the patient may be considered for atresiaplasty (Table 9.1) (Fig. 9.2a, b). Each otologic surgeon will determine their threshold for offering patients atresiaplasty.

Table 9.1 Grading system for CT evaluation of aural atresia

Jahrsdoerfer system		Modified Jahrsdoerfer system	
Anatomic structure	Points	Anatomic structure	Points
Stapes favorable	2	Stapes favorable	2
Oval window open	1	Oval window open	1
Middle ear well pneumatized	1	Middle ear well pneumatized	1
Facial nerve favorable	1	Incus/malleus favorable	1
Incus/malleus favorable	1	Incus/stapes connected	1
Incus/stapes connected	1	Mastoid well pneumatized	1
Mastoid well pneumatized	1	Round window open	1
Round window open	1	Auricle normal	1
Auricle normal	1	Tegmen mastoideum normal, mildly low, severely low	1–2
Maximum score possible	10	Malleus-incus vs stapes position	1
		Facial nerve at oval window normal	1
		Facial nerve posterior or lateral to middle ear	1
		Maximum score possible	14

Data from Jahrsdoerfer et al. [21], Yellon and Branstetter [22], Dedhia et al. [23]

Modifications of the Jahrsdoerfer grading system for atresiaplasty candidacy have since been reported (Table 9.1) [22, 23]. Additional anatomic considerations include a low-lying tegmen, enlarged and laterally positioned malleus-incus complex compared with the usual anterolateral position, and facial nerve overlying the oval window or obstructing the lateral surgical approach. Each feature is awarded one point for favorability with the exception of tegmen position, which is graded two points for normal positions, one for low-lying, and zero for severely low-lying. The grading of the facial nerve at two sites encourages systematic assessment of CN VII anatomy. If anomalies are present at either of these sites, atresiaplasty becomes very difficult to perform due to the risk of facial nerve injury [22].

Management of Children with Aural Atresia

Children with bilateral conductive hearing loss and aural atresia require amplification, early intervention (birth to 3 years), and special school services (over 3 years of age). Management recommendations for children with unilateral hearing loss have evolved over the last 10 years. Unilateral aural atresia is most commonly associated with normal hearing in the contralateral ear. Recent studies have found associations between unilateral conductive hearing loss and educational impairment. Kesser and colleagues reported that 65% of school-aged children with unilateral atresia required extra services in school [24]. Jensen and colleagues also found that children with unilateral aural atresia have significant speech and language difficulties [25]. Explanation for the difficulties seen in UHL is based on the significant

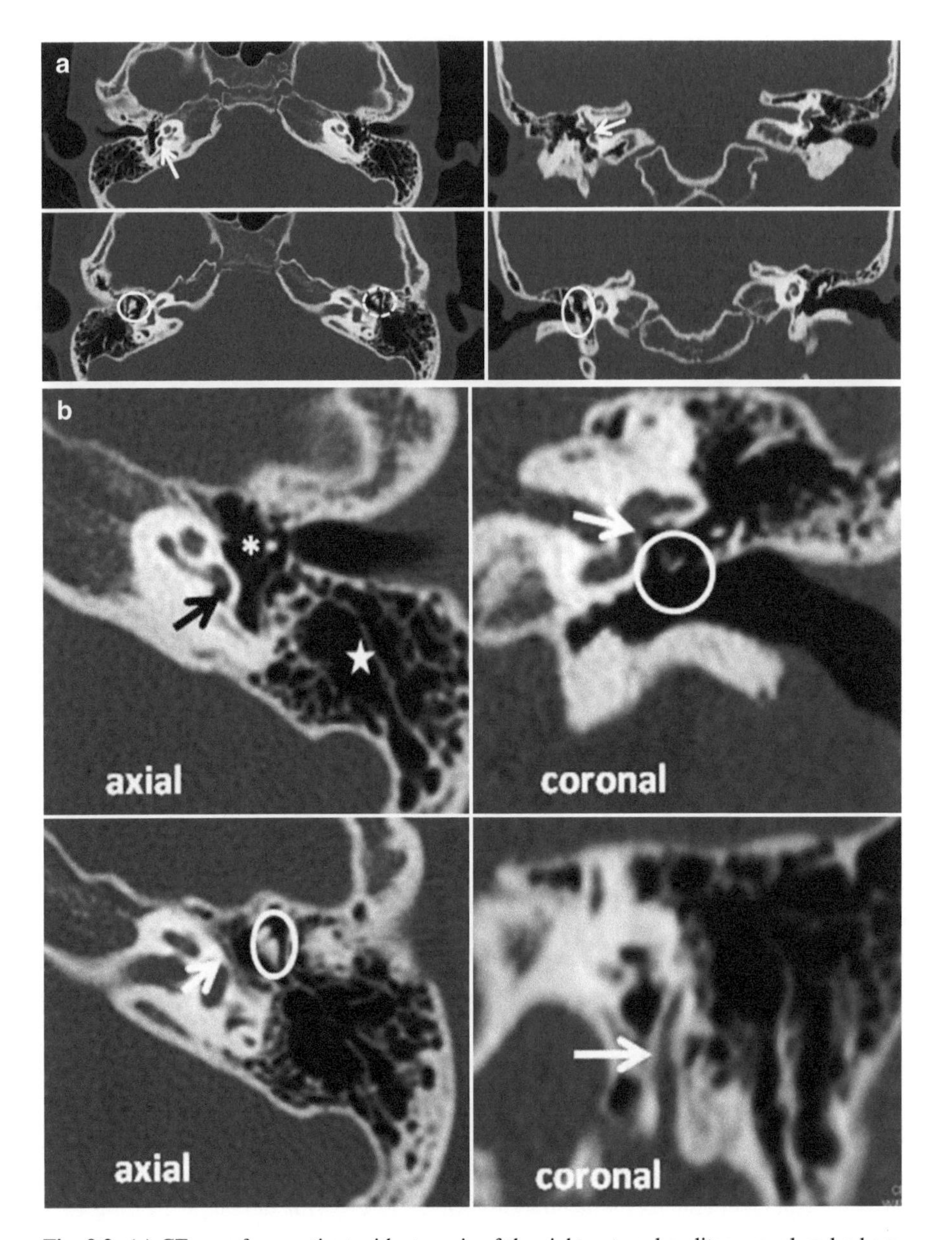

Fig. 9.2 (**a**) CT scan from patient with stenosis of the right external auditory canal and a bony atretic plate at the level of the tympanic membrane. The left panels show axial CT images of the temporal bone with stenosis of the EAC. (a) The middle ear is aerated and the round window niche is patent (arrow). (b) The right incudomalleal joint (solid circle) is fused compared to the normal left side (dotted circle). The right panels show coronal CT images from the same patient. (c) The right oval window is patent (arrow). (d) The bony atretic plate attaches to the malleus (oval). (**b**) CT images from a normal temporal bone demonstrating the structures included in the Jahrsdoerfer scale. The outer ear is not shown. Features best demonstrated on axial images include (a) round window (black arrow), mastoid pneumatization (star), and aerated middle ear (asterisk) and (b) *malleus* incus complex (circle) and tympanic segment of the facial nerve (white arrow). Features best seen on coronal images include (c) oval window (arrow) and stapes suprastructure and incudostapedial joint (circle) and (d) vertical segment of facial nerve (arrow)

disadvantage of monaural hearing in noisy environments, such as classrooms. Children with unilateral hearing loss may have issues with sound localization and understanding speech in noise and difficulties with maintaining auditory attention. This lack of attention may be interpreted by teachers as behavior problems of different etiologies than hearing loss.

The benefits of binaural hearing include improved sound localization, binaural summation, elimination of the head shadow effect and the squelch effect [26]. Most providers recommend amplification for the affected side, typically with soft-band-retained BCSP [27].

Amplification Options

Amplification recommendations are made by the audiologist and otolaryngologist based upon results of the audiological testing. Because the hearing loss associated with aural atresia is most commonly a maximal conductive hearing loss, we will focus on management of conductive hearing loss. However, it is important to understand that patients with aural atresia and sensorineural or mixed hearing loss will require different audiological management.

Bone Conduction Sound Processors

The hearing aid option for individuals with conductive hearing loss associated with aural atresia is the bone conduction sound processor (BCSP). These devices consist of a microphone, an amplifier, and a bone transducer that stimulates the cranial bone to propagate sound into the inner ear, bypassing the ear canal, tympanic membrane, and middle ear. We will use the term (BCSP) to apply to all bone stimulating devices that aid in sound amplification. There are three such devices approved by the Food and Drug Administration, the Baha® made by Cochlear Corporation (Macquarie University, NSW, Australia), the Ponto® made by Oticon (Kongebakken, Denmark), and the Sophono™ made by Medtronic (Dublin, Ireland). The options for retention of BCSPs are nonsurgical using a band or surgical using implants.

In patients less than 5 years of age with aural atresia and conductive hearing loss a band-retained BCSP is the main option for adequate access to sound to allow for speech and language learning. All three devices (Cochlear™ Baha®, the Oticon™ Ponto®, and the Medtronic Sophono™) have soft-band options.

Osseointegrated Implant-Retained BCSP

There are two brands of osseointegrated implant-retained BCSP that are FDA approved: the Cochlear Corporation™ Baha® system and the Oticon™ Ponto® bone-anchored hearing system. These osseointegrated implant retention systems are placed surgically and comprised of an osseointegrated implant and an attached retention system, either a percutaneous abutment or a subcutaneous magnet. The

Sophono device is a similar system using a surgically placed internal system secured with bone implants. This system uses a magnetic retention system and does not have an option for percutaneous retention.

Percutaneous abutments can be placed as a single-stage procedure in which the osseointegrated implant and abutment are placed. However, the patient must wait for 2–3 months for the implant to osseointegrate before using the BCSP. Ideally, the abutment would not be disturbed during the osseointegration phase. For young children there may be a concern about trauma to the exteriorized abutment during this period. In these cases, two-stage surgery should be considered. The first stage involves placement of the osseointegrated implant followed by placement of the percutaneous abutment 2–3 months later. Classically, the two-stage procedure was the procedure of choice in young children; however, recently, single-stage procedures have become an acceptable and safe option in the pediatric population [26].

Following placement of the abutment, either in one or two stages, the external processor can be used. This is usually 2–3 months following placement of the implant to allow enough time for osseointegration. The percutaneous abutments require routine maintenance. Children using the abutments are at risk for skin issues, such as granulation tissue and skin overgrowth, around the abutment. Most of these can be managed with conservative measures in the outpatient setting.

The main surgical challenge with placement of osseointegrated implants for hearing devices is to identify a region with adequate bone thickness, 3–4 mm, to accommodate the osseointegrated implants. In the normally developed skull, the suggested site for placement is 5.5 mm posterosuperior to the EAC. This position can be modified if microtia reconstruction is anticipated to avoid interference with auricle placement and blood supplies for reconstructive flaps. Alternatively placement of the implants can be performed at the same time as microtia reconstruction.

In 2013, Cochlear Corporation received FDA approval for the Baha® Attract. This retention system requires surgical placement of an osseointegrated implant and a magnet attached to the implant so that the entire system is subcutaneous. This system is placed in a single surgical procedure. The patient can start using the BCSP 4–6 weeks later since the implant is not directly loaded. This low maintenance, magnetic retention system is associated with fewer and less severe skin complications [28]. Unfortunately, the amplification in high frequencies is compromised by skin attenuation between the magnet and sound processor. In children, there are also concerns about retention of the BCSP with the magnetic system. Dimitriadis and colleagues concluded that the Attract™ device offers a good hearing solution in the appropriate patient, is cosmetically acceptable, requires minimal maintenance, and carries a low complication rate [28] (Fig. 9.3).

The Sophono® Alpha 2 MPO Bone Anchored Hearing System by Medtronic is another BCSP that can be used with a band retention system or with a bone-anchored transcutaneous magnetic retention system. This device is comprised of an internal plate that houses two magnets within a titanium case and is secured with five implants. The bone oscillator is housed in the external sound processor, which uses a metal disc and spacer to magnetically couple to the internal component. This delivers the auditory signal transcutaneously.

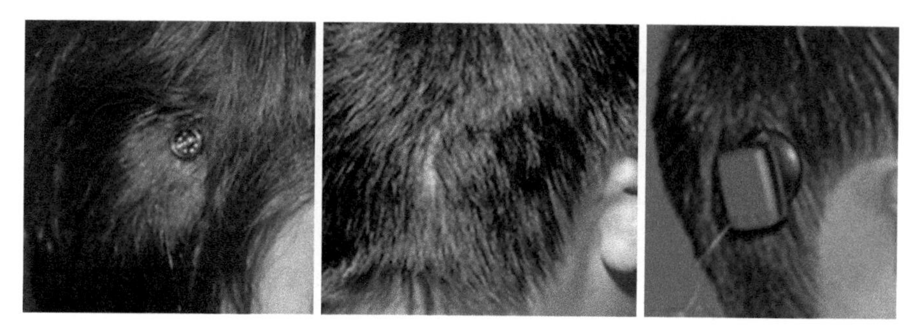

Fig. 9.3 Left panel shows a percutaneous abutment placed for retention of a bone conduction sound processor. The middle panel shows the scar associated with placement of an osseointegrated implant with magnetic retention system. The right panel shows the bone conduction sound processor worn with the magnetic retention system

There have been significant technological advances in all of the BCSPs. Features such as automated bidirectional hearing, noise reduction systems to improve sound quality and clarity, as well as learning volume control have improved the utility and patient benefit for these devices [29].

Other Devices Requiring Surgery

A number of other devices and middle ear implants are available and used outside of the United States. The Vibrant® Soundbridge™ (VSB) (MED-EL, Innsbruck, Austria) middle ear implant involves a floating mass transducer (FMT) that is placed in the round window niche or crimped onto either the long process of the incus or the stapes. This system is FDA approved for adults with moderate to severe sensorineural hearing loss. The VSB is a viable option for adults with CAA and viable middle ear anatomy. Consensus guidelines have extended the candidacy indications for the device, at least in Europe, to include mixed and conductive hearing loss, as well as sensorineural hearing loss. Placement of this device requires a preoperative CT scan to assess candidate locations for attaching the transducer. Unfortunately, there is no trial device that can be tested prior to placement. This device is also not MRI compatible, as an MRI can cause dislocation of the FMT [30].

Ear-Level Hearing Aids

Ear-level hearing aids should be considered for patients with a patent EAC and a pinna sufficiently well-formed to accommodate the hearing aid. Many patients with uncorrected aural atresia and microtia are unable to accommodate this type of hearing aid. However, patients with aural stenosis, patients with milder degrees of microtia, or those who have undergone surgical reconstruction may be candidates for ear-level amplification. There are several systems available to these patients.

Standard behind-the-ear (BTE) hearing aids may be an option for patients with an adequate ear canal and pinna. BTE hearing aids require an ear mold that attaches to the microphone and hearing aid worn in the superior aspect of the postauricular sulcus. This allows for stimulation of the affected ear potentially conferring the advantages of binaural hearing to the user. This option may require creative fitting techniques by the audiologist.

Contralateral Routing of Signal (CROS)

Contralateral routing of signal (CROS) systems require that the patient use a microphone worn on the ear with hearing loss and a receiver on the normal hearing ear. Because only the microphone is worn at the involved ear, patients do not require a patient external auditory meatus. But they require a well-defined postauricular sulcus on the involved side. The system uses Bluetooth technology to deliver the signal from the ear with hearing loss to the normal hearing ear. This provides the patient with awareness of sound on the side of the worse hearing ear. Because CROS systems deliver the signal to the normal hearing ear, instead of stimulating the involved ear, they do not provide sound localization.

Frequency Modulation (FM) Systems

Another option for hearing improvement is an FM system. This system requires that a speaker, usually the teacher or parent, wears a microphone. The patient uses a sound field or personal receiver that can be coupled to a hearing aid. The purpose of these systems is to bring the talker's voice closer to the child and to optimize the signal to noise ratio. These devices are not hearing aids in that the device does not amplify sound but rather transfers the speaker's voice into the end user's device.

Aural Atresia Repair

Another option for improving hearing is surgical correction of the anatomical malformation. Atresiaplasty was first described by Thomson in 1843. Many others have changed and improved his technique over the past 175 years [31]. Schuknecht [32] described early atresiaplasty performed via a canal-wall-down mastoidectomy; however, hearing results and potential chronic mastoid cavity disease led to changes in preferred techniques. The transmastoid approach followed with good hearing results and this is still in use. However, today most surgeons favor the modified anterior approach, initially described by Jahrsdoerfer [33].

The degree of hearing improvement obtained with atresiaplasty is associated with higher Jahrsdoerfer scores [34]. Patients with craniofacial syndromes, such as Treacher Collins or craniofacial microsomia, are often poor surgical candidates due to poorly developed middle ear structures reflected in lower

Jahrsdoerfer scores. Selection of appropriate surgical candidates for atresiaplasty and meticulous surgical technique is essential to achieving optimal patient outcomes.

For patients who are favorable candidates for atresiaplasty based on hearing and radiographic assessments, the goals of atresiaplasty, expected outcomes, and anticipated postoperative care should be discussed. The main goals of atresiaplasty are to create a skin-lined ear canal and a mobile tympanic membrane that is coupled to a mobile ossicular chain. Hearing may improve in cases of favorable anatomy, but normal hearing is not typically obtained. Postoperatively, patients with a patent ear canal and a well-defined postauricular sulcus can potentially be fit with ear-level amplification. Patients who undergo atresiaplasty will typically require ongoing otologic management to clean the ear canal.

Patients and parents need to consider their options for hearing management in the context of their preferences for microtia management. Parents should be informed about the staged nature of microtia and atresia reconstruction and that 25–50% of cases require revision [35].

When patients have aural atresia and microtia, timing of atresiaplasty is controversial. Historically, surgeons preferred to complete microtia reconstruction before atresiaplasty. Brent felt that atresiaplasty would disrupt surgical planes and vascular supply for microtia reconstruction with autologous costochondral reconstruction. He recommended that microtia surgery should precede atresia repair. For decades, the standard approach was to defer atresiaplasty until after microtia reconstruction. Due to concerns of auditory system plasticity [36] and development of complex auditory processing [37] and newer surgical techniques, some surgeons have advocated for earlier atresiaplasty in order to capture the benefit of binaural hearing during the critical development period.

Atresiaplasty prior to microtia reconstruction has gained favor particularly in patients undergoing alloplastic microtia reconstruction. This technique can be offered at a younger age compared to cartilage reconstruction. Some surgeons perform combined atresiaplasty and microtia reconstruction during a single anesthetic. Figure 9.4 provides a diagnostic and interventional timeline for aural habilitation and atresia/microtia reconstruction.

Candidacy/Indications

As described previously, Jahrsdoerfer and colleagues developed a preoperative grading system based on temporal bone CT scans to assess favorability for atresiaplasty [21]. This has been modified to improve patient selection [23]. Based on proper patient selection using these scoring systems, the degree of hearing improvement is positively correlated with higher Jahrsdoerfer scores [34]. Often patients with craniofacial syndromes, such as Treacher Collins or CFM, are poor surgical candidates due to associated poorly developed middle ear anatomy as reflected by low Jahrsdoerfer scores.

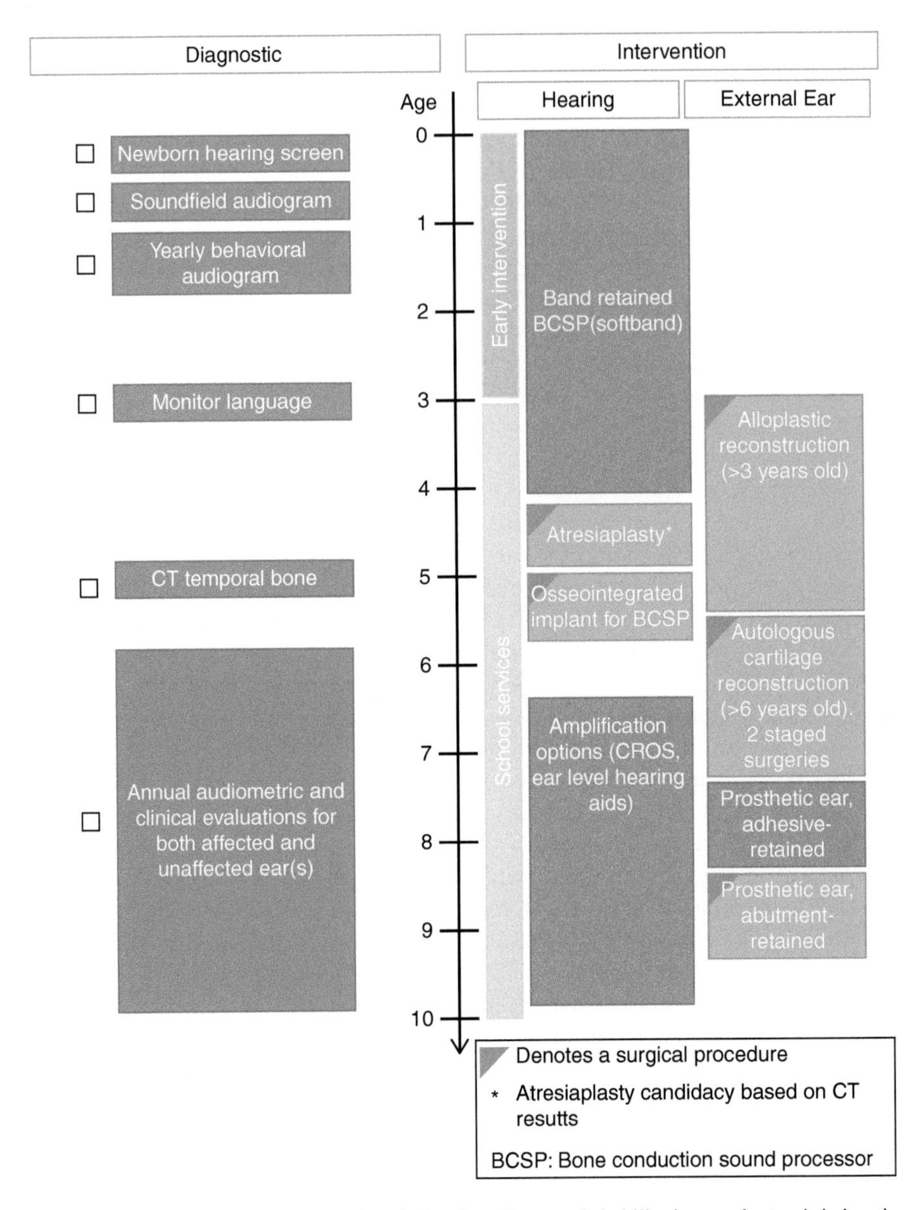

Fig. 9.4 Diagnostic and interventional timeline for aural habilitation and atresia/microtia reconstruction

Optimal age of atresiaplasty is controversial. Some parents and practitioners believe that atresiaplasty should be delayed until the child is old enough to have input into the decision-making process. Others would argue that unilateral atresia repair should proceed on a schedule similar to bilateral atresia with intervention at age 5–7 years [40]. The surgeon must weigh the risks and benefits of using a BCSP (either soft-band-retained or osseointegrated) versus atresiaplasty. In cases of bilateral atresia, the more favorable ear, determined by CT scan, should be selected for the initial surgery [31].

Patients and parents should be counseled and provided with realistic expectations for both hearing and cosmesis. A thorough discussion on hearing results is important, specifically that hearing may improve in cases of favorable anatomy, but normal hearing is not typically obtained. An understanding that amplification with hearing aids may be necessary is important. Parents should be informed about the staged nature of microtia and atresia reconstruction and that 25–50% of cases require revision [35]. Other risks of surgery include facial palsy, aural stenosis, sensorineural hearing loss, cholesteatoma, and chronic otorrhea.

All patients should be followed postoperatively to monitor the operated ear as well as the contralateral ear.

Timing of Atresiaplasty Relative to Microtia Reconstruction

CAA and microtia are associated in at least 70% of cases. When present together, timing of atresiaplasty is controversial. Historically, atresia repair was performed through an incision overlying the mastoid cortex, in an area that potentially compromised the flaps utilized in autologous costochondral microtia reconstruction. Therefore, surgeons strongly preferred to complete microtia reconstruction before atresiaplasty.

However, there has been a gradual change in sentiment over the last decade. Due to concerns of auditory system plasticity [36] and development of complex auditory processing [37], atresiaplasty is being performed earlier in order to capture the benefit of binaural hearing during the critical development period. This sequence has become more in favor due to the increasing number of alloplastic microtia reconstructions, which involve a vascularized temporoparietal flap harvested some distance from the region of atresia repair and changes in technique that do not require the traditional mastoid incision. Historical arguments regarding incomplete mastoid pneumatization as a reason to delay atresia repair are of not pertinent, as modern anterior atresiaplasty does not include the mastoid in creation of the neocanal [38, 39]. For all these reasons, current practice ranges from those who believe in early atresiaplasty, as young as 3 years of age, to later atresiaplasty. In a large case series, a combined canaloplasty and microtia reconstruction demonstrated practical hearing improvement, as well as cosmetic improvement, with a decrease in frequency of operating and overall medical costs [41].

Goals of Atresia Repair

Aural atresia repair is a technically challenging surgery with functional and cosmetic goals. The surgery should only be undertaken if the otologic surgeon feels that there is a likelihood of hearing improvement, ideally to a level no longer requiring amplification, if not to a threshold that can be easily improved with ear-level hearing aids. While some families may seek atresia repair for the cosmetic benefit of the ear canal, this procedure should only be undertaken if there is a reasonable chance for hearing improvement with minimal risk.

Surgical Approach and Details of Surgery

Atresiaplasty is performed with the patient under general anesthesia without neuromuscular blockade. Facial nerve function is monitored. The external auditory meatus must be created with excision of the soft tissue between the mastoid periosteum and the skin. The incision defines the external auditory meatus. The presence of the external auditory meatus helps to define the conchal bowl.

The external canal will be created posteriorly to the TMJ. In this region, there is often a small depression or cribriform area that correlates to the atretic canal and can be compared with CT imaging. There may be a soft tissue atretic plug present that can be followed directly into the atretic plate toward the atretic tympanic ring. If no landmarks are present to indicate the location of the EAC, drilling should be initiated as close to the glenoid fossa and tegmen as possible. Care should be taken to preserve bone between the TMJ and the anterior canal. Additionally, drilling should be confined to the atretic canal to avoid entering the mastoid air cells. Mastoid air cells that are entered during initial drilling are obliterated to prevent cholesteatoma formation. Care is taken to maximize the size of the newly created tympanic ring that will define the dimensions of the neotympanic membrane.

The location of the facial nerve should be carefully reviewed and anticipated throughout the surgery. The most common anomalies in the atretic ear are anterior and lateral displacement of the vertical segment.

Once the atretic plate is identified, the plate is skeletonized and lifted from the fibrous remnants of the TM. The ossicular mass, often malformed or fused components of malleus and incus, is freed from the atretic plate. The middle ear anatomy is identified. The stapes is inspected and palpated to check for mobility. If fusion of the malleus-incus complex is identified or fibrous incudostapedial connections are encountered, the incus must be sharply removed from the stapes and set aside for ossiculoplasty. If the incus is too anomalous to be used as an ossicular graft or the middle ear anatomy is unfavorable, a partial ossicular reconstruction prosthesis (PORP) or a total ossicular reconstruction prosthesis (TORP) can be used.

The stapes suprastructure may be discontinuous, and footplate fixation occasionally occurs though this is usually discernable on preoperative CT scans. A laser may be used to lyse soft tissue adhesions and bony attachments to minimize the risk of sensorineural hearing loss from ossicular chain manipulation.

The tympanic membrane is reconstructed using temporalis fascia. If a PORP or TORP is used, cartilage is required to reinforce the fascial graft in order to prevent extrusion of the prosthesis. The fascia is draped onto the bony annulus, and a small portion is tucked into the hypotympanum and anteriorly to the protympanum to prevent lateralization. The fascia must remain in contact with the ossicular mass to maintain hearing benefit.

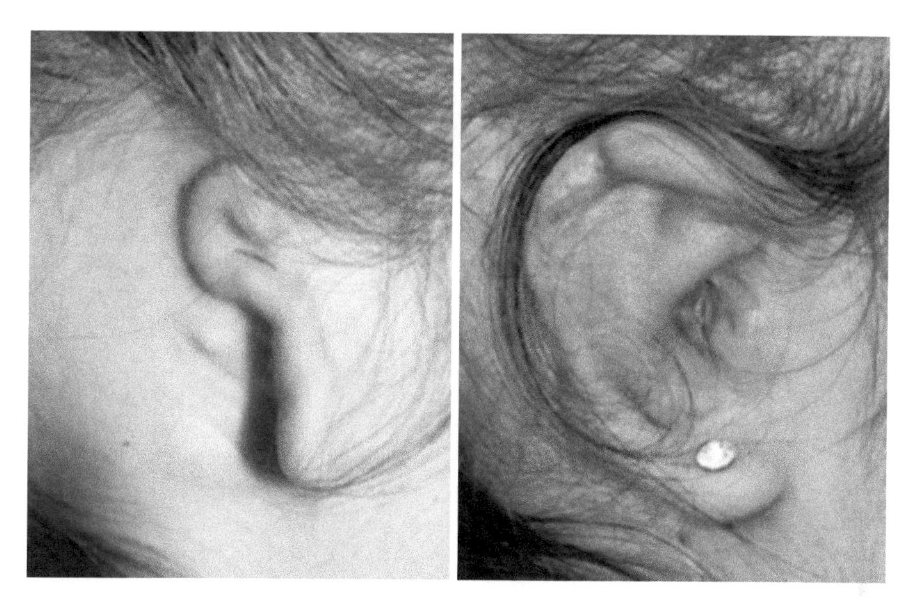

Fig. 9.5 Left panel shows patient with microtia and aural atresia. The right panel shows the same patient after completion of staged autogenous microtia reconstruction and atresiaplasty

A split-thickness skin graft (STSG) is used to line the neocanal and neotympanic membrane. This can be obtained from a number of donor sites including the arm, lateral thigh, or scalp. The graft is used to line the neocanal and tympanic membrane.

Prior to placement of the skin graft, meatoplasty is performed. Conchal skin is elevated and used to create a neotragus. If previous microtia reconstruction has been performed, overlying cartilage and soft tissue may need to be removed. The meatal opening should overlie the newly created canal and be large enough to fit the surgeon's thumb to allow expected postoperative contracture. The STSG is placed as described above. The lateral edges of the skin graft are sutured to the meatus. A nonabsorbable packing is placed in the neocanal. Most cases can be performed as an outpatient. Figure 9.5 provides a before and after example of a patient with microtia and atresia following reconstruction and atresiaplasty.

Postoperative Management

Each surgeon will have specific preferences about the postoperative care for patients undergoing atresiaplasty. The packing is typically left for 2 weeks until the follow-up appointment. The packing is gently removed and the ear canal is inspected. If the ear canal has narrowed during the postoperative period, an ear canal stent is placed with a merocel pack or ear mold impression material. The patient is seen back every 2 weeks to inspect the canal and ensure the skin graft is integrating. Small layers of granulation tissue may develop, which requires debridement and possibly cauterization of the tissue. Ototopical steroids may also be helpful for treating small amounts of granulation tissue.

Audiogram is performed 6–12 weeks postoperatively. Most patients experience immediate improvement in their hearing; however, this initial result may deteriorate over time. Case series have reported improvement of speech reception thresholds of 30 dB or better [21, 42]. If hearing does not improve to this level, patients should be re-evaluated for aural habilitation options including hearing aids, once the canaloplasty is well-healed and following revision surgery.

Complications

Common postoperative complications include canal stenosis, lateralization of the tympanic membrane, persistent conductive hearing loss, tympanic membrane perforation, and otorrhea. Less common intraoperative complications include sensorineural hearing loss, facial nerve injury, and cerebrospinal fluid leak.

Special Services for Children with Hearing Loss

Early Intervention (EI)

Children with hearing loss are at risk for speech and language delays. In the United States, EI is the system of providing necessary services, education, and support to infants and toddlers (birth to 3 years of age) who have been diagnosed with disability or developmental delay. These services are mandated by Part C of the Individuals with Disabilities Education Act (IDEA). Hearing loss is a prime example of such a condition. Multiple studies have demonstrated the benefit that EI can have on deaf and hard of hearing children [43, 44]. The 2007 American Academy of Pediatrics Position Statement on early identification and intervention for hearing loss recommends that all infants with permanent hearing loss receive EI services as soon as possible and no later than 6 months of age [45]. Further guidelines and suggestions describe the types of specialists and degree of support indicated by degree and type of hearing loss. Lieu recommends considering the child with UHL in the same context as a child with mild to moderate bilateral hearing loss [46]. Availability of these services for infants and toddlers with normal hearing in one ear is variable.

School-Based Services

Children with disabilities or developmental delays over 3 years of age are served by their local school districts. Academic accommodations such as preferential seating and use of FM systems in the classroom are described in 504 plans. Special services, such as speech therapy, are described in individualized education plans (IEP).

Multiple studies have shown the negative effects of hearing loss on academic performance [47]. Quigley and Thomure identified a correlation between degree of hearing loss and severity of academic delay [48]. Children with hearing loss may benefit from either 504 accommodations or IEP services. Some patients may benefit from exposure to sign language.

Bilateral Versus Unilateral Aural Atresia and Conductive Hearing Loss

Bilateral Hearing Loss

For children with bilateral aural atresia and associated conductive hearing loss, early introduction of sound amplification is essential to provide exposure to spoken language. These patients are unable to accommodate traditional ear-level hearing aids. Historically these children used bone conduction hearing aids. These devices are becoming obsolete and have been replaced by soft-band-retained bone conduction sound processors [49]. A soft-band BCSP is typically the mainstay of adequate access to sound for children with bilateral aural atresia for the first 5 years of life. Both the Baha® and the Ponto® provide options for implantable osseointegrated devices or for use with a soft band as described earlier in this chapter. The Medtronic Sophono is an implantable device that allows for bone conduction amplification.

Once temporal bone radiographic information is obtained, then the patient and families are counseled on additional options for hearing management. Specifically, the CT scan will allow the surgeon to assess the child's candidacy for aural atresia repair. Most children over 5 years of age with aural atresia and associated conductive hearing loss are candidates for osseointegrated implant retention systems.

Unilateral Hearing Loss

Unlike bilateral CAA, unilateral aural atresia has classically been understood to be associated with normal contralateral hearing and, therefore, normal speech and language development. Early intervention and appropriate accommodations are necessary to avoid speech and language delay and age-appropriate school performance.

Unlike children with bilateral aural atresia, the need for amplification in infants with unilateral aural atresia with a soft-band BCPS is controversial [27]. Although there has been evidence to demonstrate the impact of unilateral hearing loss on language and cognitive development and academic performance, we are not yet certain that early intervention and amplification favorably affect these outcomes. There is little evidence to demonstrate a significant benefit of BCSP in terms of speech perception in noise or sound localization; both interventions provided subjective improvement in speech and communication. Lieu recommend considering the child with UHL in the same context as a child with mild to moderate bilateral hearing loss [46]. These children may be eligible for early intervention services and school services typically provided for children who are deaf or hard of hearing.

Summary

Congenital aural atresia is a result of embryological anomalies and typically results in maximal conductive hearing loss. Treatment recommendations for patients with unilateral and bilateral atresia, although previously different, now follow similar paradigms with regard to types and timing of interventions. All patients should have audiological evaluations and should be counseled about amplification and early intervention/school services. Consideration should be given to use of band-retained BCSP until the patient is old enough to consider surgical hearing management options that include osseointegrated implant or bone-anchored retention systems and atresiaplasty.

Candidacy for atresia repair is determined based on radiographic and audiological findings. The goals of atresiaplasty are to improve hearing thresholds and create a canal that can accommodate hearing aids as necessary. Repair of aural atresia can occur before, after, or concomitantly with microtia reconstruction depending on surgeon preference. The otologic surgeon should communicate with the reconstructive surgeon to coordinate the surgical procedures.

References

1. Mitchell RM, Saltzman BS, Norton SJ, Harrison RG, Heike CL, Luquetti DV, et al. Hearing loss in children with craniofacial microsomia. Cleft Palate Craniofac J. 2017;54(6):656–63.
2. Heike CL, Luquetti DV, Hing AV. Craniofacial microsomia overview. In: Pagon RA, Adam MP, Ardinger HH, Wallace SE, Amemiya A, Bean LJH, Bird TD, Ledbetter N, Mefford HC, Smith RJH, Stephens K, editors. GeneReviews®. Seattle: University of Washington; 1993.
3. Vento AR, LaBrie RA, Mulliken JB. The O.M.E.N.S. Classification of hemifacial microsomia. Cleft Palate Craniofac J. 1991;28:68–76; discussion 77.
4. Roberson JB Jr, Goldsztein H, Balaker A, Schendel SA, Reinisch JF. HEAR MAPS a classification for congenital microtia/atresia based on the evaluation of 742 patients. Int J Pediatr Otorhinolaryngol. 2013;77:1551–4.
5. Bly RA, Bhrany AD, Murakami CS, Sie KC. Microtia reconstruction. Facial Plast Surg Clin North Am. 2016;24:577–91.
6. Abdel-Aziz M. Congenital aural atresia. J Craniofac Surg. 2013;24:e418–22.
7. Dougherty W, Kesser BW. Management of conductive hearing loss in children. Otolaryngol Clin N Am. 2015;48:955–74.
8. Qin FH, Zhang TY, Dai P, Yang L. Anatomic variants on computed tomography in congenital aural atresia and stenosis. Clin Exp Otorhinolaryngol. 2015;8:320–8.
9. Cole RR, Jahrsdoerfer RA. The risk of cholesteatoma in congenital aural stenosis. Laryngoscope. 1990;100:576–8.

10. Terzis JK, Anesti K. Developmental facial paralysis: a review. J Plast Reconstr Aesthet Surg. 2011;64:1318–33.
11. Sataloff RT. Embryology of the facial nerve and its clinical applications. Laryngoscope. 1990;100:969–84.
12. Zhao S, Han D, Wang Z Li J, Qian Y, Ren Y, et al. An imaging study of the facial nerve canal in congenital aural atresia. Ear Nose Throat J. 2015;94:E6–13.
13. Jahrsdoerfer RA. The facial nerve in congenital middle ear malformations. Laryngoscope. 1981;91:1217–25.
14. Jahrsdoerfer RA. Transposition of the facial nerve in congenital aural atresia. Am J Otol. 1995;16:290–4.
15. Hitier M, Zhang M, Labrousse M, Barbier C, Patron V, Moreau S. Persistent stapedial arteries in human: from phylogeny to surgical consequences. Surg Radiol Anat. 2013;35:883–91.
16. Moreano EH, Paparella MM, Zelterman D, Goycoolea MV. Prevalence of facial canal dehiscence and of persistent stapedial artery in the human middle ear: a report of 1000 temporal bones. Laryngoscope. 1994;104:309-320.
17. Caughey RJ, Jahrsdoerfer RA, Kesser BW. Congenital cholesteatoma in a case of congenital aural atresia. Otol Neurotol. 2006;27:934–6.
18. Abdel-Aziz M. Congenital cholesteatoma of the infratemporal fossa with congenital aural atresia and mastoiditis: a case report. BMC Ear Nose Throat Disord. 2012;12:6.
19. Kosling S, Omenzetter M, Bartel-Friedrich S. Congenital malformations of the external and middle ear. Eur J Radiol. 2009;69:269–79.
20. Altmann F. Congenital atresia of the ear in man and animals. Ann Otol Rhinol Laryngol. 1955;64:824–58.
21. Jahrsdoerfer RA, Yeakley JW, Aguilar EA, Cole RR, Gray LC. Grading system for the selection of patients with congenital aural atresia. Am J Otol. 1992;13:6–12.
22. Yellon RF, Branstetter BFT. Prospective blinded study of computed tomography in congenital aural atresia. Int J Pediatr Otorhinolaryngol. 2010;74:1286–91.
23. Dedhia K, Yellon RF, Branstetter BF, Egloff AM. Anatomic variants on computed tomography in congenital aural atresia. Otolaryngol Head Neck Surg. 2012;147:323–8.
24. Kesser BW, Krook K, Gray LC. Impact of unilateral conductive hearing loss due to aural atresia on academic performance in children. Laryngoscope. 2013;123:2270–5.
25. Jensen DR, Grames LM, Lieu JE. Effects of aural atresia on speech development and learning: retrospective analysis from a multidisciplinary craniofacial clinic. JAMA Otolaryngol Head Neck Surg. 2013;139:797–802.
26. Saliba I, Froehlich P, Bouhabel S. One-stage vs. two-stage BAHA implantation in a pediatric population. Int J Pediatr Otorhinolaryngol. 2012;76:1814–8.
27. Heubi C, Choo D. Updated optimal management of single-sided deafness. Laryngoscope. 2017;127(8):1731–2.
28. Dimitriadis PA, Carrick S, Ray J. Intermediate outcomes of a transcutaneous bone conduction hearing device in a paediatric population. Int J Pediatr Otorhinolaryngol. 2017;94:59–63.
29. Doshi J, Sheehan P, McDermott AL. Bone anchored hearing aids in children: an update. Int J Pediatr Otorhinolaryngol. 2012;76:618–22.
30. Cremers CW, O'Connor AF, Helms J, Snik ADFM. International consensus on vibrant Soundbridge® implantation in children and adolescents. Int J Pediatr Otorhinolaryngol. 2010;74:1267–9.
31. Declau F, Cremers C, Van de Heyning P. Diagnosis and management strategies in congenital atresia of the external auditory canal. Study Group on Otological Malformations and Hearing Impairment. Br J Audiol. 1999;33:313–27.
32. Schuknecht HF. Congenital aural atresia. Laryngoscope. 1989;99:908–17.
33. Jahrsdoerfer RA. Congenital atresia of the ear. Laryngoscope. 1978;88:1–48.
34. Yeakley JW, Jahrsdoerfer RA. CT evaluation of congenital aural atresia: what the radiologist and surgeon need to know. J Comput Assist Tomogr. 1996;20:724–31.
35. Glasscock ME 3rd, Schwaber MK, Nissen AJ, Jackson CG. Management of congenital ear malformations. Ann Otol Rhinol Laryngol. 1983;92:504–9.

36. Sharma A, Dorman MF, Spahr AJ. A sensitive period for the development of the central auditory system in children with cochlear implants: implications for age of implantation. Ear Hear. 2002;23:532–9.
37. Johnson KL, Nicol T, Zecker SG, Kraus N. Developmental plasticity in the human auditory brainstem. J Neurosci. 2008;28:4000–7.
38. James AL, Papsin BC. Cochlear implant surgery at 12 months of age or younger. Laryngoscope. 2004;114:2191–5.
39. Service GJ, Roberson JB Jr. Current concepts in repair of aural atresia. Curr Opin Otolaryngol Head Neck Surg. 2010;18:536–8.
40. Roberson JB Jr, Reinisch J, Colen TY, Lewin S. Atresia repair before microtia reconstruction: comparison of early with standard surgical timing. Otol Neurotol. 2009;30:771–6.
41. Zhao S, Wang D, Han D, Gong S, Ma X, Li Y, et al. Integrated protocol of auricle reconstruction combined with hearing reconstruction. Acta Otolaryngol. 2012;132:829–33.
42. Teufert KB, De la Cruz A. Advances in congenital aural atresia surgery: effects on outcome. Otolaryngol Head Neck Surg. 2004;131:263–70.
43. Yoshinaga-Itano C, Coulter D, Thomson V. Developmental outcomes of children with hearing loss born in Colorado hospitals with and without universal newborn hearing screening programs. Semin Neonatol. 2001;6:521–9.
44. Moeller MP. Early intervention and language development in children who are deaf and hard of hearing. Pediatrics. 2000;106:E43.
45. American Academy of Pediatrics. Year 2007 position statement: principles and guidelines for early hearing detection and intervention programs. Pediatrics. 2007;120:898–921.
46. Lieu JE. Management of children with unilateral hearing loss. Otolaryngol Clin N Am. 2015;48:1011–26.
47. Culbertson JL, Gilbert LE. Children with unilateral sensorineural hearing loss: cognitive, academic, and social development. Ear Hear. 1986;7:38–42.
48. Tharpe AM. Unilateral and mild bilateral hearing loss in children: past and current perspectives. Trends Amplif. 2008;12:7–15.
49. Verhagen CV, Hol MK, Coppens-Schellekens W, Snik AF, Cremers CW. The Baha Softband. A new treatment for young children with bilateral congenital aural atresia. Int J Pediatr Otorhinolaryngol. 2008;72:1455–9.

Chapter 10
Combined Atresia Microtia (CAM) Repair: A New Method of Reconstruction of Form and Function in Congenital Aural Atresia and Microtia

Joseph B. Roberson Jr.

Introduction

I first met Dr. John Reinisch in 2004 after inviting him to a yearly conference I have organized since 1994 focused on congenital aural atresia and microtia (CAAM) and other types of hearing impairment in the pediatric population. After watching his technique of alloplastic reconstruction of the microtia defect for several years from afar, I became very intrigued by the results. Over the ensuing years, a professional relationship and friendship developed that would eventually lead into the enhancement of options available to patients with CAAM.

During the first years of my professional life, I was very fortunate to work closely with Dr. Burt Brent, perhaps the most experienced surgeon in the history of the United States who expertly performed microtia repair via the rib graft technique. In observing the hearing function and talking to our patients about their hearing challenges in everyday life, it became obvious that patients undergoing rib graft outer ear reconstruction were experiencing similar limitations and habilitation of both form and function. We now understand these limitations are, namely, due to the lack of binaural hearing during the critical period of hearing development. This observation is well described by Kaplan and colleagues in a recent publication:

> Recent studies have shown another alarming phenomenon: Long-term hearing deficits may remain after asymmetric hearing loss has been treated if the correction was not completed within a critical time window [1].

The concept is further amplified in comments made after studying a population of patients who had hearing correction surgery between 11 and 20 years by Breir and colleagues stating:

J. B. Roberson Jr. (✉)
California Ear Institute, Global Hearing – International Center for Atresia and Microtia Repair, East Palo Alto, CA, USA
e-mail: execadmin@calear.com

© Springer Nature Switzerland AG 2019

J. F. Reinisch, Y. Tahiri (eds.), *Modern Microtia Reconstruction*,
https://doi.org/10.1007/978-3-030-16387-7_10

> Despite near-normal postoperative audiograms, all patients were found to have some lasting deficits in binaural hearing, particularly in complex processing tasks such as speech comprehension [in noise] and sound localization. Results suggest that a sensitive and critical period of development is [nearly] complete by 5 years of age [2].

This concept of a critical period of auditory development has been evident to those working with the hearing impaired for many years. It became more obvious to me two decades ago as I put together a group through the Let Them Hear Foundation, a foundation started by my wife and I in 2002 that established a cochlear implant advocacy program eventually responsible for achieving insurance coverage for bilateral cochlear implants in the United States after several years of legal action against insurance companies. Research data and empiric evidence defining the critical period of auditory development as well as critical two-ear function during this developmental time zone with hearing aids, cochlear implants, or corrective surgery are very strong, and the principle applies to unilateral hearing loss seen with atresia and microtia as well.

> In short, normal human development requires independent, two-ear function within the critical period of auditory development.

The surgical techniques required for the rib graft microtia repair require the canal surgery to follow all stages of the rib graft microtia repair. Immediately, upon hearing John's presentation back in 2004, it became obvious the technique used for insertion of a porous polyethelene (PPE) scaffold could occur after the surgery to construct an ear canal. The opportunity to restore hearing early in a child's life before reconstruction of the pinna now seemed to be a plausible possibility. I was incredibly excited thinking about the marked effect this may have in alleviating the issues patients were experiencing after undergoing hearing restoration surgery at much later ages in life.

I performed the first ear canal surgery prior to microtia repair and published about my first 70 patients in 2009 [3]. Figure 10.1 shows an ear canal created in this way 1 month after the procedure. This new technique allowed for creation of an ear canal to restore hearing prior to PPE microtia repair. For the first time, binaural hearing was accomplished in patients with CAAM at 3 years of age, within the critical period of development of auditory development.

After several years of separate canal and microtia surgeries following these methods, it was a patient's parent who first asked why everything could not be done in one surgery. After extensive collaboration between Dr. Reinisch, myself, and our surgical teams, the first combined atresia microtia (CAM) repair was performed in the California Ear Institute's facilities in Palo Alto, California. Since that time, I have performed over 400 CAMs with three different surgeons in the California Ear Institute's facilities in Palo Alto. The vast majority of these procedures have been performed with Dr. Reinisch who kindly travels from Los Angeles to our facility for each of these surgeries so that we are able to extend this unique, comprehensive service to patients.

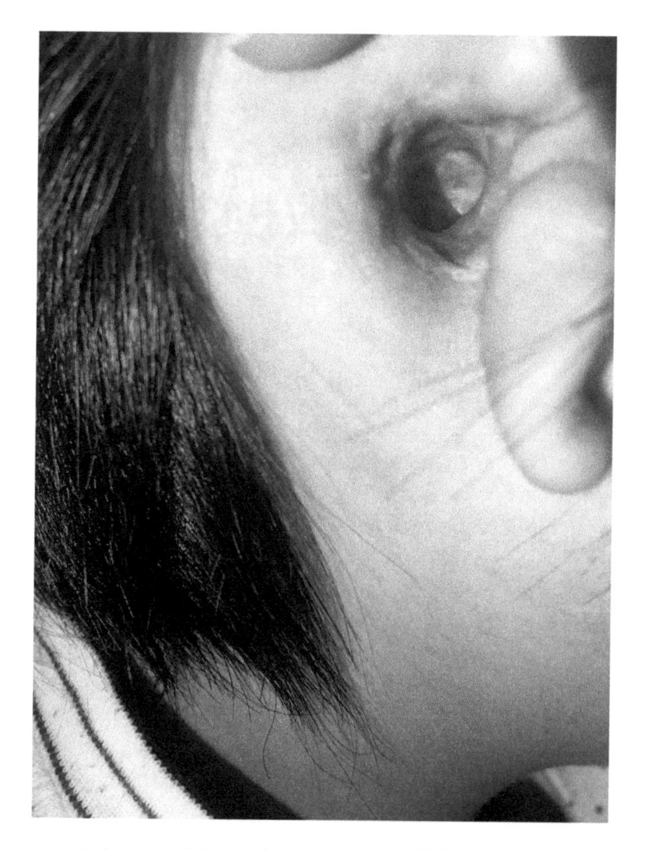

Fig. 10.1 Reconstructed ear canal 1 month post-op, before PPE microtia repair

The average age of ear canal surgery for children following rib graft microtia repair is 12.2 years in our clinic. The average age of ear canal surgery prior to or at the same time as PPE microtia repair is 4.1 years of age. The impact on auditory development has become a strong reason for parents to choose PPE for microtia reconstruction.

Hearing

Patients and parents now look for restoration of form *and* function when selecting options for treatment of congenital aural atresia and microtia. Our understanding of hearing function and auditory development has improved over the past two decades and sheds light on the inadequacies of our early strategies for treatment of the hearing component of this condition.

My medical training improperly taught me (and many others) that unilateral hearing is adequate for normal function. We now know this is wrong: *single-sided hearing loss is a disability*. Perhaps the strongest data supporting this fact is the ten-time increase of having to repeat a grade for children with unilateral hearing loss and the average income levels of those with unilateral hearing loss, which is one-third less than that of their two-ear hearing peers [4]. Adults with single-sided deafness will readily testify to the situations in which they have difficulty: directional hearing and hearing in noise.

Parents were told (and still are by many well-intentioned providers) that one-ear hearing is enough. This statement is undoubtedly not intended to harm but it is false and misleading. Directional hearing will always be impossible when hearing from only one ear. It is important to understand that an observer (such as a parent or uniformed physician) watching a one-eared hearing child or adult in a quiet room will see function and understanding appear to be normal. However, when the same child or adult is placed in normal, everyday situations where background noise is present, the deficits are significant.

Alarmingly, the system of complex function of the auditory system develops before its dysfunction becomes readily apparent, which may be beyond the time period during which intervention can improve function, since it is beyond the critical period of auditory development. Since many of the deficits produced by single-sided hearing loss cannot be reversed after the critical period of auditory development has passed, statements like "one ear is adequate for hearing" run the risk of withholding from a child adequate development that cannot be restored later in life.

As this becomes more widely understood and backed by more data, I believe lack of hearing restoration with treatment of CAAM will be viewed more strongly as negligence on the part of the provider should the patient and/or his or her parent not be provided with all the options available regarding both form and function.

Critical Period of Auditory Development

Human auditory development is a very active process that occurs almost solely within the first decade of life and mainly in the first 5 years of life. First, we develop the ability to understand spoken language (called receptive language) during the first 3 or 4 years of life. Next, expressive language ensues and continues up to about 5 years of age. Lastly, complex auditory functions begin development at birth and continue to about 10 years of age. While the development of each of these areas of hearing and communication function improves slightly with age, the vast majority of development occurs in the first years of life. Once a person is beyond those years of development, the functions cannot be altered significantly, as you know this is the definition of a critical period. Other body systems have similar developmental paradigms; for example, amblyopia must be corrected early in life or function of the lazy eye can never be restored.

Importantly, for the complex function to develop normally, two-ear hearing *must* be achieved at an early age. Each ear's data stream must be *independent*, allowing the brain to process the auditory signal needed for these functions. Three examples are illustrative:

- Language development: Both the number of words and the complexity of speech composition in patients with unilateral hearing loss are reduced [5].
- Directional sound: To understand where sound is coming from, the brain takes the time the sound arrives at each ear and performs a geometry calculation to determine the azimuth from which the sound originates. If only one ear has sound input, we cannot localize sound. This is very easily understood by anyone associated with unilateral CAAM patients. For the system to develop correctly, binaural sound input must be supplied during early auditory development.
- Hearing in noise: Our inner ears deliver to the brain all the sound from our environment. It is the brain that focuses on spoken language filtering out unwanted noise. To perform this function – and to learn to perform this function during the critical period auditory development – the brain must have two separate and independent sound streams, one from each ear. If these two sound streams are not supplied early in life, the system does not develop normally, and the individual will never be able to process sound in noise normally. An example we all can understand is a busy restaurant. When the surrounding sounds begin to increase as dinner progresses, we have all had the experience where we "lean in" to understand someone at our table. With two ears, our speech understanding will drop from 100% in a quiet setting into 90–99% in this situation. That can be annoying and challenging as we all have experienced. People with one ear will experience a drop in speech understanding to 50–60% understanding range. That is a disability.

If the system does not develop normally during the critical period of development, it will not develop later in life, and the patient will be left with this dysfunction in noise throughout life. Children in the classroom with single-sided hearing impairment experience this phenomenon, which can lead to poor performance and withdrawal, anger issues, poor concentration, and similar behavioral issues.

Box 10.1 lists hearing habilitation options from most to least desirable in terms of mimicry of normal hearing physiology. It should be noted that single or bilateral implantable and non-implantable bone conduction hearing devices do not provide binaural independent data streams and sound input, do not allow the brain performance or development of hearing in noise, do not provide directional sound, and therefore do not improve hearing in noise.

Box 10.1. Rank of Hearing Habilitation Options Closest to Normal Hearing

1: Canal
2: Canal + hearing aid
3: Vibrant Soundbridge (MED-EL, Innsbruck, Austria)
4: Bone conduction implant

- BAHA® (Cochlear Corporation, Macquarie University, NSW, Australia)
- Ponto® (Oticon, Kongebakken, Denmark)
- BoneBridge (MED-EL, Innsbruck, Austria)

Patient Selection

Every patient is not a candidate for surgical creation of an ear canal. A solid understanding of “when to say no” is critical for surgeons to develop in advising their patients. Communication among CAAM team specialists such as plastic surgeons, craniofacial surgeons, orthodontic surgeons, audiologist, anesthesiologists, and otologic surgeons is critical to determining what practical experience has shown to be unique individualized treatment plans for each patient.

We use a classification system published in 2013 [6] named “HEAR MAPS” to fully evaluate each patient. Use of this system also helps us to study our results and outcomes. Each letter corresponds to a characteristic of the patient of interest. Two of the letters require objective test data – H with a hearing test and A with an atresia score from a CT scan of the temporal bone – while the others are gained during the physical examination. See Fig. 10.2.

Patients who are adequate candidates for canal creation can have an ear canal and an eardrum created either as a separate procedure from PPE microtia repair – we suggest at least 4 months between atresia repair and microtia repair in this choice – or simultaneously with PPE microtia repair, combined atresia repair, or CAM, the subject of this chapter.

Of note, I have performed a few dozen canal surgeries following PPE microtia repair in which the implant was situated favorably, but I do not recommend this. Canal surgery following PPE placement puts the implant at risk of exposure and/or infection and is best avoided if possible.

Two of the eight data points in HEAR MAPS are test data (the hearing test or audiogram and the CT scan). The remainder can be determined by physical

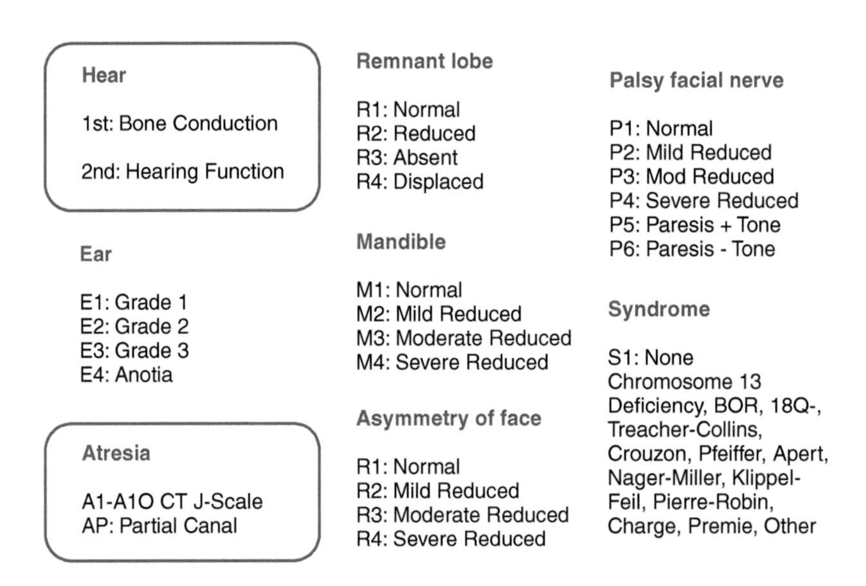

Fig. 10.2 HEAR MAPS. Grading system

Box 10.2. Surgical Candidacy Grading

<5: Rarely reconstruct (unless for HD)
5: Reconstruct for some bilateral
6–7: Adequate chance of success
8–10: Very good chance of success

examination of the patient. The CT scan should *only* be read by the otologic surgeon and not radiology if a decision is being made for a patient with regard to potential surgery. I use the 10-point scale originally developed by Jahrsdoerfer [7], while other surgeons use different evaluation scales. As seen in Box 10.2, patients with a score of 6–10 on their CT scans (using a 10-point scale of grading) are candidates for surgical creation of an ear canal. Patients with a score of 5 with bilateral CAAM are occasionally candidates for ear canal surgery as well. Scores of 5 or less produced hearing infrequently enough that other methods of hearing provision are better options.

Nearly all patients who have an ear canal created under these guidelines enjoy an improved hearing percent chance of successful restoration into the normal range, increasing with a higher CT score (the "A" in HEAR MAPS). While hearing can be brought into normal ranges with canal surgery, we cannot yet achieve 100% function of a normally formed ear. The hearing we do achieve, however, is close to normal, allowing for both development and function of the auditory system, such as directional hearing and hearing in noise as noted above.

Cholesteatoma

Every child must have a CT scan before treatment for CAAM, even those who are not canal candidates or those who do not want a canal surgically created. The reason is a rare condition of canal cholesteatoma. As the ear canal develops, a small pit forms, and a cell tract dissolves toward the future ear canal. In some individuals, this process never starts and CAAM results, while in others the process starts and then arrests, leading to a buried skin cyst within the temporal bone or soft tissue called a cholesteatoma. The condition is present in 4% of the 3300 patients evaluated by me in my database. In multiple examples, I have encountered patients who did not have a CT prior to microtia repair. Later, after undergoing microtia repair with either rib graft or PPE techniques, the cyst slowly enlarges, erodes bone, and may become infected. Loss and infection of both rib graft microtia repair and PPE microtia repair have occurred. In some patients, loss of inner ear function, facial nerve injury, and/or meningitis may result. We have found the presence of cholesteatoma *cannot* be excluded by physical examination alone. Importantly, patients should not have microtia repair of any type over a small ear canal as cholesteatoma can develop as a result. See Fig. 10.3a, b.

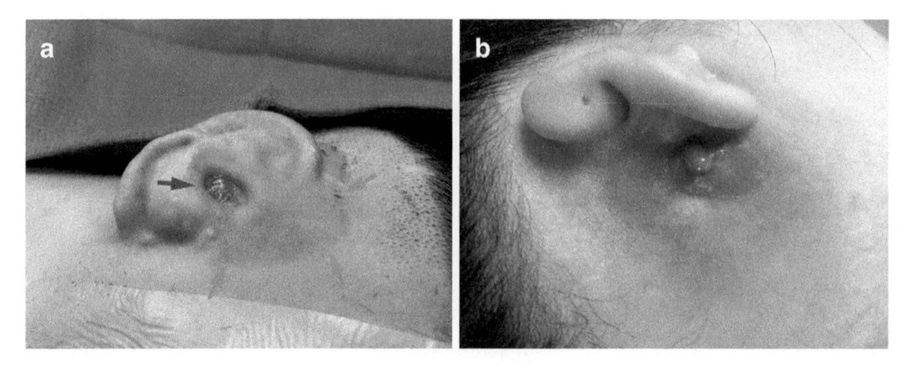

Fig. 10.3 (**a**) Patient with cholesteatoma following microtia repair. Red arrow: external auditory canal meatus with infected cholesteatoma. Blue arrows: margin of cholesteatoma extending under microtia repair. (**b**) Infected cholesteatoma with fistula presurgical repair

Some patients can have congenital canal cholesteatoma removed and a full ear canal and eardrum created, with the intention of hearing restoration (either as separate procedures or in some instances as part of the CAM procedure). Others should have these conditions resected and treated with removal of all components of the cyst or canal by an otologic surgeon prior to microtia repair with either PPE or rib graft surgery. Small car canals may also progress to canal cholesteatoma if microtia repair is performed over them. Consultation with a CT by the otologic surgeon on your team will determine if a cholesteatoma or an inadequately small ear canal is present and how to handle it.

Age of CAM

Children should be 3 years of age and 15 kg or more in weight. Two factors determine the earliest age we perform CAM for CAAM. The first is safety. As the procedure takes 7–8 hours, anesthetic considerations for 3-year-olds are paramount. Pediatric anesthesiologists are engaged, and minimal inhalational agents are used due to injection of dilute solutions of both lidocaine and bupivacaine before the procedure begins and ends. Three years of age has become a dividing line for risk of general anesthesia in young children. All CAMs performed at our institution have been accomplished on an outpatient basis with same-day discharge.

Coincidentally, at 3 years of age, a significant amount of growth toward the adult size of the head and the ear has already occurred. Figure 10.4 is illustrative of this growth pattern. As can be seen, the outer ear has reached 88% of adult size at 3 years of age and 92% of adult size by 7 years of age. Both rib and PPE surgical techniques require implant size estimation based on anticipated final pinna size after growth has occurred by approximately 18 years of age.

As the middle ear bones are fully formed at birth, middle ear structures can be repaired or augmented as needed without risk of future growth requiring prosthesis

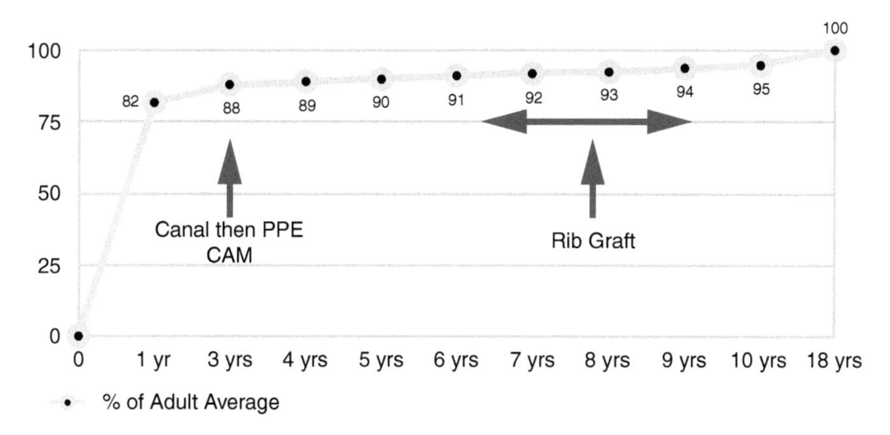

Fig. 10.4 Head growth by age. Note: Outer ear (Pinna) is 85% of adult size at 3 years of age. (Used with permission of CEI Medical Group from Farkas et al. [13])

change, for example. After performing several dozen canal reconstructions prior to PPE, a panel of surgeons at the California Ear Institute blindly viewed intraoperative video and attempted to estimate the age of the patient. No predictive ability was noted in patients preselected with adequate HEAR MAPS scores for the procedure.

Surgical Technique and Setup

CAM surgery is performed in a dedicated operating room in our facility with a hand-selected anesthesiologist staff comfortable and adept with children and long procedures. As the procedure involves many steps, an OR team needs significant training to efficiently provide the environment as well as the equipment and the supplies necessary for successful outcomes.

Specialized equipment necessary to the performance of CAM surgery includes otologic and neurotologic micro-instrumentation (some of which has been custom-designed for the CEI Otology Surgery Center), high speed otologic drills, an operating microscope with attached high definition video and recording equipment, facial nerve monitoring, laser (CO_2 or visible wavelength lasers such as KTP or argon suffice), split-thickness skin graft dermatome capable of submillimeter thickness harvest, and custom titanium ossicle reconstruction prostheses of multiple sizes and types. Each of these is needed for the ear canal creation portion of the procedure. See Fig. 10.5. Plastic surgical instrumentation, eye level magnification in the form of loupes, smoke evacuation, and handheld battery-operated cautery devices used to form and place the PPE implant should also be on hand. Anesthesia needs are discussed elsewhere in this book.

After successful induction of general anesthesia, endotracheal intubation is accomplished. The endotracheal tube is sewn in, securing it to the teeth in the maxilla. The patient is rotated 180 degrees on an OR bed that allows side to side rotation and allows the otologic surgeon to sit with legs under the table with the microscope

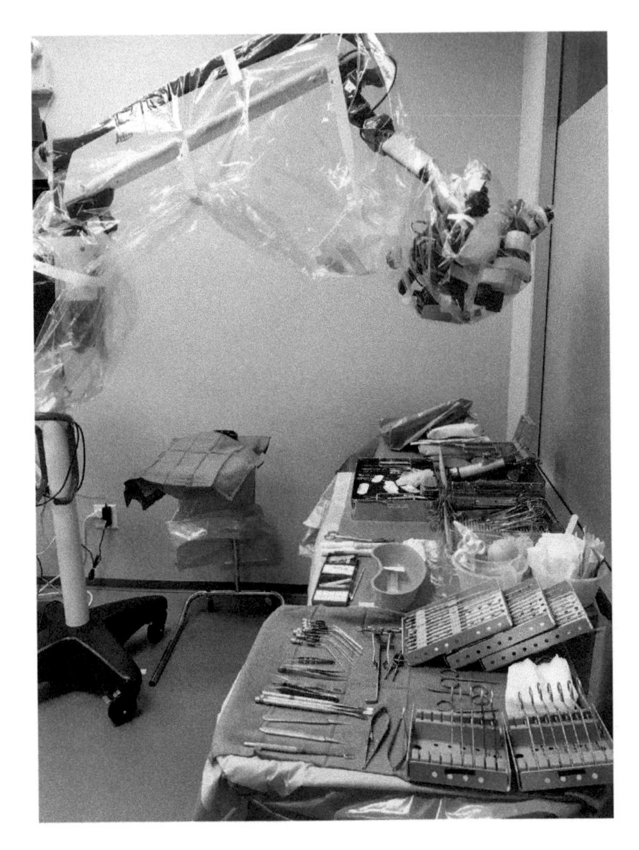

Fig. 10.5 OR equipment setup

in place for his or her portion of the procedure. Facial nerve monitoring electrodes are placed in the orbicularis oris and the orbicularis oculi ipsilateral to the ear being reconstructed and covered with a sterile adhesive drape which is later prepped within the field. See Fig. 10.6. Continuous monitoring is performed throughout the case with the exclusion of the temporoparietal flap elevation. A Foley catheter and temperature probe are placed. Sterile clear plastic drapes are used to drape off the face including the nose/mouth/eyes and facial nerve monitoring electrodes. The endotracheal tube position is confirmed with anesthesia and further secured with the same.

Hair is removed around the ear as well as the contralateral scalp where the partial thickness skin graft is to be harvested. Using palpation and Doppler if needed, the temporoparietal artery is located and marked with an indelible marker. See Fig. 10.7. Care is taken at the area of the proposed ear canal to ensure the artery is adequately anterior. In some cases, the artery is directly over the proposed canal site and must be relocated anteriorly [8]. See Fig. 10.8. Preservation of this artery is critical to PPE success.

In unilateral cases, the contralateral ear is used as a model, and X-ray or clear cellophane is used to trace the ear for use when constructing the PPE implant.

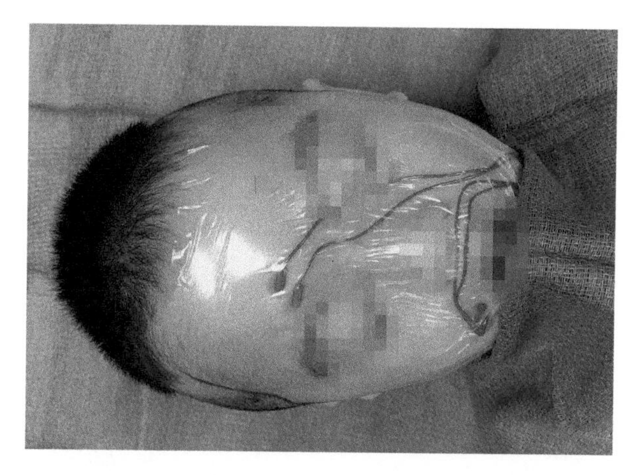

Fig. 10.6 Facial nerve monitor

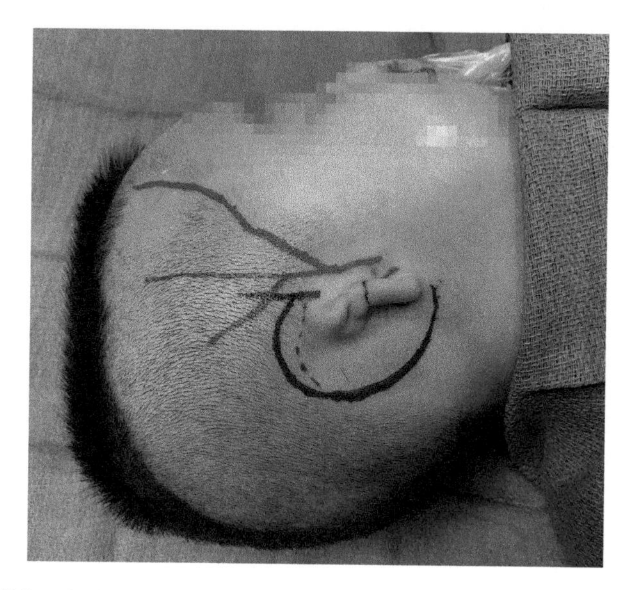

Fig. 10.7 CAM marked

Measurements in an anterior-posterior direction from the lateral canthus of the ipsilateral eye and superior-inferior positioning are calculated, and the final position of the ear is marked with an indelible marker. See Figs. 10.9 and 10.10.

Local anesthesia is infiltrated in the areas of future dissection to minimize the depth of general anesthesia needed over the ensuing hours. Additional injections may be needed during the procedure. Careful tracking of the total amount injected is recommended to remain well under potentially toxic dosing. Hair is braided if long and a potential impediment to the procedure. Prophylactic antibiotics (vancomycin) are administered intravenously.

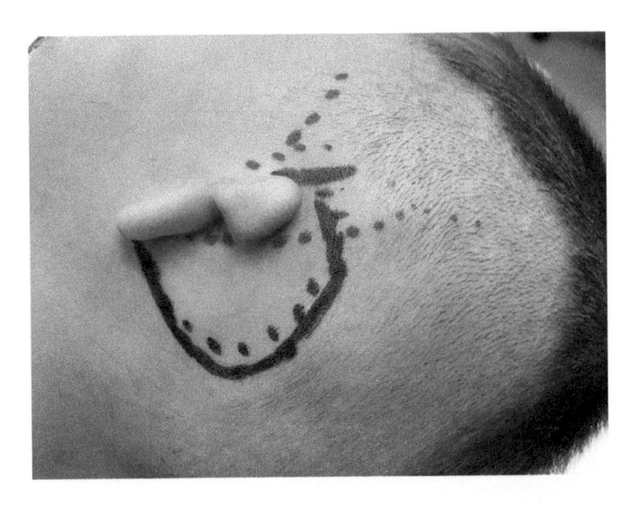

Fig. 10.8 CAM posterior vessel

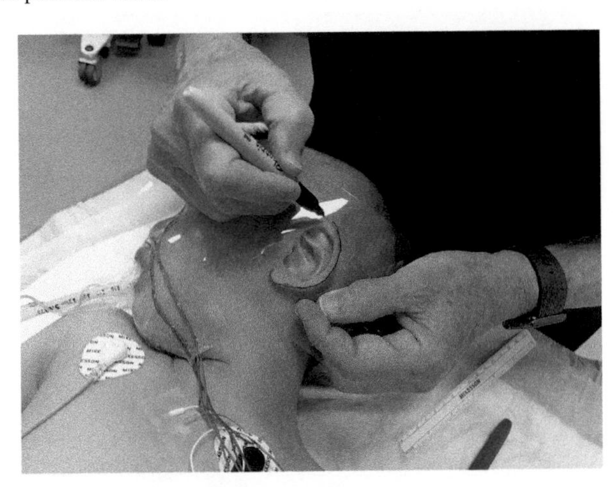

Fig. 10.9 CAM template

Chlorhexidine prep of the entire head is performed, and sterile drapes are positioned, leaving the head completely exposed, as the contralateral ear will be important for positioning of the microtia repair, partial thickness skin graft, and full-thickness skin graft harvest on the contralateral side on unilateral cases. The endotracheal tube is placed within a sterile endoscopy sleeve and allowed to rest on top of the sterile drapes. See Figs. 10.11 and 10.12. The area of full-thickness skin graft harvest in the groin previously marked is included in the skin preparation and draping process but covered with a drape to be cut through later in the procedure when the skin is harvested and wound closed.

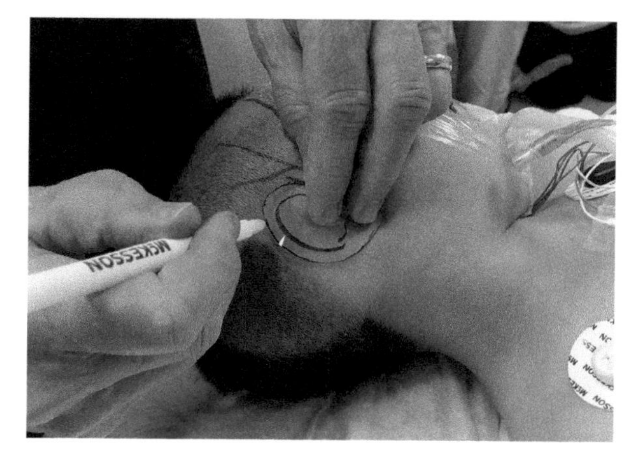

Fig. 10.10 CAM template 2

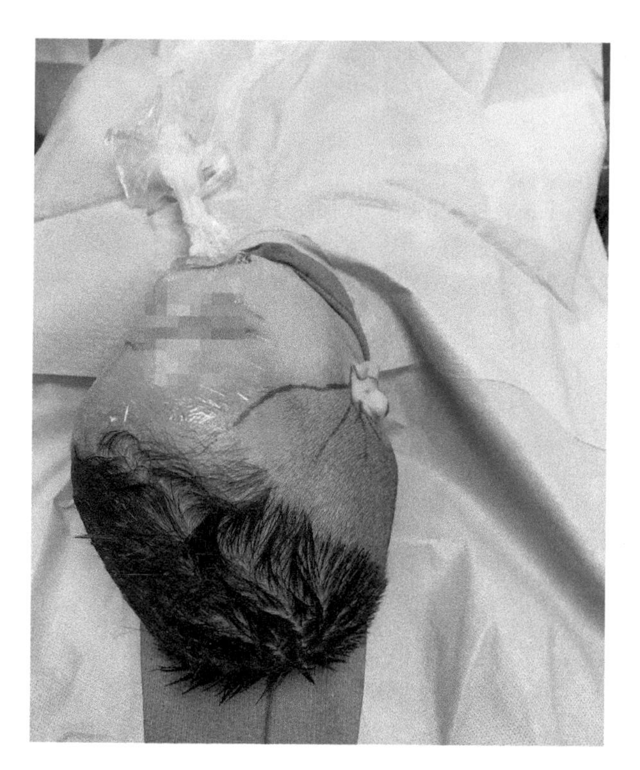

Fig. 10.11 CAM drape 1

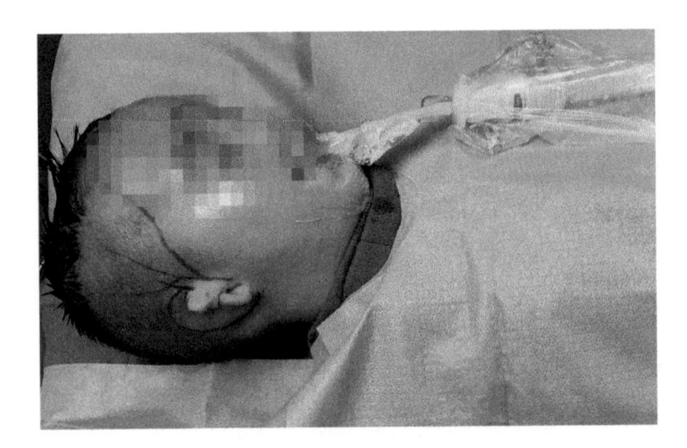

Fig. 10.12 CAM drape 2

Surgery begins with removal of the cartilaginous auricular remnant, maintaining the overlying skin pedicled and anteriorly maintaining its blood supply. This flap is later divided into two vascularized anteriorly based flaps. The inferior one becomes the tragus, and the superior flap lines the concha as well as the superior and posterior meatus of the opening of the ear canal. The lobule is mobilized by severing it from the auricular remnant while retaining its vascularity anteriorly. It is held in a steri strip until later in the procedure, inferior to the dissection field. The cartilage is retained on the back table in saline for later use.

Previous marked vessels of the temporoparietal fascia layer are noted, and the flap is elevated. Care must be taken to avoid injury to the overlying skin and hair follicles while maintaining the blood supply of the flap. Secondary incision is not needed as retractors and headlights allow work through the bed of the microtia cartilage resection. After the lateral plane of the temporoparietal flap is dissected to an adequate size, the deep layer of dissection is accomplished over the temporalis fascia, completely mobilizing the flap for later use. It is left in situ until needed later in the procedure.

Attention is turned to the ear canal; the microscope is draped and placed within the surgical field. The facial nerve monitoring is tested to ensure normal operation. A superiorly based u-shaped flap of periosteum is created with both deep and superficial layers. The base of the flap is at 1:30, with its inferior resection at 7:30 in a right ear in anatomic position. In a left ear, the flap is based at 10:30 extending toward 4:30. The purpose of the flap is to support the PPE implant once inserted to prevent inferior displacement over time. The bone over the area of proposed ear canal is exposed with elevation of the flap.

Using continuous suction irrigation and progressively smaller cutting and diamond burrs, the bone is removed, meanwhile sculpting an ear canal while maintaining bone over the tegmen, the temporomandibular joint, and the facial nerve inferiorly. Dissection is stopped just short of the ossicles to avoid sound transmission from drill contact. Care is made to open as few mastoid air cells as necessary for ear canal size.

The laser is then placed within the field, and the remaining boney fixation of the ossicles is removed. A shelf is created for placement of the new tympanic membrane. Careful inspection of the ossicles, their attachments, and supporting ligaments is made to ensure their mobility. A careful inspection of the stapes footplate and the incudostapedial joint is made with endoscopes if not seen adequately through the operating microscope.

Should ossicular reconstruction be needed, measurements are taken, and a prosthesis is custom-created for the patient's anatomy. A bed of antibiotic-soaked methyl cellulose is placed in the middle ear.

Attention is turned to the temporal fascia. After moving the temporoparietal flap, the temporal fascia is incised in a shape and size needed for transplantation and formation of an eardrum. The fascia is prepared on a block under the microscope and fashioned to the correct size for the individual patient.

The scalp is infiltrated with hydro-dissection fluid of dilute bupivacaine and flattened over the area of split-thickness skin graft harvest on the opposite occipital scalp. A dermatome is used to harvest a skin graft of 0.25 mm thickness, leaving the hair follicles in the scalp without damage as we have previously published [9]. See Fig. 10.13. A nonstick dressing is coated with antibiotic ointment and sewn in position as a dressing. The skin is cleaned of every hair under magnification.

The prepared fascia is placed over the ossicular mass and placed directly on the boney ledge. The previously harvested skin graft is trimmed to size to be placed as a single graft covering the boney walls and the surface of the newly placed temporal fascia, thereby creating the tympanic membrane. The medial lumen of the newly created ear canal is filled with pieces of antibiotic-soaked methyl cellulose, supporting the eardrum reconstruction and the skin graft against the vascularized bone of the ear canal. Lateral portions of the skin graft are folded into the canal in a "rosebud" pattern and covered with a Silastic disc to protect it from being moved until late in the procedure sequence.

Skin is harvested from the groin (or inner upper arm in some cases) in an elliptical donor site. The site is closed in layers and sealed with cyanoacrylate. The full-thickness skin graft is thinned using scissors and preserved for later surfacing of the

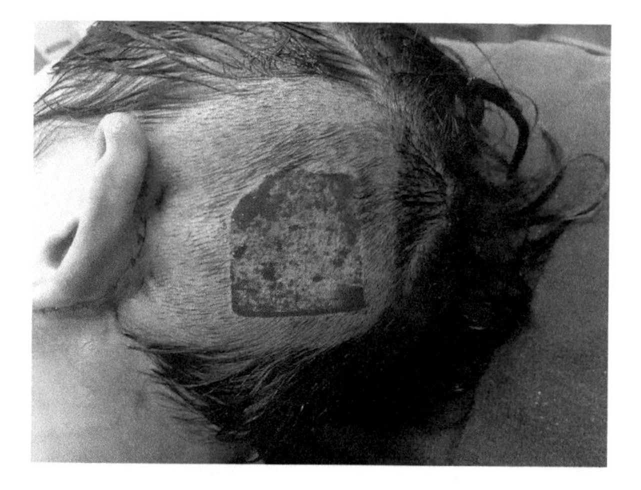

Fig. 10.13 Split-thickness skin graft donor site

microtia reconstruction. In unilateral cases, a second piece of full-thickness skin is harvested from the post-auricular sulcus contralateral to the reconstruction, and the skin over the mastoid is advanced, and the wound is closed. In bilateral cases, this second skin graft can be harvested from the upper inner arm. It is thinned as well and provides an excellent color match for any of the anterior surface of the new ear not covered by the superior retained flap originally covering the microtic remnant.

Using the previously prepared template, the PPE implant is designed and welded with a handheld cautery unit. The implant is placed in antibiotic solution for later use.

The PPE implant is placed within the field and secured with the superiorly based periosteal flap. The temporoparietal flap is removed from under the scalp and draped over the PPE implant to be secured with resorbable sutures, making sure its blood supply remains intact. The posterior skin is advanced slightly from over the mastoid and sutured to the deep fascia in the retro-auricular area.

After the entire PPE implant is covered with a vascularized layer, the skin grafts are applied and trimmed to fit. Five and six chromic interrupted sutures are placed in all skin grafts to produce an air tight seal in all suture lines. The groin graft covers the posterior surface of the ear, while the pedicled graft as the skin graft from the contralateral ear covers the lateral surface of the ear.

The lobule remnant is freed and dissected to fit in the anatomic position, where it is held in place with resorbable sutures. The cartilage remnant is used to harvest a cartilage tragal implant. The inferior flap from over the microtic remnant is sewn to the periosteum at the edge of the mandibular fossa using the operating microscope. The cartilage graft is slipped inside the skin flap, and a tragus is created with through and through sutures.

The inferior edge of the superior flap which covered the microtic remnant is sewn to retained periosteum at the posterior, inferior, and superior edges of the ear canal opening. The "rose bud" STSG is unfurled and trimmed to meet the edge of the full-thickness skin grafts laterally. The ear canal is packed with a merocel sponge which is inflated with antibiotic solution. See Figs. 10.14, 10.15, 10.16, and 10.17. Two previously inserted drains in the area of dissection are connected

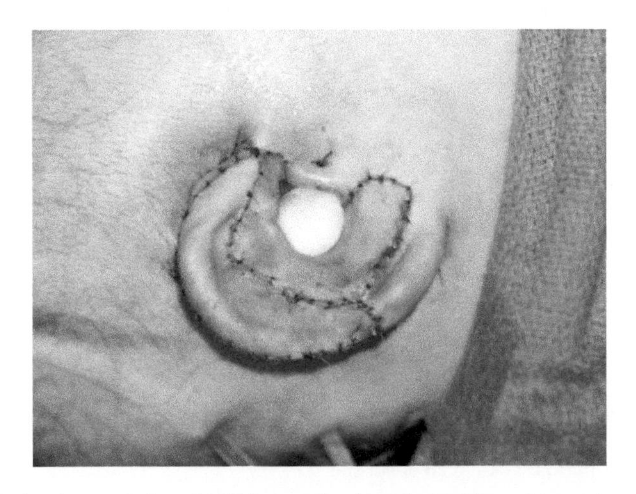

Fig. 10.14 Patient1, completion of CAM procedure in girl with bilateral microtia

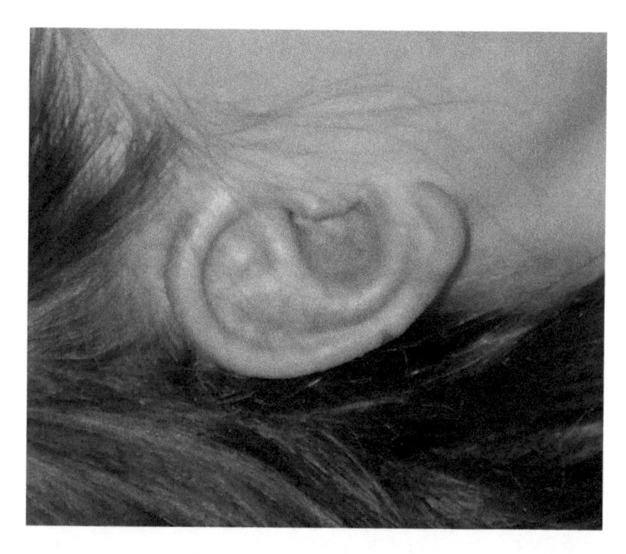

Fig. 10.15 Same patient as in Fig. 10.14, 10 months post-op

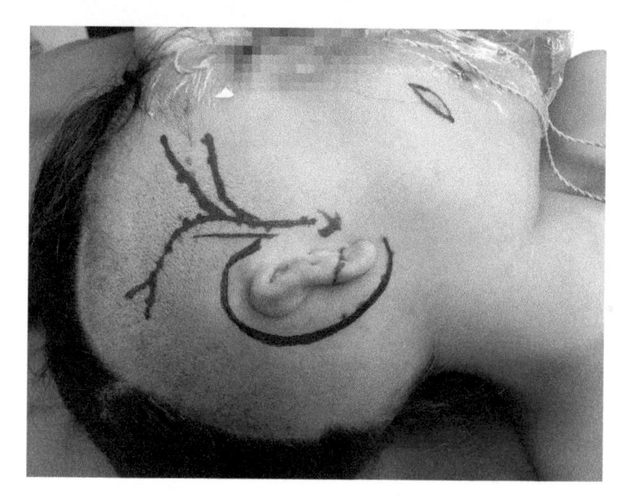

Fig. 10.16 Patient 2: OR

to suction, allowing the tissue layers to be pulled together over the PPE implant. A soft material used for ear canal impressions that cures over 2 minutes – Azoft – is mixed and placed over the reconstruction and allowed to set into a firm but mildly flexible covering around the reconstruction. Prolene® (Ethicon, Somerville, NJ, USA) sutures are used to sew the Azoft mold to the surrounding skin, protecting it from inadvertent removal. See Fig. 10.18. After securing the mold, the drains are removed. The skin graft sites contralaterally are dressed, and a head wrap and covering are applied to provide mild pressure in the areas of dissection.

All areas of dissection are injected with a mix of short- and long-acting anesthetic solution (including the IV site and the suture in the maxilla holding the ET in place) in order to allow the child to awake without pain from general anesthesia.

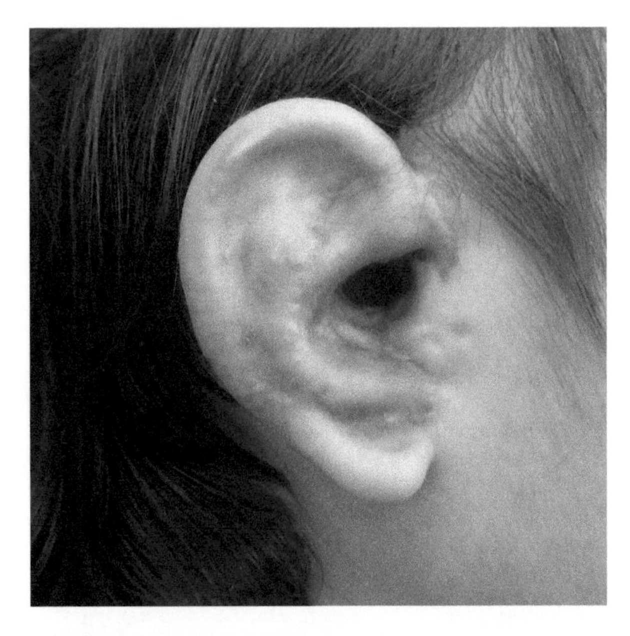

Fig. 10.17 Patient 2: 8 months post-op

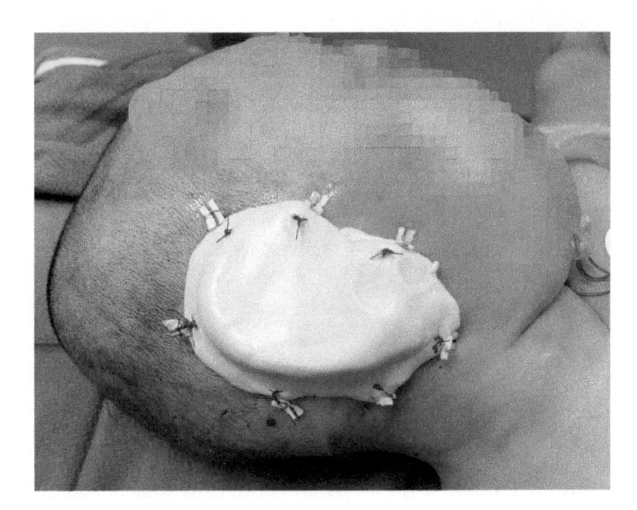

Fig. 10.18 Post-op mold dressing

Surgical time averages approximately 7.5 hours. All patients have been discharged the day of surgery as outpatients, a tribute to the quality of anesthetic care as described elsewhere in this work by Dr. Novak, one of our CEI anesthesiologists.

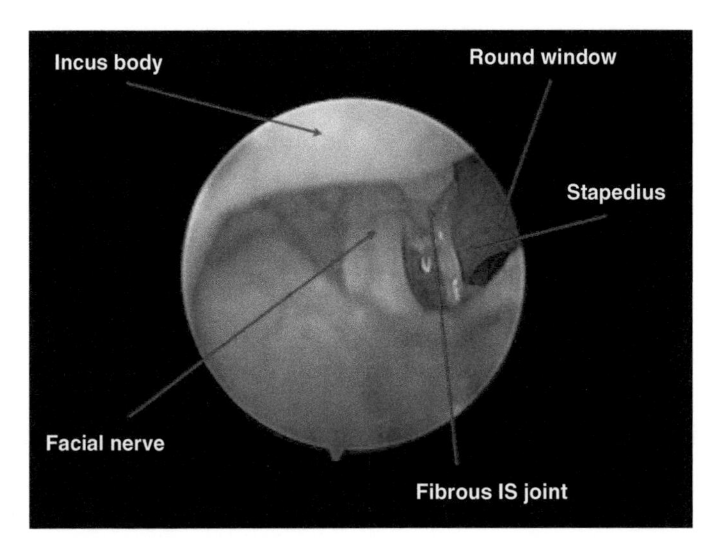

Fig. 10.19 Fibrous incudostapedial joint

Ossicular Reconstruction

Previously unrecognized, we have reported a 32% incidence of malformation of the joint between the incus and stapes [10]. See Fig. 10.19. In a significant percentage of cases, this congenital anatomic abnormality has reduced hearing results in past patients. By reconstructing the ossicular chain with customized prostheses, the impact on hearing loss can be alleviated or reduced, achieving marked improvement in postoperative outcomes. Care must be used, as, over 50% of the time, the facial nerve is exposed congenitally just above the stapes and oval window and is at risk for injury [11].

In some patients, reconstruction of the ossicular abnormality is best accomplished with immediate reconstruction, while, in a small percentage of patients, it is best to check the postoperative audiogram 5 months or more after surgery when the hearing results stabilize. In 6 percent of patients, revision surgery is indicated to raise the created eardrum and performed ossicular reconstruction due to inadequate postoperative hearing results. Using this strategy as outlined in the above reference, 94 percent of patients require only one surgery.

In selected patients, reconstruction with an active middle ear implant is an option. Placement of a Vibrant Soundbridge (MED-EL, Innsbruck, Austria), attached to either the ossicles or placed against the round window, can return hearing to functionally adequate levels [12]. See Fig. 10.20.

Results

Microtia repair results utilizing CAM repair are nearly identical to PPE results without ear canal creation, with the following exceptions:

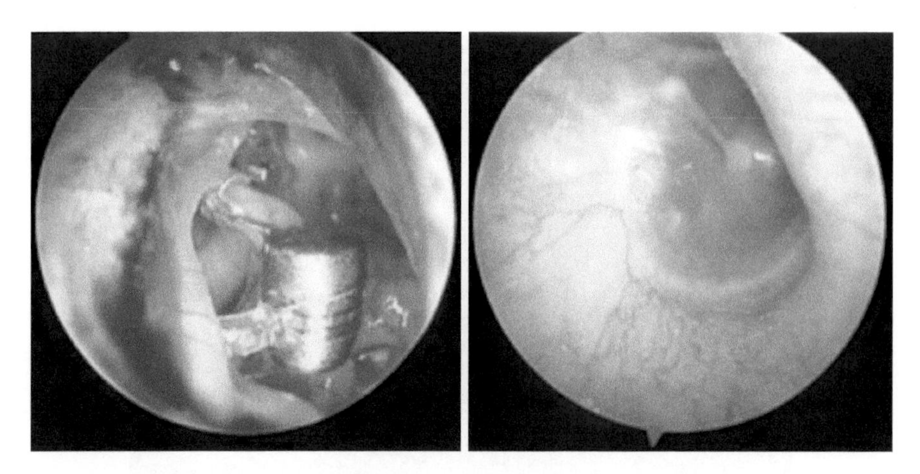

Fig. 10.20 Vibrant Soundbridge (MED-EL, Innsbruck, Austria) vibroplasty

- Due to the mastoid periosteal flap used to suspend the PPE scaffold in CAM repair, the PPE implant is more prone to fracture due to a blow to the ear. Early results showed fracture in just over 5% of patients. After instituting more significant welding of the connection points of the PPE scaffold, this complication has been virtually eliminated.

Microtia repair results utilizing CAM repair differ from separate atresia repair and microtia repair surgery as:

- CAM patients are less likely to see the PPE scaffold descend over time compared to patients who have atresia repair and microtia repair at different times. Presumably, this is due to the more vigorous suspension of the PPE with the mastoid periosteum, a significantly stronger tissue than other suspension techniques applied in microtia repair following atresia repair.
- CAM patients are less likely to experience canal stenosis than patients with separate surgeries.

Microtia repair results using rib graft compare to microtia repair results using PPE in the following way:

- Canal stenosis following rib graft microtia repair is more likely to occur than when PPE technique is utilized; both CAM repair and separate canal/microtia technique have lower incidence of stenosis.

Hearing results following microtia repair using rib graft, PPE in CAM technique, and PPE in separate canal and microtia repair are identical. See Fig. 10.21.

Long- and short-term complications occur in less than 10% of patients, requiring re-operating in less than 3% of patients. At this time, 9 years after the first CAM, we see no difference in immediate or delayed complication rates compared to other techniques and ages of surgery in my practice.

Infection in the perioperative period can occur and has been limited to PPE infection in two patients early in the series. A change to intravenous vancomycin from

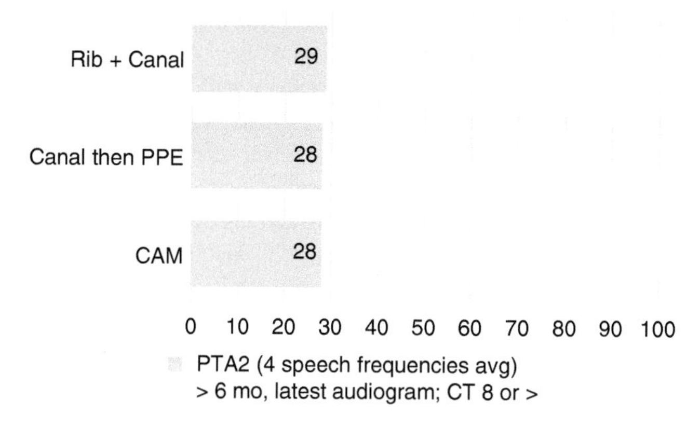

Fig. 10.21 Hearing results: average hearing results following rib graft, CAM, and separate microtia repair. (Data from Roberson et al. [3])

cefazolin has eliminated PPE infections in the last 175+ patients. No case of ear canal infection has occurred.

Eardrum movement away from the ossicles may occur late or early. Usually, a pressure from the middle ear – such as otitis media – has been responsible. In the last several years, securing the fascia graft used for tympanic membrane reconstruction has decreased this problem to just under 3% of patients. If hearing loss accompanies eardrum lateralization, revision surgery may be indicated.

Stenosis has been the largest and most devastating complication of atresia repair and may occur in up to 30% of patients. Using minimally traumatic technique, skin graft coverage, as well as other surgical techniques, we have been successful in markedly reducing this complication. Since 2012, addition of a custom-made ear canal mold made 3–4 weeks post-op and worn for 4 months during sleep only (and discontinued thereafter) has reduced canal stenosis to under 2%.

Sensorineural hearing loss may occur with any ear surgery but has not been experienced in our CAM series. Similarly, facial nerve injury with resultant paresis or paralysis can occur from atresia repair but has not been experienced in CAM patients.

Skin graft loss may also cause mucosa to resurface the ear canal surface and may create a moist ear canal. Inadequate healing or lack of hygiene of the ear canal after healing can allow damaged skin to heal disruptively in 2% of patients. Resurfacing of the ear canal is needed in a small percentage of this 2% as most can be managed with surface-applied preparations and treatment.

Further Considerations

More than 275 patients have selected combined atresia microtia repair for reconstruction of the congenital form and function deficits associated with congenital aural atresia and microtia since first performed in February 2008. These cases represent just under 10% of the canal reconstruction surgeries I have performed to date on patients from 49 different countries.

In the first decades of my career, children with atresia and microtia treated surgically required multiple procedures over several years. This was almost always psychologically traumatic to children. Additionally, surgery was done after school age and had effects on confidence and psychological adjustment. CAM repair performed at 3 or 4 years of age alleviates many of the ill effects of prior treatment protocols.

Undoubtedly, the future will see advances in biomaterials and autogenous tissue growth outside the patient for future implantation. Quite easily, a carved autogenous cartilage scaffold could be used with this technique currently. A more biocompatible and flexible scaffold than PPE will be a further advance to be enjoyed by future patients. The current CAM technique should be, with potentially small modifications, amenable to other types of implant material.

Plastic surgeons and otologists both have important skills to contribute when seeking to provide both form and function for patients they are privileged to treat. I have enjoyed a wonderful professional relationship with and have learned much from the senior editor of this book, with several advances to show for our collaboration. I expect the junior editor of this work and others will help to achieve further advancements in the state of the art as well.

Summary

The opportunity for a "one and done" surgical procedure with CAM repair is extremely attractive to parents, especially to those travelling a long distance for services. A cooperative effort among pediatric plastic surgery, otology, and anesthesia is necessary to achieve excellent results in this complicated and long surgical procedure. To date, surgical results and complication rates similar or better than other forms of atresia and microtia repair make combined atresia microtia (CAM) repair – a new surgical procedure for treatment of congenital aural atresia and microtia – an option for properly selected patients.

References

1. Kaplan AB, Kozin ED, Remenschneider A, Eftekhari K, Jung DH, Polley DB, Lee DJ. Amblyaudia: review of pathophysiology, clinical presentation, and treatment of a new diagnosis. Otolaryngol Head Neck Surg. 2016;154(2):247–55.
2. Breir J, Hiscock M, Jahrsdoerfer RA, Gray L. Ear advantage in dichotic listening after correction for early congenital hearing loss. Ear advantage in dichotic listening after correction for early congenital hearing loss. Neurophsycologia. 2003;36(3):209–16.
3. Roberson JB, Reinisch J, Colen TY, Lewin S. Atresia repair before microtia reconstruction: comparison of early with standard surgical timing. Otol Neurotol. 2009;30(6):771–6.

4. Kochkin S. The Impact of Untreated Hearing loss on Household Income, August 2005, Better Hearing Institute, Alexandria, VA, viewable at http://www.betterhearing.org/PDFs/MarkeTrak7_ImpactUntreatedHLIncome.pdf.
5. Lieu JEC, Tye-Murray N, Karzon RK, Piccirillo JF. Unilateral hearing loss is associated with worse speech-language scores in children. Pediatrics. 2010;125(6):e1348–55.
6. Roberson JB Jr, Goldsztein H, Balaker A, Schendel SA, Reinisch JF. Int J Pediatr Otorhinolaryngol. 2013;77(9):1551–4.
7. Jahrsdoerfer RA, Yeakley JW, Aguilar EA, Cole RR, Gray LC. Grading system for the selection of patients with congenital aural atresia. Am J Otol. 1992;13:6–12.
8. Imran F-H, Yong HK, Das S, Huei YL. Anatomical variants of the superficial temporal artery in patients with microtia: a pilot descriptive study. Anat Cell Biol. 2016;49(4):273–80.
9. Goldsztein H, Ort S, Roberson JB Jr, Reinisch J. Scalp as split thickness skin graft donor site for congenital atresia repair. Laryngoscope. 2013;123(2):496–8.
10. Balaker AE, Roberson JB, Goldsztein H. Fibrous Incudostapedial joint in congenital aural atresia. Otolaryngol Head Neck Surg. 2014;150(4):673–6.
11. Goldsztein H, Roberson JB. Anatomical facial nerve findings in 209 consecutive atresia cases. Otolaryngol Head Neck Surg. 2013;148(4):648–52.
12. Service GJ, Roberson JB. Alternative placement of the floating mass transducer in implanting the MED-EL Vibrant Soundbridge. Oper Tech Otolaryngol Head Neck Surg. 2010;21(3):194–6.
13. Farkas LG, Posnick JC, Hreczko TM. Anthropomorphic growth study of the head. Cleft Palate Craniofac J. 1992;29(4):303–8.

Chapter 11
Bilateral Microtia Reconstruction

Claire van Hövell tot Westerflier, Youssef Tahiri, and John F. Reinisch

Introduction

Bilateral microtia is an uncommon condition. It differs significantly from unilateral microtia. In addition to being less common than unilateral microtia (1:9 ratio), the presence of a bilateral conductive hearing loss can have a marked impact on a child's future potential if untreated [1–4]. Therefore, early intervention to restore hearing is the first priority in patients with bilateral microtia [5–16]. Although seen as an isolated deformity, bilateral microtia is more commonly associated with syndromes such as Treacher Collins, Goldenhar, CHARGE, and Bixler syndromes [1, 2, 17, 18]. These patients have several different anomalies apart from their microtia, which makes their treatment plan more complex than patients with isolated unilateral microtia.

In this chapter, we will focus on the differences between unilateral and bilateral microtia. We will also show how these differences will affect ear reconstruction, including size and positioning of the ears, skin graft harvest, timing of surgery, and performing atresia repair.

Electronic Supplementary Material The online version of this chapter (https://doi.org/10.1007/978-3-030-16387-7_11) contains supplementary material, which is available to authorized users.

C. van Hövell tot Westerflier
University Medical Center Utrecht, Department of Pediatric Plastic Surgery,
Utrecht University, Utrecht, The Netherlands

Y. Tahiri (✉)
Plastic and Reconstructive Surgery, Cedars-Sinai Medical Center, Los Angeles, CA, USA
e-mail: Youssef.Tahiri@cshs.org

J. F. Reinisch (✉)
Keck School of Medicine, University of Souther California, Los Angeles, CA, USA

Craniofacial and Pediatric Plastic Surgery, Cedars Sinai Medical Center,
Los Angeles, CA, USA

© Springer Nature Switzerland AG 2019

J. F. Reinisch, Y. Tahiri (eds.), *Modern Microtia Reconstruction*,
https://doi.org/10.1007/978-3-030-16387-7_11

Epidemiology

Microtia is a rare anomaly with a prevalence that varies geographically, which suggests some genetic component to its etiology. The condition is seen with a higher frequency in Asia and the western regions of both North and South America [19]. Bilateral microtia is seen in approximately 10% of microtia patients [1, 3, 4, 20–27]. Reported prevalences vary between studies, as different definitions for bilateral microtia are used. Most studies define the bilateral condition as microtia/anotia on both sides. However, in some reports, patients were considered to have bilateral involvement if there were any clinical signs (such as preauricular tags or mandibular hypoplasia) on the contralateral side [28]. Studies that have focused on bilateral microtia as microtia/anotia on two sides report prevalences varying between 7% and 23% [2, 17, 20, 21, 22, 29]. Canfield and colleagues found significant associations between the occurrence of bilateral microtia and a maternal age above 40, Hispanic maternal ethnicity, and Mexico as maternal birthplace [3]. However, when adjusting for other characteristics, only maternal age above 40 was associated with bilateral microtia.

Hearing

The most significant problem in patients with bilateral microtia is the fixed, congenital, conductive hearing loss [2, 22, 30]. Bilateral hearing loss can have a negative impact on speech and language development, academic achievements, self-esteem, and income [31, 32]. Although the great majority of microtia children have a normal cochlea and normal bone conduction hearing, the absence of air conduction significantly reduces their hearing threshold to the 65–70 dB range. This is above the 40–45 dB range of normal speech [5, 11–15, 33]. A number of parents are convinced that their young infant or child with bilateral microtia has normal hearing. This is seen more frequently in families where their child is the first or only child, since these parents do not have the experience of seeing normal hearing or speech development in an older sibling. Some parents are conditioned unconsciously to speak louder and closer to their child. However, without early intervention, most children with bilateral microtia will not develop normal speech. It is well known that the first two years of life are critical in language acquisition. During this period, hearing ability is crucial for learning spoken language. There is growing evidence that the early absence of sounds and access to language lead to cognitive delay, mental health difficulties, a higher possibility of traumatic accidents, and limited literacy. Therefore, it is essential to provide early hearing in young patients with bilateral microtia [5–16, 31].

Options to improve hearing include atresiaplasty or the use of a bone conduction hearing aid [34–39]. These options are further explained in Chap. 9 on "Management of Conductive Hearing Loss Associated with Aural Atresia and Microtia." According to a study on the vibratory patterns of bone-conducted sound, sound vibrations from

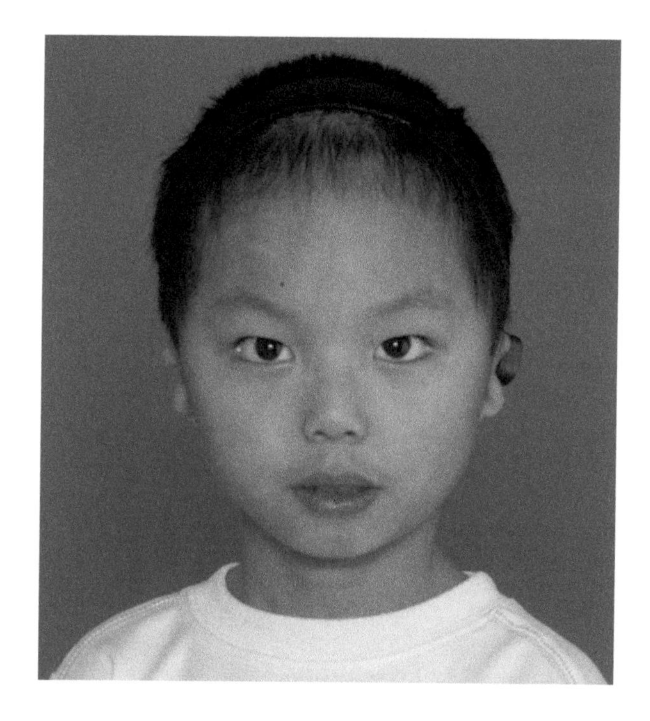

Fig. 11.1 A 3-year-old boy with bilateral microtia. He is wearing a BAHA with a headband. Early hearing restoration is crucial in patients with bilateral microtia. Hearing ability is a crucial component in learning spoken language

a bone conduction hearing aid (BCHA) are transmitted via the skull bone to both the ipsilateral and the contralateral cochlea. Therefore, in patients with bilateral atresia, placement of a unilateral BCHA is usually sufficient (Fig. 11.1) [40]. The type of auditory rehabilitation should be individualized. Several factors should be taken into account, such as patients' and families' wishes, their socioeconomic situation, the anatomy of the middle ear determined by CT scan, and age of the patient. According to the Jahrsdoerfer grading system of candidacy for atresiaplasty, patients with a score of 6 or lower are not a candidate for atresiaplasty/canalplasty [41]. However, when considering bilateral atresia, patients with lower scores may still benefit from canalplasty, especially in situations such as sleeping, swimming, bathing, or sports where a BCHA may not be worn. In patients with bilateral atresia, the ear with the most favorable score should be selected for the initial surgery [36].

Speech

High rates of speech difficulties are reported for children with bilateral microtia. Jensen and colleagues found that 86% of patients with bilateral microtia had received speech therapy, starting at a mean age of 2.8 years [42]. In-clinic evaluation by the speech pathologist demonstrated mainly articulation errors (86%) and language errors (71%) in this group. This was significantly higher than in the unilateral groups (respectively, 21–35% and 16–31%).

Whether these speech issues are caused by the conductive hearing loss remains unclear, since all the included patients received some form of aural intervention at different ages (0.5–5 years). In patients with bilateral microtia, other issues also contribute to the development of speech problems. A prospective cohort study demonstrated that almost all patients with microtia have ipsilateral soft palate muscular dysfunction (96%), resulting in velopharyngeal insufficiency (VPI) in 70% of the patients [43]. However, most patients with unilateral microtia can compensate with their non-affected side, and, therefore, nasality is only noticeable in a quarter of these patients. This is different in the bilateral group, where both sides of the soft palate are affected, resulting in almost a complete paralysis in 59% of the studied group. Therefore, the rate of hypernasal speech is higher in bilateral patients (81%) than in unilateral patients. Also, more severe grades (70% grade 2 and 3 VPI) are seen in the bilateral group compared to the unilateral group (12.5% grade 2 and 3 VPI).

This emphasizes the importance of including speech assessments as a part of the examination of all microtia patients. In patients with VPI, assessment by a speech therapist familiar with cleft children is recommended. If required, a specialized cleft palate team should determine further intervention for severe VPI.

Academic Achievements

Many studies have focused on the academic achievements of patients with sensorineural hearing loss (SNHL), showing that children with both unilateral and bilateral SNHL have more problems in school compared to children with intact binaural hearing [44–49]. However, the academic consequences of conductive hearing loss due to aural atresia have been less well studied. Therefore, it is unclear if the results of these studies can be extrapolated to children with microtia. Only one study has reported the prevalence of problems in school of patients with bilateral microtia [42]. They found that 43% of the patients with bilateral microtia had received school intervention, meaning that they were enrolled in a school for the deaf. None of the bilateral patients had learning difficulties in school nor problems with discipline and attention. All of these patients had received some form of a hearing aid. Their numbers were, however, based on parental reports and a small group of patients.

Jaw Deformity

Given the common embryologic origin of portions of the external/middle ear and mandible, it is not surprising that maxillofacial malformations may coexist with microtia. Reports show that approximately 40% of patients with microtia show manifestations of hemifacial microsomia (HFM) [50, 51]. In patients with HFM, the mandible is always involved to some degree [52, 53]. This can vary from mild flattening of the condylar head to a complete agenesis of the condyle, ascending ramus, and glenoid fossa. In some cases, there is secondary involvement of skeletal structures like the temporal and zygomatic bones [50].

The mild to moderate hypoplasia of the jaw seen with unilateral microtia rarely causes functional limitations in these children. In patients with unilateral microtia and ipsilateral jaw deformity, mandibular distraction or orthognathic surgery is usually delayed to mid or late teenage years. However, in patients with bilateral microtia, the jaw hypoplasia of both sides may have more adverse effects. Some patients with bilateral microtia have significant retrognathia, which can cause obstructive sleep apnea and failure to thrive at a young age. These patients might require tracheostomy or early mandibular distraction. The bilateral jaw deformity also poses challenges for anesthesia. Uezono and colleagues prospectively examined the difficulty of visualization of the larynx in school-aged patients with microtia undergoing reconstructive surgery [54]. They found that there was a significantly higher incidence of difficulty in larynx visualization in bilateral patients (43%) compared to unilateral patients (2%). Therefore, it is important to decide preoperatively if it is necessary to operate a patient with bilateral jaw hypoplasia in a hospital instead of an outpatient surgical center.

Syndromes

In the clinical assessment of a patient with microtia, looking for associated anomalies and syndromes is important. Around 15–60% of patients with microtia have additional abnormalities [4, 17, 22, 55]. The most common accompanying dysmorphic features are vertebral anomalies, macrostomia, oral clefts, facial asymmetry, renal abnormalities, cardiac defects, microphthalmia, holoprosencephaly, and polydactyly [1, 17, 21]. Associated malformations or syndromes are more common in bilateral cases. Approximately 90% of patients with bilateral microtia have an associated anomaly (in contrast to 40% in unilateral microtia). However, not all of these are part of a syndrome. Most studies report that 40–50% of patients with bilateral microtia are syndromic [1]. This figure may be artificially high because non-syndromic children with bilateral microtia may not be referred to a genetic clinic for evaluations.

A wide range of disorders has been reported with microtia as a clinical feature, mostly as case reports. Disorders due to abnormalities in branchial arch development include HOXA1 deficiency, HOXA2 deficiency, oculo-auricular syndrome, branchio-oto-renal (BO/BOR) syndrome, Treacher Collins syndrome, DiGeorge deletion syndrome, and Nager syndrome [56]. Of these, Treacher Collins syndrome (TCS) is most commonly seen in patients with microtia. TCS is an autosomal dominant disorder of craniofacial development, characterized by hypoplastic facial bones, microtia, or severe malformation of the pinna, micrognathia, auditory pits, hearing loss, and cleft palate. Figure 11.2 shows a 4-year-old patient with TCS and bilateral microtia. She successfully underwent bilateral polyethylene ear reconstruction as well as fat grafting to both malar areas.

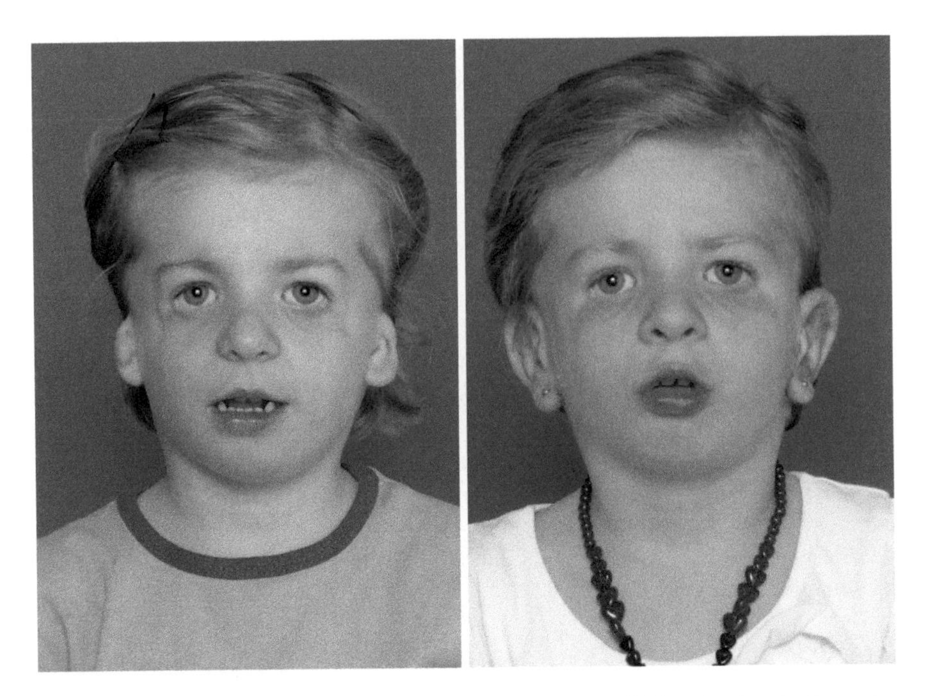

Fig. 11.2 A 4-year-old female with Treacher Collins syndrome and bilateral microtia. She underwent successful bilateral polyethylene ear reconstruction as well as fat grafting to both malar areas

Fibroblast growth factor signaling defects include fibroblast growth factor 3 deficiency and lacrimo-auriculo-dento-digital (LADD) syndrome. Microtia-associated syndromes with other molecular mechanisms are CHARGE syndrome, Walker-Walburg syndrome, Klippel-Feil syndrome, Meier-Gorlin syndrome, Bixler syndrome, Muenke syndrome, and Wildervanck syndrome [1, 2, 17, 18, 56].

Bilateral Ear Reconstruction

The published literature contains relatively little information about auricular reconstruction in patients with bilateral microtia. Overall, a similar procedure to unilateral microtia is performed. However, it is important to note some differences. Most of the literature about bilateral reconstruction describes the use of costal cartilage on both sides [57–61]. Most surgeons prefer to reconstruct each ear at a different time, whereas others prefer to reconstruct both ears simultaneously. However, reconstructing both ears at the same time poses postoperative issues for the patient while resting and sleeping, since pressure on the newly reconstructed ears has to be avoided [58]. Besides these postoperative issues, other disadvantages of autologous reconstruction, such as having surgery after starting school, hospitalization for discomfort, multiple procedures, visible chest scars, lack of ear projection, and potential rib cage deformity, are compounded in bilateral reconstruction. Furthermore, most surgeons consider a prior, early atresiaplasty as a contraindication for traditional autologous ear reconstruction because its scarring jeopardizes the viability of the mastoid skin when elevated to place the costal framework.

The fact that alloplastic reconstruction, without discomfort and the need for multiple surgeries, can be combined with atresiaplasty and can be done before school are advantages that are readily understood and appreciated by parents. The benefits of an implant reconstruction in children with bilateral microtia are even more obvious (bilateral microtia [62, 63]) (Fig. 11.3a–g and Video 11.1).

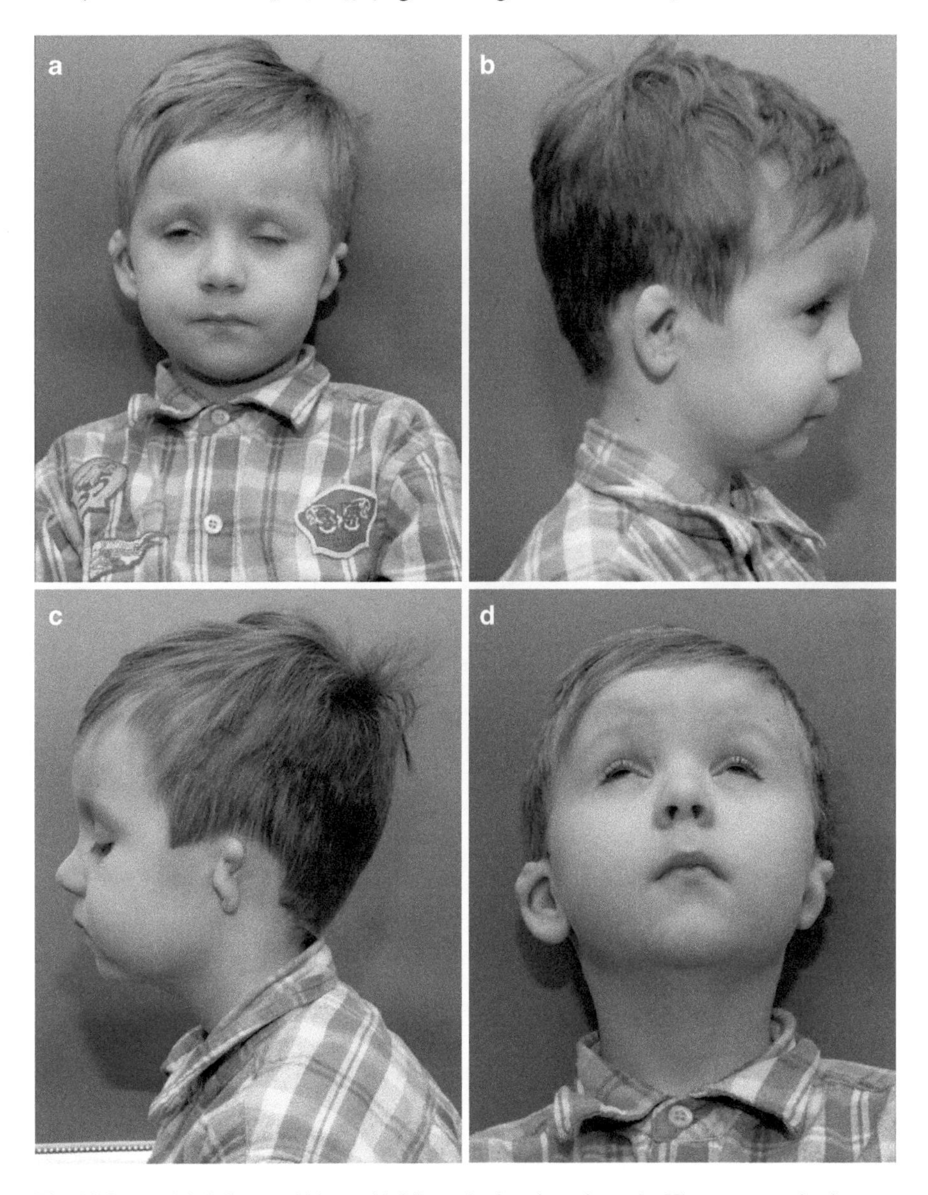

Fig. 11.3 **(a–g)** A 3.5-year-old boy with bilateral microtia and atresia. His reconstructive journey involved only two surgeries, 5 months apart. He underwent successful bilateral combined atresia microtia reconstruction

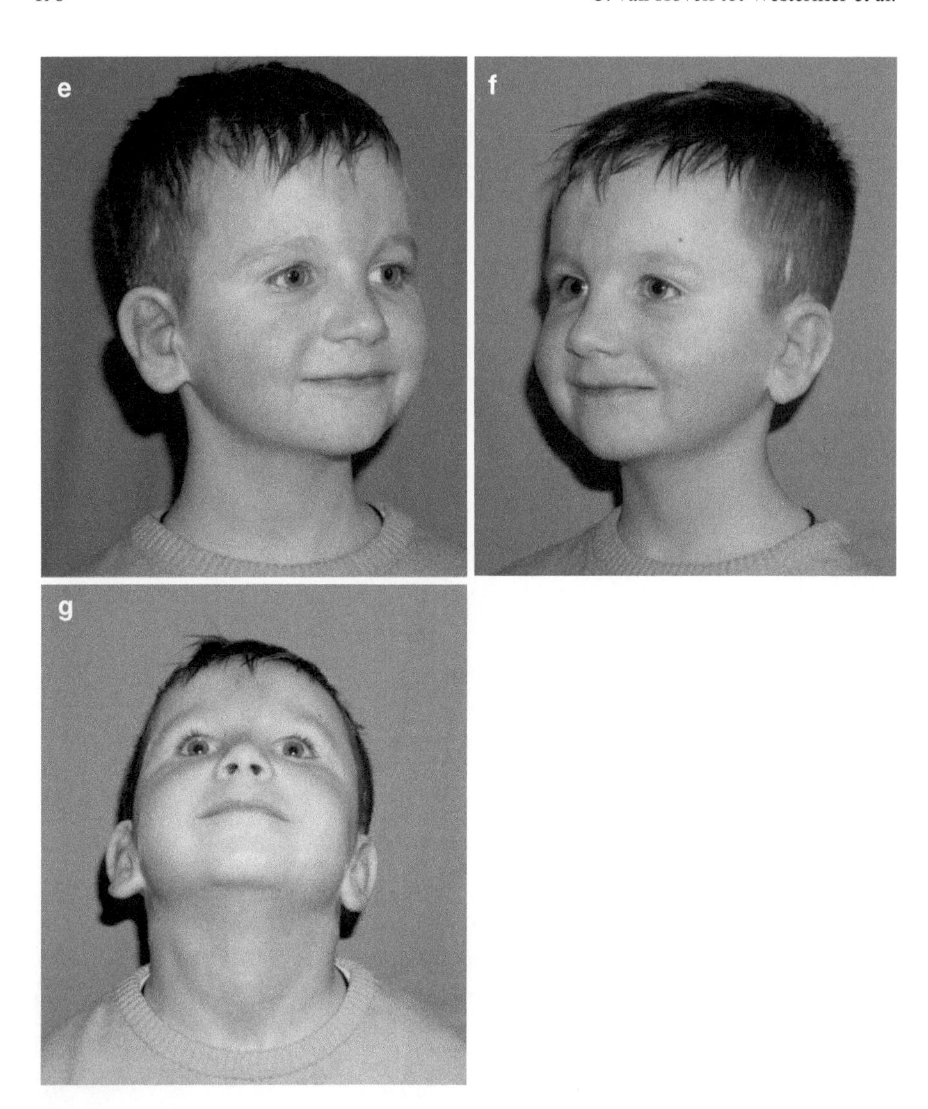

Fig. 11.3 (continued)

Staging and Planning of Surgeries

For auricular reconstruction in patients with bilateral microtia, it is important to start with a good plan for both surgeries. Bilateral alloplastic ear reconstruction cannot be performed simultaneously because of the surgical time required and the fact that pressure would be placed on the initial ear when performing the reconstruction on the opposite side. Another reason why both surgeries should not be performed together is that it would be difficult to keep pressure off of both ears during sleep during the first 2 weeks after surgery. A minimum of 4 months should be allowed between the first and the second ear reconstruction. Prolonged pressure on a newly reconstructed ear can result in flap necrosis and eventual framework exposure. Furthermore, waiting a minimum of 4 months between surgeries allows the first reconstructed ear to heal. If revision surgery for any aesthetic imperfection is necessary, this will be more apparent after the swelling has gone down and can be addressed at the time of the second ear reconstruction.

Another factor that should be taken into account when planning the reconstruction of the auricle is whether a canalplasty will be performed. There are several combinations possible when both bilateral canalplasty and bilateral outer ear reconstruction are indicated. The first option consists of starting with an early canalplasty as early as 3 years of age. The initial ear reconstruction can be done either after the first canalplasty or after the second canalplasty. This approach requires a total of four procedures and may be preferable for less experienced surgeons, when the expected time of simultaneous procedures would be excessive, or if the surgeons doing the ear reconstruction and canalplasty are in different locations.

The second option consists of three procedures to complete the bilateral atresia and ear reconstructions. We call this option a hybrid combined atresia microtia repair (CAM). It starts with a canalplasty in the ear with the best atresia score. After 4 months or more, an alloplastic ear reconstruction of the ipsilateral ear and simultaneous canalplasty of the contralateral ear are performed. The third and final stage consists of ear reconstruction of the contralateral ear. The hybrid CAM allows complete ear reconstruction in only three procedures. It is a good option when one would like to provide natural hearing as soon as possible and for surgeons with good speed but who are not yet comfortable with the single ear CAM.

Finally, it is possible to perform simultaneous atresiaplasty and ear reconstruction. We call this a combined atresia microtia repair or CAM. We wait a minimum of 4 months between the two stages and protect the contralateral ear reconstruction from pressure during the surgery with doughnut padding. The option is ideal for international patients wanting to make as few trips as possible. It is best done by surgeons with significant experience who can perform each procedure rapidly (Fig. 11.4a–l).

Positioning and Size

When reconstructing the first ear in a patient with bilateral microtia, there is no contralateral ear to serve as a model for the size and position of the ear. The surgeon has some leeway when making the initial ear, as long as the second ear is symmetric in size and position. Unless the ear lobe is absent or markedly displaced, it can serve as a landmark to help outline the lower extent of the ear. In some syndromic patients with bilateral microtia, the postauricular hairline is low reducing the amount of the available non-hair-bearing mastoid skin. It is fortunate that ears, like the brain and eyes, reach their mature size much earlier than the nose or jaws. It allows for early reconstruction without the need for later revision of or early compensation for later growth.

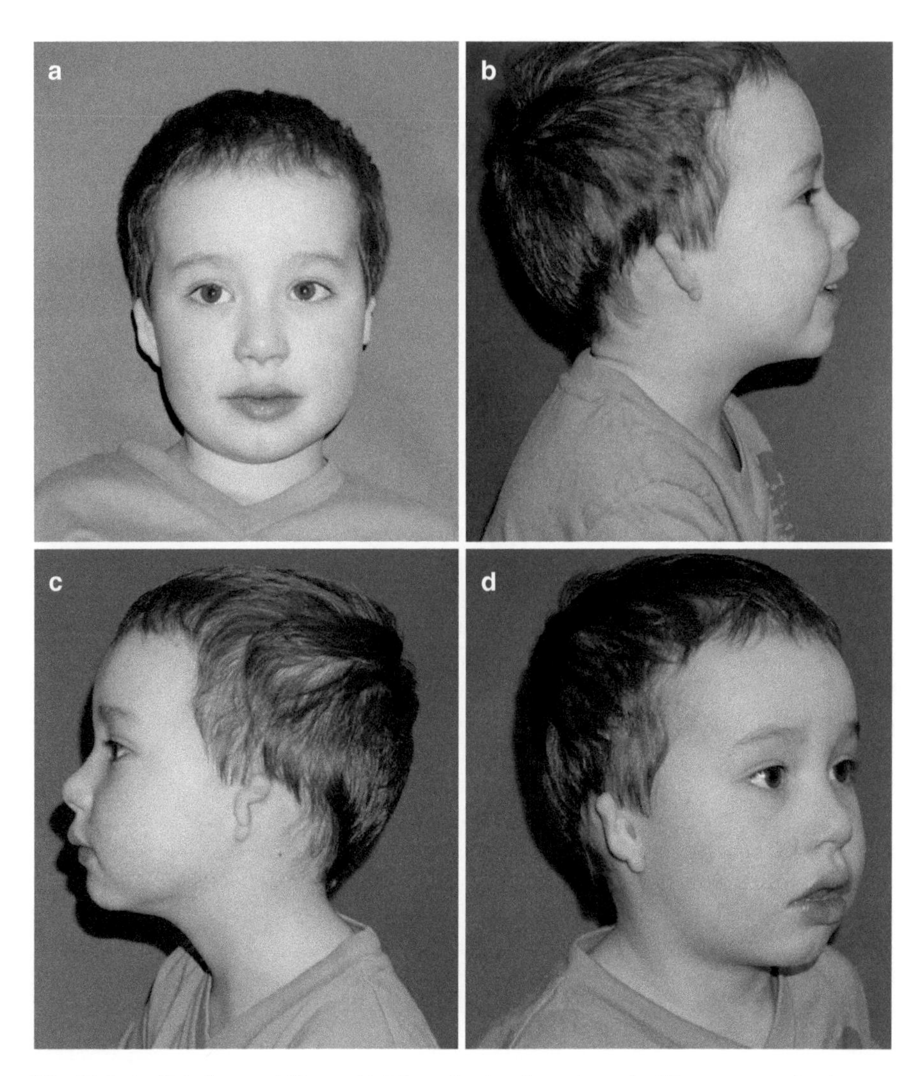

Fig. 11.4 (a–l) A 4-year-old boy with bilateral microtia and atresia. His reconstructive journey involved only two surgeries, 4 months apart. He underwent successful bilateral combined atresia microtia reconstruction

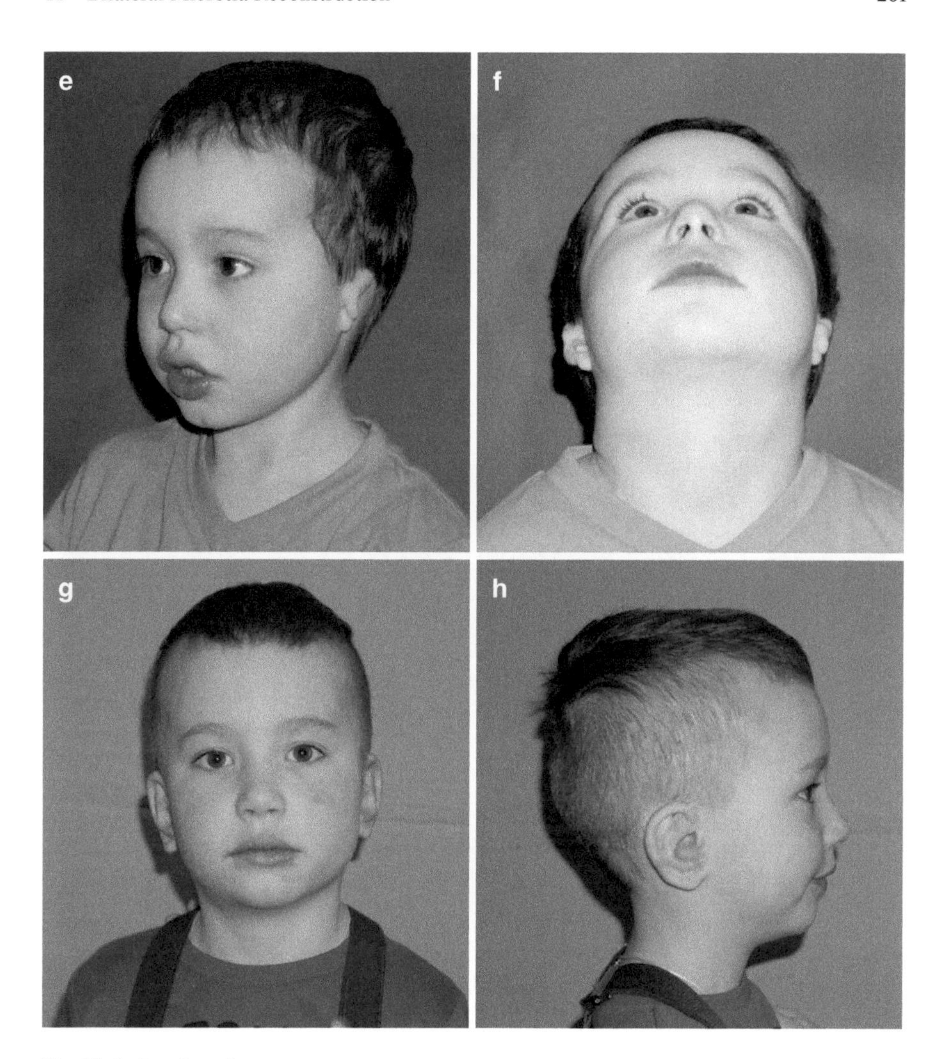

Fig. 11.4 (continued)

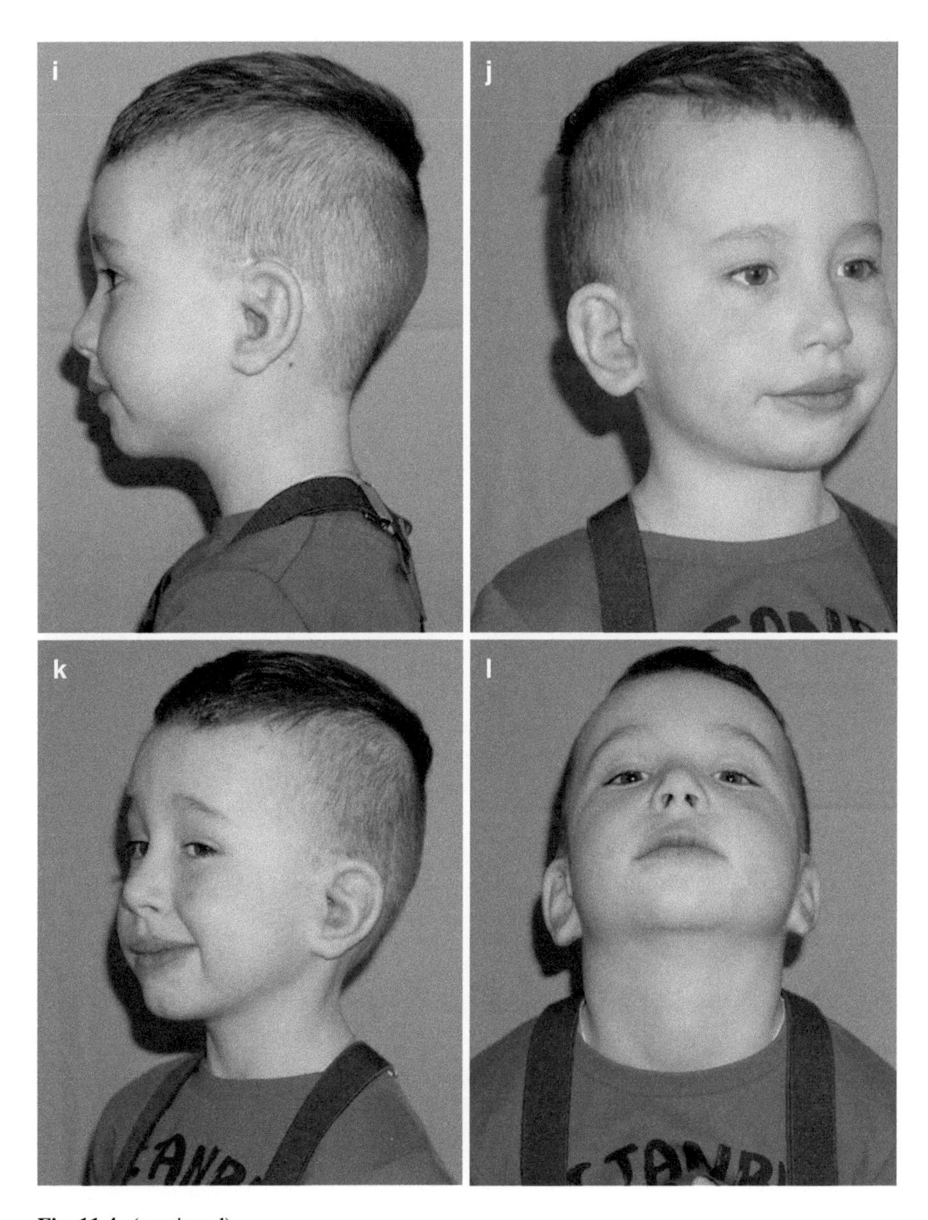

Fig. 11.4 (continued)

Skin Grafts

The lateral surface of the reconstructed auricle should match the color of the adjacent cheek and ear lobe. In most unilateral microtia patients, the skin of the ear remnant and non-hair-bearing mastoid usually will cover only a portion of the lateral surface reconstructed ear. Unless the ear remnant is very large, one will need to harvest the postauricular skin of the contralateral ear to obtain additional full-thickness skin to have a uniform color of the lateral surface of the reconstructed ear. In patients with bilateral microtia, this skin is not available for grafting. Therefore, other donor sites with reasonable color match are needed for coverage of the lateral surface of the ear. Alternative areas with reasonable color and thickness are the upper inner arm and clavicular. Another option is a split-thickness skin graft from the scalp. These grafts can result in inclusion cyst even when the hair shafts are removed and contract more than full-thickness skin grafts.

Other Considerations

Since the two ears are reconstructed in a staged fashion, the first ear will swell from being dependent during the contralateral procedure. The swelling is temporary and will resolve within 1–2 days after surgery.

Other considerations are the frequent presence of other anomalies since many patients with bilateral microtia have a syndrome. Many patients have retrognathia, making intubation more difficult. The placement of bone-anchored hearing implants, removal of cheek remnants, placement of fat grafts, correction of macrostomia, and lateral canthopexy can be combined with ear reconstruction to reduce the number of additional surgeries in these children.

Conclusion

Bilateral microtia is significantly different than unilateral microtia. It should not be seen as two unilateral microtias in the same patient. The most significant difference is the bilateral conductive hearing loss, which has to be treated at an early age with the use of a bone conductive hearing aid device to provide adequate hearing for proper speech and language development. Other differences are the higher incidence of syndromes in bilateral patients and the bilateral jaw hypoplasia causing sleep apnea and difficult intubation. An early atresia repair by an experienced otologists can be extremely rewarding when children stop wearing their bone conduction hearing device. Alloplastic ear reconstruction using a porous polyethylene implant is the ideal method in patients with bilateral microtia, because it allows for early atresia repair and significantly reduces the number of surgical interventions needed (Figs. 11.5a–c and 11.6).

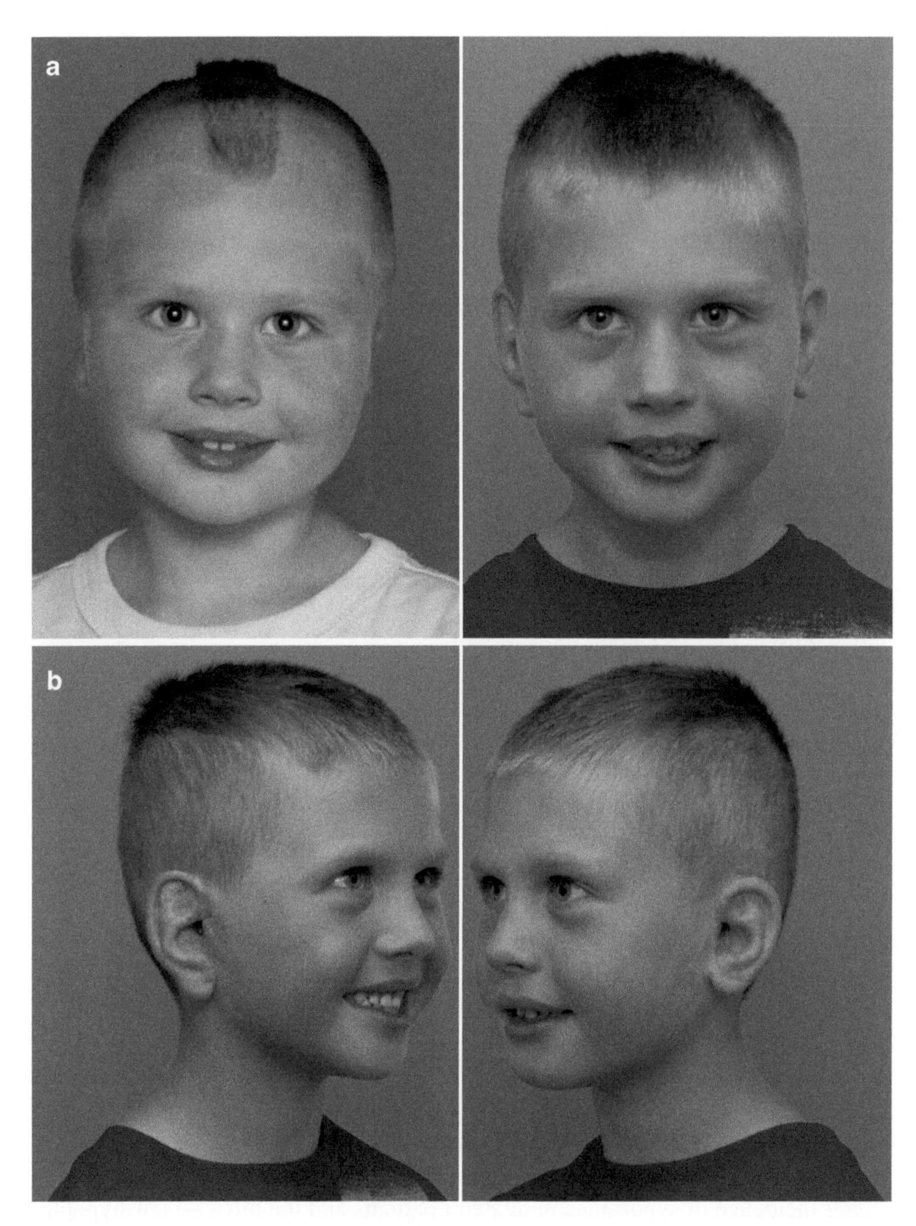

Fig. 11.5 (**a–c**) A 3.5-year-old boy with bilateral microtia and atresia. His reconstructive journey involved four surgeries because of scheduling conflicts. He had two early atresia repairs followed by two microtia reconstruction. All four out-patient surgeries were completed in a single calendar year

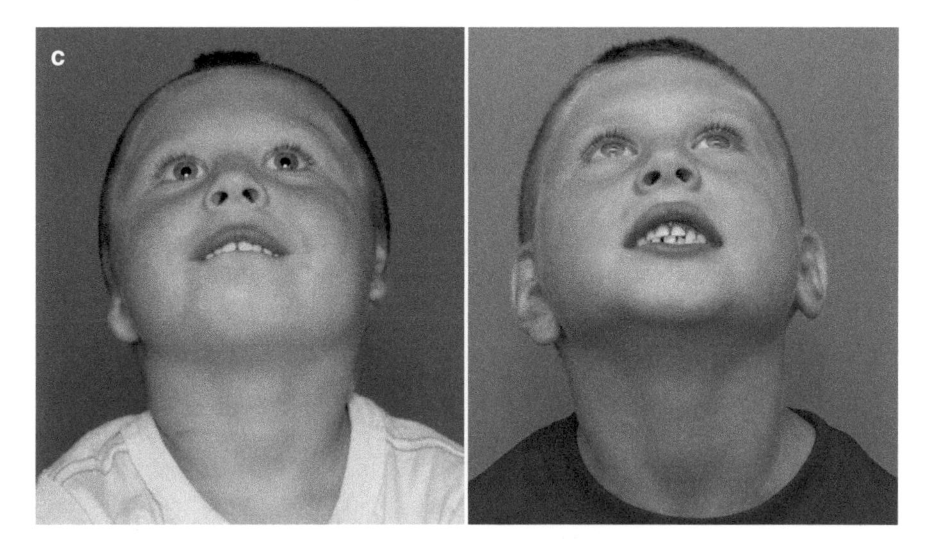

Fig. 11.5 (continued)

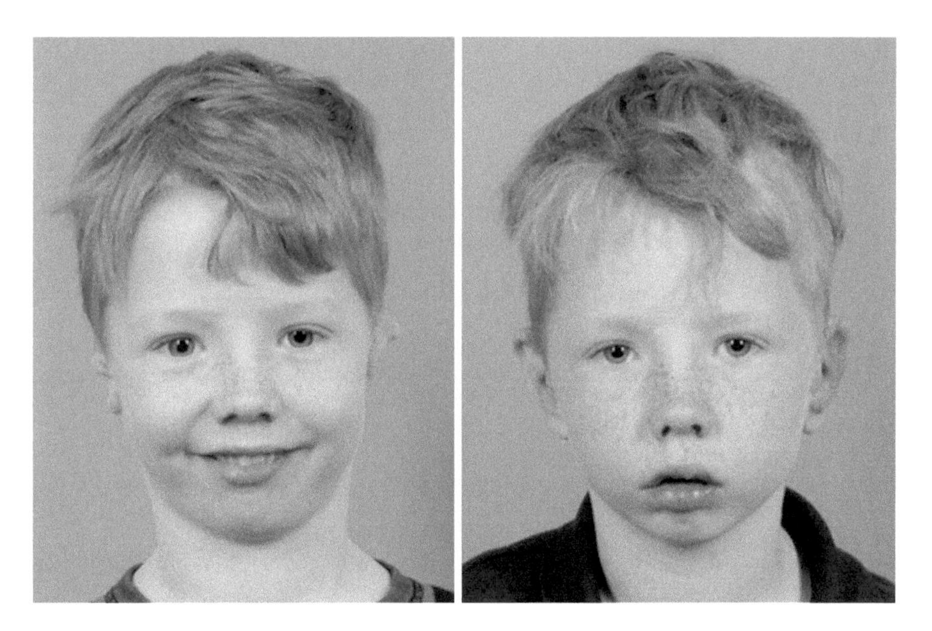

Fig. 11.6 A 4-year-old boy with bilateral microtia who underwent successful bilateral external ear reconstructions. He was not a candidate for atresia reconstruction

References

1. Luquetti DV, Heike CL, Hing AV, Cunningham ML, Cox TC. Microtia: epidemiology and genetics. Am J Med Genet A. 2012;158 A(1):124–39.
2. Klockars T, Rautio J. Embryology and epidemiology of microtia. Facial Plast Surg. 2009;25(3):145–8.
3. Canfield MA, Langlois PH, Nguyen LM, Scheuerle AE. Epidemiologic features and clinical subgroups of anotia/microtia in Texas. Birth Defects Res A Clin Mol Teratol. 2009;85(11):905–13.
4. Castilla EE, Orioli IM. Prevalence rates of microtia in South America. Int J Epidemiol. 1986;15(3):364–8.
5. Wang Y, Fan X, Fan Y, Chen X. Hearing improvement with softband and implanted bone-anchored hearing devices and modified implantation surgery in patients with bilateral microtia-atresia. Int J Pediatr Otorhinolaryngol. 2018;104:120–5.
6. Verhagen CVM, Hol MKS, Coppens-Schellekens W, Snik AFM, Cremers CWRJ. The Baha Softband. A new treatment for young children with bilateral congenital aural atresia. Int J Pediatr Otorhinolaryngol. 2008;72(10):1455–9.
7. van der Pouw KTM, Snik FM, Cremers CWRJ. Audiometric results of bilateral bone-anchored hearing aid application in patients with bilateral congenital aural atresia. Laryngoscope. 1998;108(4):548–53.
8. Jovankovičová A, Staník R, Kunzo S, Majákova L, Profant M. Surgery or implantable hearing devices in children with congenital aural atresia: 25 years of our experience. Int J Pediatr Otorhinolaryngol. 2015;79(7):975–9.
9. Hol MKS, Cremers CWRJ, Coppens-Schellekens W, Snik AFM. The BAHA Softband: a new treatment for young children with bilateral congenital aural atresia. Int J Pediatr Otorhinolaryngol. 2005;69(7):973–80.
10. Fuchsmann C, Tringali S, Disant F, Buiret G, Dubreuil C, Froehlich P, Truy E. Hearing rehabilitation in congenital aural atresia using the bone-anchored hearing aid: Audiological and satisfaction results. Acta Otolaryngol. 2010;130(12):1343–51.
11. Frenzel H, Hanke F, Beltrame M, Wollenberg B. Application of the vibrant Soundbridge in bilateral congenital atresia in toddlers. Acta Otolaryngol. 2010;8:966–70.
12. Fan Y, Zhang Y, Wang S, Chen X. Auditory development after placement of bone-anchored hearing aids Softband among Chinese Mandarin-speaking children with bilateral aural atresia. Int J Pediatr Otorhinolaryngol. 2014;78(1):60–4.
13. Fan Y, Zhang Y, Wang P, Wang Z, Zhu X, Yang H, Chen X. The efficacy of unilateral bone-anchored hearing devices in Chinese Mandarin-speaking patients with bilateral aural atresia. JAMA Otolaryngol Head Neck Surg. 2014;140(4):357–62.
14. Fan X, Wang Y, Wang P, Fan Y, Chen Y, Zhu Y, Chen X. Aesthetic and hearing rehabilitation in patients with bilateral microtia-atresia. Int J Pediatr Otorhinolaryngol. 2017;101:150–7.
15. de Brito R, Pozzobom Ventura LM, Jorge JC, Oliveira EB, Manzoni Lourencone LF. An implantable hearing system as rehabilitation for hearing loss due to bilateral aural atresia: surgical technique and audiological results. J Int Adv Otol. 2016;12(3):241–6.
16. Asma A, Ubaidah MA, Hasan SS, Wan Fazlina WH, Lim BY, Saim L, Goh BS. Surgical outcome of Bone Anchored Hearing Aid (Baha) implant surgery: a 10 years experience. Indian J Otolaryngol Head Neck Surg. 2010;65(3):251–4.
17. Mastroiacovo P, Corchia C, Botto LD, Lanni R, Zampino G, Fusco D. Epidemiology and genetics of microtia-anotia: a registry based study on over one million births. J Med Genet. 1995;32:453–7.
18. Wang RY, Earl DL, Ruder RO, Graham JM. Syndromic ear anomalies and renal ultrasounds. Pediatrics. 2001;108(2):E32.
19. Reinisch J. Modern Microtia Reconstruction, Linton Whitaker Lecture, American Society of Craniofacial Surgeons. Tuscon. 2019;12.

20. Forrester MB, Merz RD. Descriptive epidemiology of anotia and microtia, Hawaii, 1986-2002. Congenit Anom. 2005;45(4):119–24.
21. Harris J, Kallen B, Robert E. The epidemiology of anotia and microtia. J Med Genet. 1996;33(10):809–13.
22. Shaw GM, Carmichael SL, Kaidarova Z, Harris JA. Epidemiologic characteristics of anotia and microtia in California, 1989-1997. Birth Defects Res A Clin Mol Teratol. 2004;70(7):472–5.
23. Suutarla S, Rautio J, Ritvanen A, Ala-Mello S, Jero J, Klockars T. Microtia in Finland: comparison of characteristics in different populations. Int J Pediatr Otorhinolaryngol. 2007;71(8):1211–7.
24. Yang J, Carmichael SL, Kaidarova Z, Shaw GM. Risks of selected congenital malformations among offspring of mixed race-ethnicity. Birth Defects Res A Clin Mol Teratol. 2004;70(10):820–4.
25. González-Andrade F, López-Pulles R, Espín VH, Paz-y-Miño C. High altitude and microtia in Ecuadorian patients. J Neonatal-Perinatal Med. 2010;3(2):109–16.
26. Aase JM, Tegtmeier RE. Microtia in New Mexico: evidence for multifactorial causation. Birth Defects Orig Artic Ser. 1977;13(3A):113–6.
27. Llano-Rivas I, Gonzalez-del Angel A, del Castillo V, Reyes R, Carnevale A. Microtia: a clinical and genetic study at the National Institute of Pediatrics in Mexico City. Arch Med Res. 1999;30(2):120–4.
28. Tasse C, Bohringer S, Fischer S, Ludecke HJ, Albrecht B, Horn D, Janecke A, Kling R, Konig R, Lorenz B, Majewski F, Maeyens E, Meinecke P, Mitulla B, Mohr C, Preischl M, Umstadt H, Kohlhase J, Gillessen-Kaesbach G, Wieczorek D. Oculo-auriculo-vertebral spectrum (OAVS): clinical evaluation and severity scoring of 53 patients and proposal for a new classification. Eur J Med Genet. 2005;48(4):397–411.
29. Sanchez O, Mendez JR, Gomez E, Guerra D. Clinico-epidemiologic study of microtia. Invest Clin. 1997;38(4):203–17.
30. Reed R, Hubbard M, Kesser BW. Is there a right ear advantage in congenital aural atresia? Otol Neurotol. 2016;37(10):1577–82.
31. Li D, Chin W, Wu J, Zhang Q, Xu F, Xu Z, Zhang R. Psychosocial outcomes among microtia patients of different ages and genders before ear reconstruction. Aesthet Plast Surg. 2010;34(5):570–6.
32. Kaga K, Asato H, editors. Microtia and atresia combined approach by plastic and otologic surgery. Basel: Karger; 2013.
33. Wang D, Zhao S, Zhang Q, Ma X, Ren R. Vibrant SoundBridge combined with auricle reconstruction for bilateral congenital aural atresia. Int J Pediatr Otorhinolaryngol. 2016;l86:240–5.
34. Doshi J, Sheehan P, McDermott AL. Bone anchored hearing aids in children: an update. Int J Pediatr Otorhinolaryngol. 2012;76:618–22.
35. Declau F, Cremers C, Van de Heyning P. Diagnosis and management strategies in congenital atresia of the external auditory canal. Study Group on Otological Malformations and Hearing Impairment. Br J Audiol. 1999;33:313–27.
36. Service GJ, Roberson JB Jr. Current concepts in repair of aural atresia. Curr Opin Otolaryngol Head Neck Surg. 2010;18:536–8.
37. Roberson JB Jr, Reinisch J, Colen TY, Lewin S. Atresia repair before microtia reconstruction: comparison of early with standard surgical timing. Otol Neurotol. 2009;30:771–6.
38. Zhao S, Wang D, Han D, Gong S, Ma X, Li Y, et al. Integrated protocol of auricle reconstruction combined with hearing reconstruction. Acta Otolaryngol. 2012;132:829–33.
39. Teufert KB, De la Cruz A. Advances in congenital aural atresia surgery: effects on outcome. Otolaryngol Head Neck Surg. 2004;131:263–70.
40. Stenfelt S, Hakansson B, Tjellstrom A. Vibration characteristics of bone conducted sound in vitro. J Acoust Soc Am. 2000;107(1):422–31.
41. Jahrsdoerfer RA, Yeakley JW, Aguilar EA, Cole RR, Gray LC. Grading system for the selection of patients with congenital aural atresia. Am J Otol. 1992;13:6–12.

42. Jensen DR, Grames LM, Lieu JE. Effects of aural atresia on speech development and learning: retrospective analysis from a multidisciplinary craniofacial clinic. JAMA Otolaryngol Head Neck Surg. 2013;139:797–802.
43. Van Hövell tot Westerflier CVA, Colin Bracamontes I, Tahiri YT, Breugem CC, Reinisch J. Soft palate dysfunction in children with microtia. J Craniofac Surg. 2019;30(1):188–92.
44. Lieu JEC. Children with unilateral hearing loss. Semin Hear. 2010;31(4):275–89.
45. Tharpe AM, Bess FH. Identification and management of children with minimal hearing loss. Int J Pediatr Otorhinolaryngol. 1991;21(1):41–50.
46. Tharpe AM, Bess FH. Minimal, progressive, and fluctuating hearing losses in children: characteristics, identification, and management. Pediatr Clin N Am. 1999;46(1):65–78.
47. Rapin I. Conductive hearing loss effects on children's language and scholastic skills. A review of the literature. Ann Otol Rhinol Laryngol Suppl. 1979;88(Supplement):3–12.
48. Vila PM, Lieu JEC. Asymmetric and unilateral hearing loss in children. Cell Tissue Res. 2015;361(1):271–8.
49. Van Hövell tot Westerflier CVA, van Heteren JAA, Breugem CC, Smit AL, Stegeman I. Impact of microtia and aural atresia on academic performance: a systematic review. Int J Pediatr Otorhinolarynogol. 2018;114:175–9.
50. Gougoutas AJ, Singh DJ, Low DW, Bartlett SP. Hemifacial microsomia: clinical features and pictographic representations of the OMENS classification system. Plast Reconstr Surg. 2007;120(7):112e–20e.
51. Fu Y, Li C, Dai P, Zhang T. Three-dimensional assessment of the temporal bone and mandible deformations in patients with congenital aural atresia. Int J Pediatr Otorhinolaryngol. 2017;101:164–6.
52. Kaban JC, Mulliken JB, Murray JE. Three-dimensional approach to analysis and treatment of hemifacial macrosomia. Cleft Palate J. 1981;18(2):90–9.
53. Vento AR, LaBrie RA, Mulliken JB. The OMENS classification of hemifacial microsomia. Cleft Palate Craniofac J. 1991;28(1):68–76.
54. Uezono S, Holzman RS, Goto T, et al. Prediction of difficult airway in school-aged patients with microtia. Paediatr Anaesth. 2001;11:409–13.
55. Kelley PE, Scholes MA. Microtia and congenital aural atresia. Otolaryngol Clin North Am. 2007;40:61–80.
56. Alasti F, van Camp G. Genetics of microtia and associated syndromes. J Med Genet. 2009;46:361–9.
57. Brent B, Tanzer RC, Rueckert F, Brown FE. Auricular repair with autogenous rib cartilage grafts: two decades of experience with 600 cases. Plast Reconstr Surg. 1992;90(3):355–74.
58. Liu X, Zhang Q, Quan Y, Xie Y, Shi L. Bilateral microtia reconstruction. J Plast Reconstr Aesthet Surg. 2010;63(8):1275–8.
59. Osorno G. Autogenous rib cartilage reconstruction of congenital ear defects: report of 110 cases with Brent's technique. Plast Reconstr Surg. 1999;104(7):1951–4.
60. Osorno G. A 20-year experience with the Brent technique of auricular reconstruction: pearls and pitfalls. Plast Reconstr Surg. 2007;119(5):1447–63.
61. Wilkes G, Wong J, Guilfoyle R. Microtia reconstruction. Plast Reconstr Surg. 2014;134:464e–79e.
62. Reinisch JF, Lewin S. Ear reconstruction using a porous polyethylene framework and temporoparietal fascia flap. Facial Plast Surg. 2009;25(3):181–9.
63. Reinisch JF. Ear reconstruction in young children. Facial Plast Surg. 2015;31:600–3.

Chapter 12
Adjunct Procedures Related to Mandibular Reconstruction and Soft Tissue Facial Improvement

Daniel Mazzaferro, Sanjay Naran, and Scott Bartlett

Introduction

While microtia may occur as an isolated manifestation, it is often associated with other anomalies or syndromes including mandibular hypoplasia (unilateral or bilateral), vertebral anomalies, macrostomia, oral clefts, soft tissue hypoplasia renal abnormalities, cardiac defects, microphthalmia/orbital deformity, holoprosencephaly, and polydactyly [1–4]. Similar to that of patients with isolated microtia, those with soft tissue, mandibular, and orbital deformities experience sequelae secondary to poor aesthetic form and inadequate physiological function. Correction of such soft tissue, mandibular, and orbital deformities is therefore a critical component of treatment.

There are important planning considerations that should be noted when treating anomalies commonly associated with microtia. When planning for ear reconstruction later in life with the possible use of a temporoparietal fascia (TPF) flap and local skin, it is important to respect this local soft tissue that may be used for future reconstruction, such that it is not compromised by any of the adjunct procedures to be described. Ultimately, there should be no scar in the auricular region and no compromise of the TPF flap.

D. Mazzaferro (✉) · S. Bartlett (✉)
Division of Plastic and Reconstructive Surgery, University of Pennsylvania and The Children's Hospital of Philadelphia, Philadelphia, PA, USA
e-mail: bartletts@email.chop.edu

S. Naran (✉)
Division of Pediatric Plastic Surgery, Advocate Children's Hospital, Chicago, IL, USA

Section of Plastic and Reconstructive Surgery, University of Chicago Medicine & Biological Sciences, Chicago, IL, USA

Department of Plastic Surgery, University of Pittsburgh School of Medicine, Pittsburgh, PA, USA

© Springer Nature Switzerland AG 2019

J. F. Reinisch, Y. Tahiri (eds.), *Modern Microtia Reconstruction*,
https://doi.org/10.1007/978-3-030-16387-7_12

Common syndromes that include microtia in the majority (>50%) of patients are oculo-auriculo-vertebral spectrum disorders (i.e., craniofacial microsomia), mandibulofacial dysostosis disorders (Treacher Collins syndrome and Nager syndrome), Antley-Bixler syndrome (hypertelorism, microtia, clefting), Branchiootic syndrome, Kabuki syndrome, Meier-Gorlin syndrome (ear, patella, short-stature), and Miller syndrome. Of the syndromes, the two that are most common are craniofacial microsomia (CFM) and Treacher Collins syndrome (TCS). CFM involves varying degrees of hypoplasia of the orbit, mandible, ear, nerves, soft tissue, and extra-craniofacial features. This is often classified utilizing the OMENS + classification system. Goldenhar variant of CFM includes features of CFM in addition to epibulbar dermoids and vertebral anomalies [5]. Treacher Collins syndrome diagnosis relies on genetic testing and a variety of phenotypic expressions including hypoplasia of the mandible and zygoma, microtia or other external ear abnormalities, conductive hearing loss, coloboma, absence of lower eyelashes, and oro-ocular deformity of varying degree.

The primary focus of this chapter will be on adjunct procedures related to mandibular reconstruction and soft tissue facial improvement, both of which may apply to many of the syndromes previously mentioned.

Mandibular Reconstruction

A variety of congenital etiologies affecting the mandible may require mandibular reconstruction, including CFM and Treacher Collins syndrome. While many classification systems exist, the Pruzansky-Kaban modified classification is perhaps the most widely utilized in evaluating mandibular deformities, grouping them into one of the four categories [6, 7]. The Pruzansky-Kaban mandibular classification is incorporated in OMENS + classification system utilized for CFM.

Type 1 deformities have a small ramus with identifiable anatomy; type 2a deformities have a functioning TMJ but with an abnormal shape, yet the glenoid fossa remains in an acceptable functional position; type 2b deformities have an abnormally placed TMJ which cannot be incorporated in the surgical reconstruction; and finally type 3 deformities have an absent ramus and nonexistent glenoid fossa [7]. Due to increased uncertainty over the inter-rater reliability of this classification, our research group recently published a new classification scheme based on 3D CT imaging with an improved inter-rater reliability [8]. Surgical techniques may include various combinations of distraction osteogenesis, autologous non-vascularized rib grafts with or without distraction, and conventional orthognathic surgery at skeletal maturity. The ultimate goal of treatment is achievement of a level occlusal plane, facial symmetry, and psychosocial satisfaction.

Distraction Osteogenesis

Mandibular distraction osteogenesis allows for lengthening of native bone and, to a certain degree, soft tissue expansion. While the principles of distraction osteogenesis were introduced by Ilizarov, who employed the technique for lower

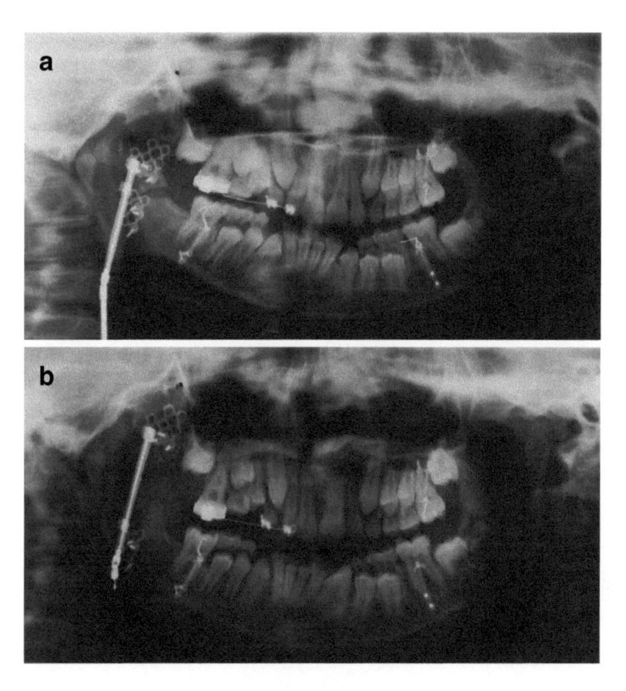

Fig. 12.1 Panoramic radiographs of patient with vertical distraction. (**a**) Two days after placement of vertical distracters. (**b**) Nine weeks after placement of vertical distracters

extremity lengthening following bony osteotomy and slow progressive distraction to facilitate new bony creation, it was McCarthy who pioneered its use in the facial skeleton [9]. Distraction vector is patient specific and dictated by the specific areas of mandibular hypoplasia. All elements of the mandible, as well as a functional and correctly positioned TMJ, are required. For example, for patients in whom a type 1 mandible is present, the occlusal plane may often be corrected with one or more rounds of vertical distraction of the ramus (Fig. 12.1a, b). Similarly, forward projection of the mandible may be improved with horizontal distraction at the body (Fig. 12.2a–d). Functional issues, including obstructive sleep apnea and difficulty feeding, are often improved following distraction. Two distraction techniques exist, osteotomy and half-pin fixation with external device versus an internal screw fixed device. The distraction phase occurs at a rate of roughly 1 mm per day followed by a consolidation phase that allows for bone healing and mineralization. The consolidation phase requires approximately 2 days for every millimeter distracted [10].

The pathologic side of the mandible grows at a slower rate than the contralateral side, because of which, overcorrection is recommended. While distraction alone improves occlusal relationships and facial aesthetics, orthognathic surgery is often still required at skeletal maturity in cases where orthodontics alone does not suffice. Scars from access incisions are hidden below the jawline when using internal devices, and the semi-buried distraction arms are brought out behind the ear; these may be revised as needed as a final stage procedure.

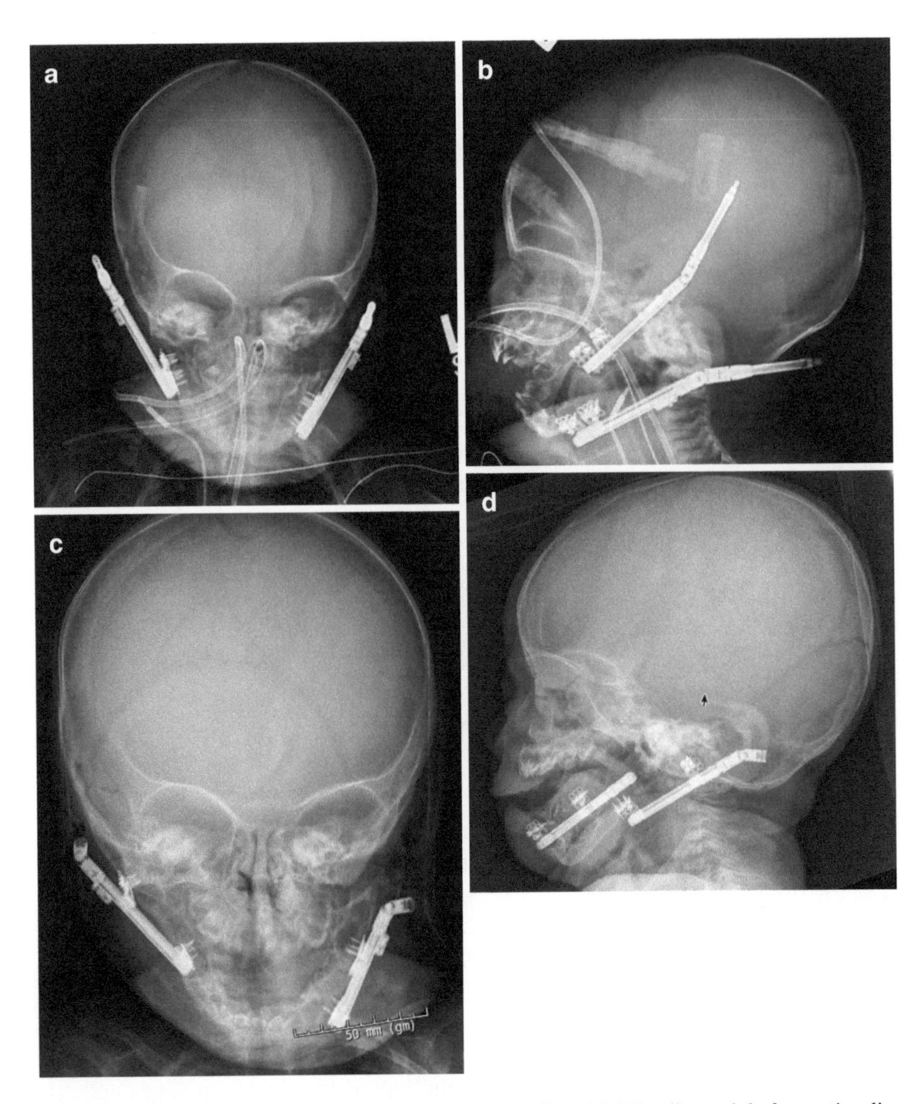

Fig. 12.2 Radiographs of patient with horizontal distraction. (**a**) AP radiograph before active distraction. (**b**) Lateral radiograph before active distraction. (**c**) AP radiograph after active distraction. (**d**) Lateral radiograph after active distraction

Currently, while curvilinear distractors are available, they are significantly limited by soft tissue constraints, and so distraction is often limited to a single vector at a time. Development of multiaxial distractors continues, which would provide the ability to change planes during active distraction [11]. This is relevant in more complex mandibular hypoplasia where there is often inferomedial displacement of the condyle/ramus. The use of a multi-vector distractor also allows for forward distraction while simultaneously adjusting the angulation. Three-dimensional surgical planning and cutting guides have gained favor in aiding improved placement of the distraction device and maximizing outcome [12, 13]. In an effort to reduce the relatively high surgical site infection rate in distraction osteogenesis, the development of fully embedded distraction devices that may be activated with external magnetics or motors is also currently being explored [14].

Distraction is not without risk, and so one must be aware of high-risk complications including infection, hardware failure, bony non-union, tooth bud injury, and damage to local structures and nerves resulting in temporary or permanent paralysis or paresthesia [15, 16]. Lip numbness, partial facial palsy, bony non-union, and hardware failure are rarer complications. Relapse may also occur to some degree.

Rib Graft

In cases of a severely hypoplastic ramus and condyle, autogenous costochondral grafting is often the method of choice, as it allows for the creation of a new ramus and pseudocondyle, coupled with the introduction of a potential "growth center" (at the cartilage/bone junction) that may result in natural growth of the construct. Type 2b and 3 mandibles may be unable to be corrected by distraction osteogenesis alone and therefore often require costochondral grafting. Costochondral grafts are preferred over vascularized bone grafts because they include a cartilaginous component that may be used to form a new TMJ, but when the deformity is severe (i.e., missing body and ramus), a vascularized fibular transfer may be preferred. Overcorrection is typically avoided because of the expected growth from the graft. Preoperative planning with orthodontics is imperative to determine final mandibular positioning with leveling of the mandibular cant and bringing the chin point in line with the midsagittal plane. A posterior open bite should be expected and accounted for in this planning stage due to the elongation of the ramus (Fig. 12.3) and can be managed with serial splinting or orthodontic bone anchors guided elongation of the maxilla guided by the orthodontist. The collaborative work of plastic surgeon and orthodontist is crucial to restore a functional occlusion.

The rib graft is typically harvested from the ipsilateral sixth or seventh costal cartilage after the affected mandible is appropriately prepped. The cartilaginous head of the rib graft is rounded off to approximately 0.5–1 cm in height. Placement of the graft on the affected side is done with the mandible in the most down and

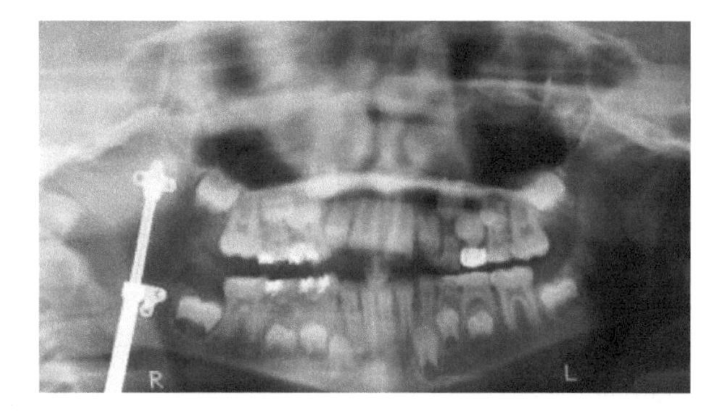

Fig. 12.3 Panoramic radiograph after active vertical distraction with posterior open bite on the right side

forward position allowed by the contralateral TMJ joint. The rib graft is loaded to the native mandible with maximal overlap using titanium screws.

Behavior of the graft may not be reliable. There are several reports of varying outcomes including graft overgrowth, graft resorption, slowed graft growth, non-union, and ankylosis [17–19]. In the author's experience, rib grafts that are unloaded typically resorb, whereas loaded grafts appear to lengthen over time and increase in volume (Fig. 12.4a, b). While this has yet to be proven volumetrically, recent analyses by the authors have revealed that rib graft growth is significantly slower than the contralateral side (Fig. 12.5a, b). Long-term ankylosis may occur, with ossification of the cartilage cap thought to be the likely etiology [18]. If this were to occur, a future TMJ release would be necessary. The authors believe the best way to prevent a high incidence of ankylosis is to harvest an adequate amount of cartilage (0.5–1 cm), perform minimal and blunt atraumatic dissection at the neocondylar level of the cranial base, and facilitate aggressive physical therapy and mobilization after an adequate immobilization period of approximately 3 weeks [20]. Again, collaborative surgical and orthodontic effort is imperative in achieving optimal facial symmetry, aesthetics, and function.

Rib Graft with Distraction Osteogenesis

There is a paucity of literature on long-term results following costochondral grafting, and as such evidence-based recommendations remain relatively anecdotal. The current trend of literature does, however, suggest that growth of costochondral grafts remains relatively unpredictable, but the graft itself does provide for a stable construct [20]. Given that graft behavior is not reliable, subsequent distraction osteogenesis is often required, something patients and parents should be properly informed of and counseled for prior to surgery.

Principles of distraction follow those utilized in distraction of the native mandible as previously described. There are three possible sites of osteotomy and subsequent distraction: within the native mandible, at the mandible-rib graft junction, or within the rib graft. There are reports of increased complication rates when distracting at the mandible-rib graft junction regardless of successful previous union [21]. The reason is believed to be due to a weak interface between two embryologically unique bones that have different growth patterns (rib graft with endochondral ossification versus native mandible with intramembranous ossification). At our institution, we have experienced successful distraction results by creating an osteotomy at the level of the native mandible and mesial to mandible-rib graft junction [20]. Distraction occurs at the same rate as previously described, 1 mm per day, continuing until overcorrection is achieved, followed by a period of consolidation and ultimately removal of hardware. Figures 12.6a–f and 12.7a–l show a long-term follow-up over 9 years in a patient with Goldenhar syndrome and a type 3 mandible treated with rib graft, distraction osteogenesis, and fat grafting.

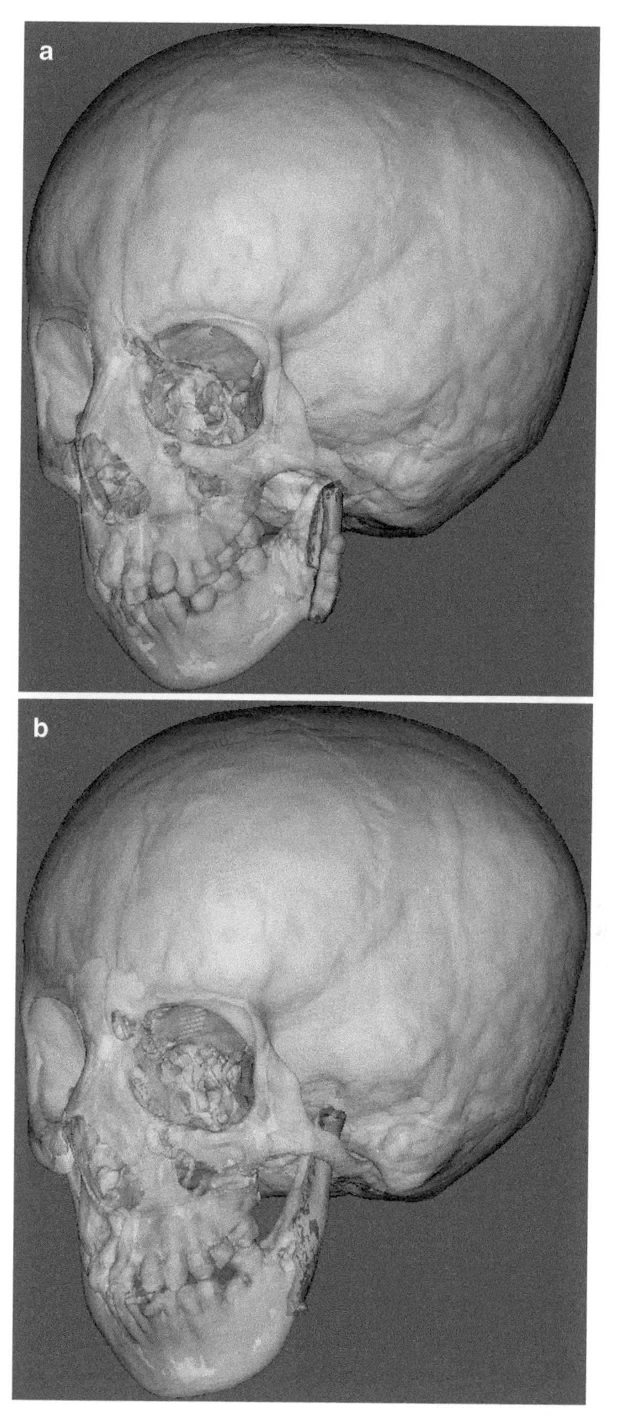

Fig. 12.4 Postoperative 3D CT of patient with rib graft. (**a**) Early postoperative. (**b**) Late postoperative

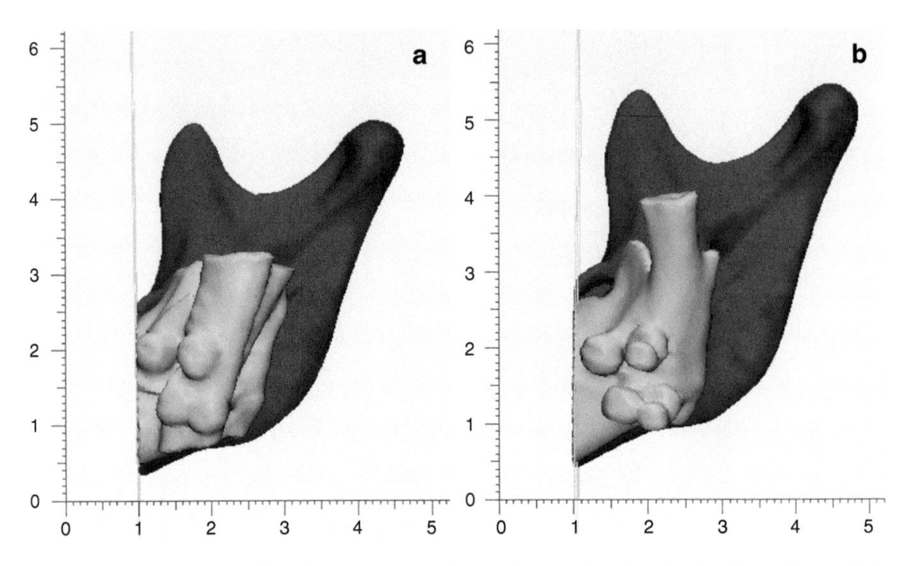

Fig. 12.5 Postoperative 3D CT comparing size and growth of patient's rib graft-mandible (aquamarine) versus native mandible (magenta). (**a**) Early postoperative. (**b**) Late postoperative

Orthognathic Surgery

Orthognathic surgery is the final bony surgical intervention performed in achievement of a correct and level dental occlusion. While skeletal alignment is the focus of orthognathic surgery in these patients, attention is placed on also achieving maximum soft tissue balance in the process. Again, surgical plans are patient- and deformity-specific and may involve isolated LeFort 1, isolated mandible bilateral sagittal split osteotomies, or a combination of the two. Furthermore, inclusion of a genioplasty may also be warranted.

In cases of type 1 deformities, orthognathic surgery alone may be all that is needed in order to achieve level dental occlusion and facial symmetry. In such cases, surgery should be performed at skeletal maturity. In the CFM patient, the ideal time for orthognathic surgery is controversial, but the authors believe it is best performed when the patient is old enough to have some degree of skeletal maturity yet young enough to prevent significant maxillary and soft tissue deformities. Also, patients who require distraction osteogenesis often require orthognathic surgery later in life on the affected side due to a decreased rate of skeletal growth [22].

Orthognathic surgery classically utilizes preoperative stone models to cut and reposition the maxilla and mandible into class I occlusion and subsequently generate a splint. While this method is accurate and reliable, it is extremely time-consuming. The development of virtual surgical planning (VSP) has significantly curtailed this time constraint while improving accuracy [13, 23]. A few limitations with using VSP are the increased costs and continued necessity of dental impressions due to

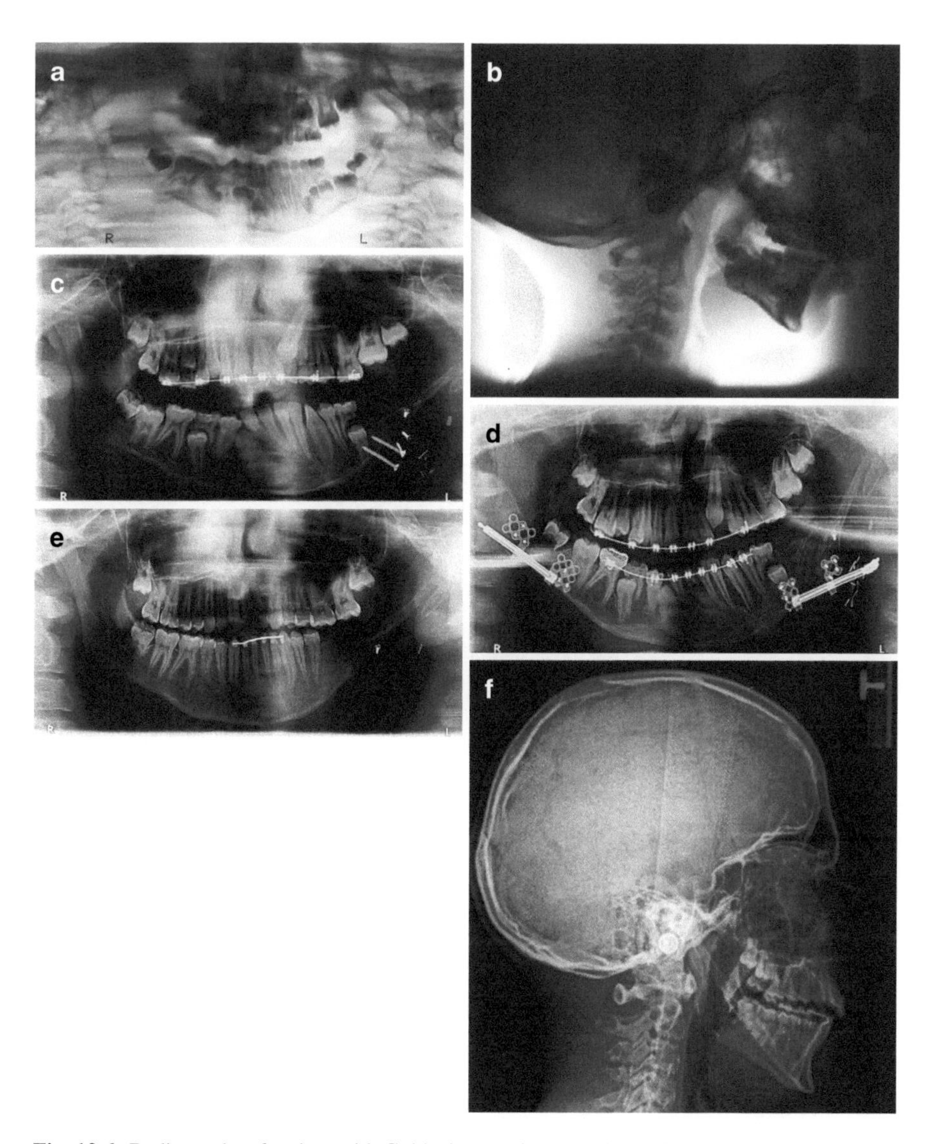

Fig. 12.6 Radiographs of patient with Goldenhar syndrome and type 3 mandible. (**a**) Panoramic before rib graft at 6 years old. (**b**) Lateral before rib graft at 6 years old. (**c**) Panoramic before distraction at 12 years old. (**d**) Panoramic after distraction at 13 years old. (**e**) Panoramic long-term follow-up at 17 years old. (**f**) Lateral long-term follow-up at 17 years old

the inability of bone beam/medical CTs to capture the maxillary mandibular occlusal surface. While some believe the simplicity and cost savings associated with the traditional modeling are best for single-jaw classic orthognathic procedures, more complex cases typically involving syndromic patients often benefit from utilization of VSP.

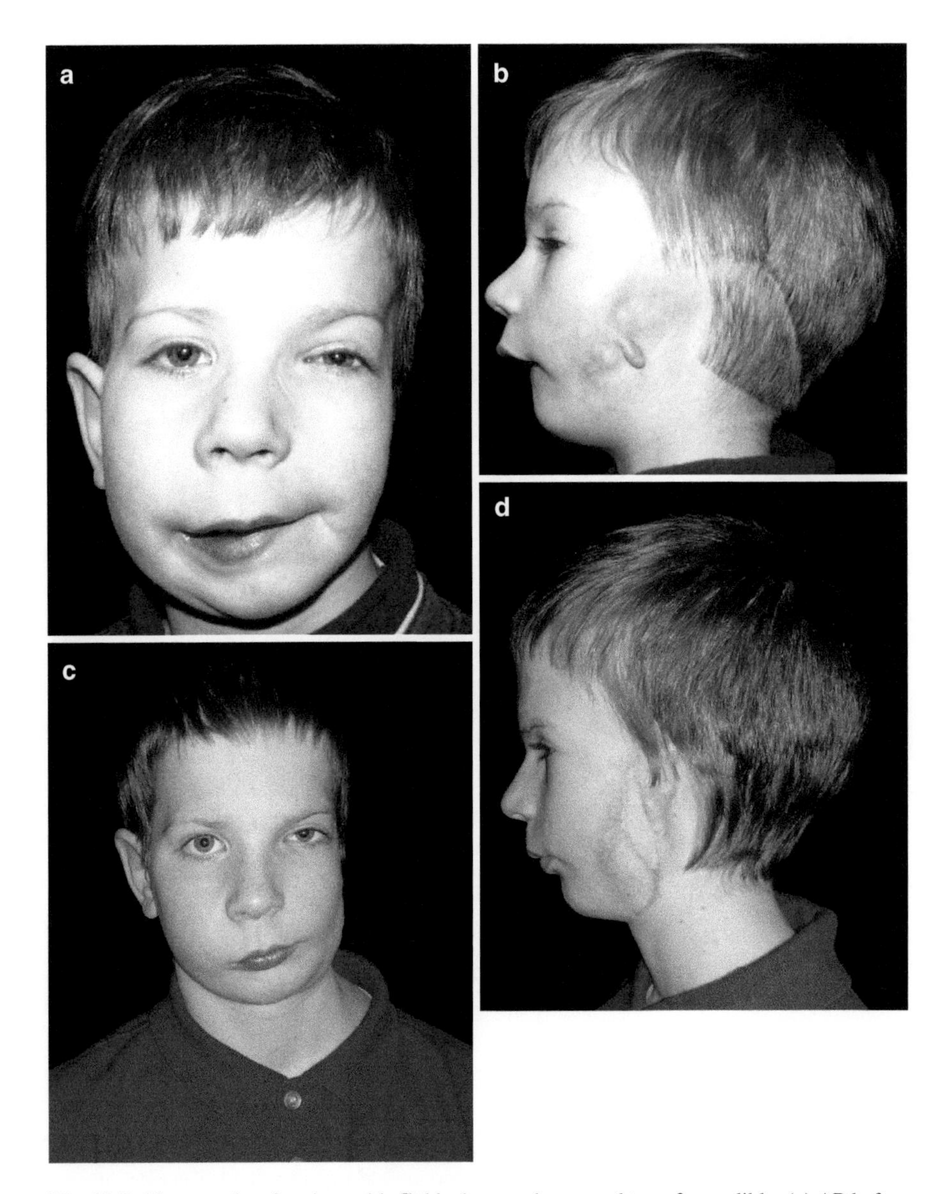

Fig. 12.7 Photographs of patient with Goldenhar syndrome and type 3 mandible. (**a**) AP before rib graft at 7 years old. (**b**) Lateral before rib graft at 7 years old. (**c**) AP after rib graft and subsequent free flap for soft tissue coverage at 11 years old. (**d**) Lateral after rib graft and subsequent free flap for soft tissue coverage at 11 years old. (**e**) AP before distraction at 12 years old. (**f**) Lateral before distraction at 12 years old. (**g**) AP after distraction at 13 years old. (**h**) Lateral after distraction at 13 years old. (**i**) AP before fat grafting at 15 years old. (**j**) Lateral before fat grafting at 15 years old. (**k**) AP after fat grafting at 17 years old. (**l**) Lateral after fat grafting at 17 years old

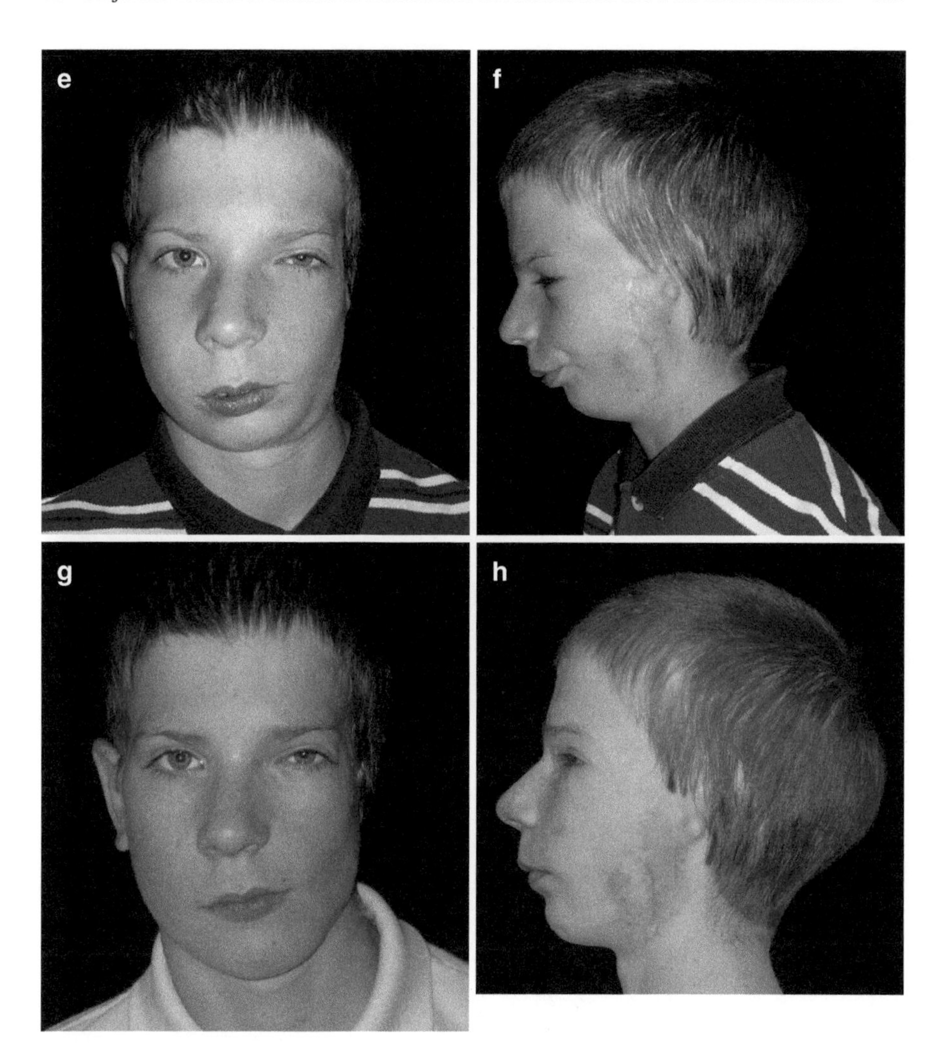

Fig. 12.7 (continued)

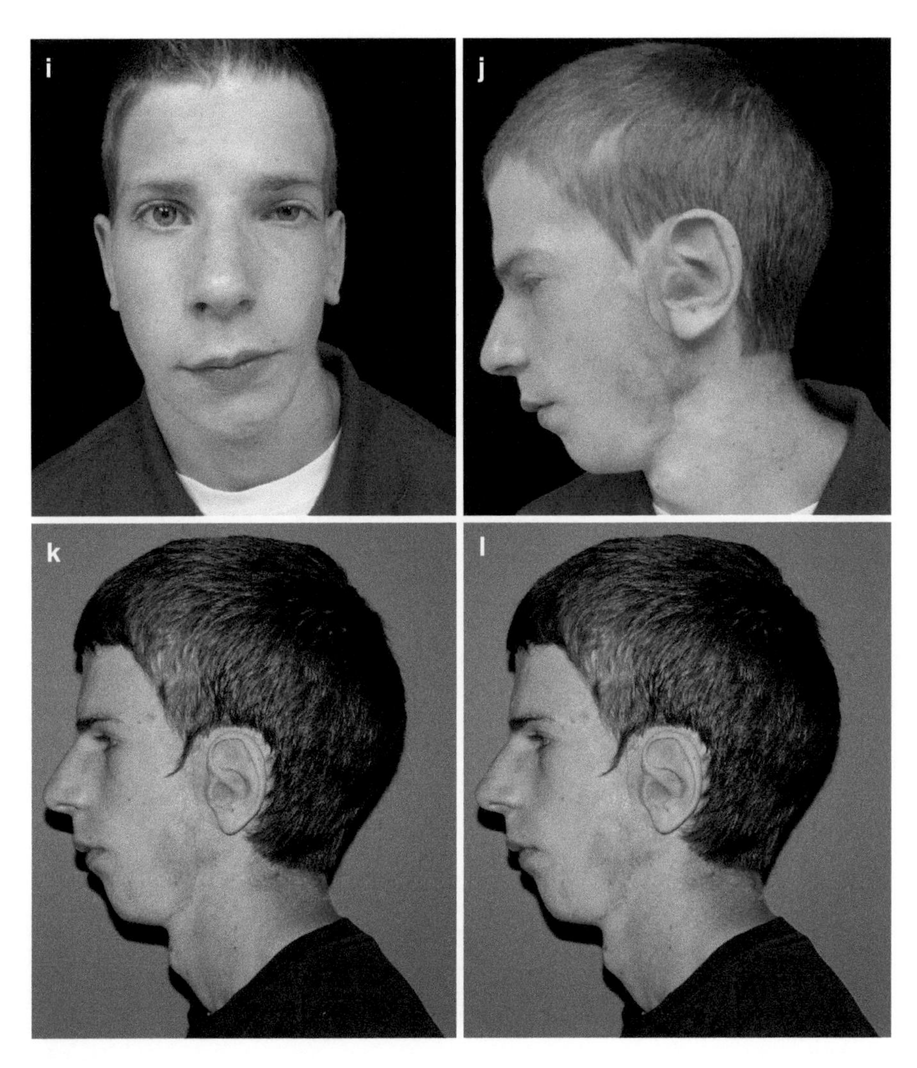

Fig. 12.7 (continued)

Fat Grafting

The first description of adipose tissue's potential benefit to correct contour irregularities and facial depression dates back to the late nineteenth and early twentieth century [24]. The technique lost popularity over the next several decades due to graft resorption and cyst formation. The creation of liposuction spurred new hope for fat utilization [25]. However, early experience saw the injected lipoaspirate resorbs almost completely. Recent advancement in technique, atraumatic harvest, purification of harvested fat, and meticulous placement of the graft has allowed for improved long-term retention and aesthetic outcomes [26].

Bony surgery alone (distraction osteogenesis, rib autograft, and orthognathic surgery) falls short of correcting soft tissue deficiencies. Fat grafting to the face is the final surgical intervention in achievement of facial soft tissue symmetry and is strongly urged in patients with severe deformity. It has replaced larger, more risky operations used to increase soft tissue volume, such as parascapular free flaps. It can be expected that approximately two-thirds of the injected fat will be revascularized and retained. This is the primary reason why sequential injections are often needed to achieve optimal results [27].

In some cases, bony surgery may not be an option. Patient compliance may be unreliable, oral hygiene may be poor, access to care may be limited, etc. [28] Despite an inability to correct skeletal symmetry and occlusal relationship, soft tissue augmentation alone may provide significant improvement in facial symmetry. Therefore, while it is typically best to first correct skeletal alignment followed by soft tissue asymmetries, fat grafting may be thought of as both primary and secondary procedures.

Fat grafting is a low-risk procedure, especially in comparison to the former standard of soft tissue augmentation, microsurgical free flap tissue transfers [27, 29]. The minimal risks of fat grafting include minor bleeding, variability of adipose volume survival, under- or overcorrection, and donor site contour irregularities. The most common complications are really an expectation, which are under correction and a need for repeat fat grafting. Rarely, long-term overgrowth of grafted fat may occur.

Additional Associations with Microtia and Surgical Considerations

Since many patients with microtia often experience comorbid craniofacial anomalies, it is important to understand the proper timing and management of surgically altering structures surrounding the ear so that optimal ear reconstruction remains possible. The TPF is commonly used for posterior auricular coverage in the Nagata and Brent staged techniques for auricular reconstruction and for implant coverage [30–33]. Therefore, craniofacial anomalies that utilize coronal incisions, which are commonly performed in patients with TCS and CFM, should be avoided prior to completion of ear reconstruction, as a unicoronal approach would burn the bridge for a future TPF flap.

Patients with TCS commonly present with a hypoplastic zygoma, inferior orbital rim, and colobomas or pseudocolobomas of the lower eyelid that are pathognomonic for TCS. The zygomatico-orbital complex is accessed and reconstructed through a coronal approach. Autologous bone graft is used to reconstruct the inferior and lateral orbital rims and for additional contouring as needed. Midface hypoplasia is corrected with bone graft reconstruction, and the notched eyelid(s) are corrected with a lateral canthopexy to reorient the axis of the palpebral fissure and correct lateral orbital dystopia.

Macrostomia is caused by clefting of the oral commissure, also known as a Tessier 7 cleft, and can occur in patients with CFM. The discontinuation of the orbicularis oris causes an abnormally wide mouth affecting oral function and aesthetics. Treatment of macrostomia involves repositioning of the oral commissure to a symmetrical alignment as the unaffected side in unilateral cases. This is accomplished by identifying the transition from cleft to non-cleft tissue, repositioning the commissure to a similar distance as the unaffected side and revising any scarring at the affected commissure to prevent contracture and lateral drift.

Conclusion

Isolated microtia is not often the only anomaly present in patients. Typical associations include varying degrees of mandibular, orbital, zygomatic, and soft tissue deficiencies that require surgical correction. The severity of each deformity determines the type of reconstruction required. There is also an important interplay in how surgery can affect neighboring structures. Therefore, it is important for a craniofacial surgeon to understand the proper timing and management of associated anomalies relative to ultimate microtia correction.

References

1. Harris J, Källén B, Robert E. The epidemiology of anotia and microtia. J Med Genet. 1996;33(10):809–13.
2. Kaye CI, Rollnick BR, Hauck WW, Martin AO, Richtsmeier JT, Nagatoshi K. Microtia and associated anomalies: statistical analysis. Am J Med Genet. 1989;34(4):574–8.
3. Mastroiacovo P, Corchia C, Botto LD, Lanni R, Zampino G, Fusco D. Epidemiology and genetics of microtia-anotia: a registry based study on over one million births. J Med Genet. 1995;32(6):453–7.
4. Luquetti DV, Heike CL, Hing AV, Cunningham ML, Cox TC. Microtia: epidemiology and genetics. Am J Med Genet A. 2012;158A(1):124–39.
5. Tuin J, Tahiri Y, Paliga JT, Taylor JA, Bartlett SP. Distinguishing goldenhar syndrome from craniofacial microsomia. J Craniofac Surg. 2015;26(6):1887–92.
6. Pruzansky S. Not all dwarfed mandibles are alike. Birth Defects. 1969;5:120–9.
7. Kaban LB, Padwa BL, Mulliken JB. Surgical correction of mandibular hypoplasia in hemifacial microsomia: the case for treatment in early childhood. J Oral Maxillofac Surg. 1998;56(5):628–38.

8. Swanson JW, Mitchell BT, Wink JA, Taylor JA, Bartlett SP. Surgical classification of the mandibular deformity in craniofacial microsomia using 3-dimensional computed tomography. Plast Reconstr Surg Glob Open. 2016;4(1):e598.
9. Ilizarov GA, Ledyaev VI. The replacement of long tubular bone defects by lengthening distraction osteotomy of one of the fragments. 1969. Clin Orthop Relat Res. 1992;280:7–10.
10. Davidson EH, Brown D, Shetye PR, Greig AV, Grayson BH, Warren SM, et al. The evolution of mandibular distraction: device selection. Plast Reconstr Surg. 2010;126(6):2061–70.
11. Ortakoglu K, Karacay S, Sencimen M, Akin E, Ozyigit AH, Bengi O. Distraction osteogenesis in a severe mandibular deficiency. Head Face Med. 2007;3:7.
12. Wu B-ZZ, Ma L, Li Y, Chen S, Yi B. Costochondral graft in young children with hemifacial microsomia. J Craniofac Surg. 2017;28(1):129–33.
13. Yu H, Wang B, Wang M, Wang X, Shen SG. Computer-assisted distraction osteogenesis in the treatment of hemifacial microsomia. J Craniofac Surg. 2016;27(6):1539–42.
14. Boisson J, Strozyk H, Diner P, Picard A, Kadlub N. Feasibility of magnetic activation of a maxillofacial distraction osteogenesis, design of a new device. J Craniomaxillofac Surg. 2016;44(6):684–8.
15. Meling TR, Høgevold H-EE, Due-Tønnessen BJ, Skjelbred P. Comparison of perioperative morbidity after LeFort III and monobloc distraction osteogenesis. Br J Oral Maxillofac Surg. 2011;49(2):131–4.
16. Nout E, Wolvius EB, van Adrichem LN, Ongkosuwito EM, van der Wal KG. Complications in maxillary distraction using the RED II device: a retrospective analysis of 21 patients. Int J Oral Maxillofac Surg. 2006;35(10):897–902.
17. Figueroa AA, Gans BJ, Pruzansky S. Long-term follow-up of a mandibular costochondral graft. Oral Surg Oral Med Oral Pathol. 1984;58(3):257–68.
18. Guyuron B, Lasa CI Jr. Unpredictable growth pattern of costochondral graft. Plast Reconstr Surg. 1992;90(5):880–6.
19. Perrott DH, Umeda H, Kaban LB. Costochondral graft construction/reconstruction of the ramus/condyle unit: long-term follow-up. Int J Oral Maxillofac Surg. 1994;23(6 Pt 1):321–8.
20. Tahiri Y, Chang CS, Tuin J, Paliga JT, Lowe KM, Taylor JA, et al. Costochondral grafting in craniofacial microsomia. Plast Reconstr Surg. 2015;135(2):530–41.
21. Wan DC, Taub PJ, Allam KA, Perry A. Distraction osteogenesis of costocartilaginous rib grafts and treatment algorithm for severely hypoplastic mandibles. Plast Reconstr Surg. 2011;127(5):2005–13.
22. Weichman KE, Jacobs J, Patel P, Szpalski C, Shetye P, Grayson B, et al. Early distraction for mild to moderate unilateral craniofacial microsomia: long-term follow-up, outcomes, and recommendations. Plast Reconstr Surg. 2017;139(4):941e–53e.
23. Hammoudeh JA, Howell LK, Boutros S, Scott MA, Urata MM. Current status of surgical planning for orthognathic surgery: traditional methods versus 3D surgical planning. Plast Reconstr Surg Glob Open. 2015;3(2):e307.
24. Hirschberg M. Ueber die Wiederanheilung vollständig vom Körper getrennter, die ganze Fettschicht enthaltender Hautstücke. 1893;46:183.
25. Illouz YG. The fat cell "graft": a new technique to fill depressions. Plast Reconstr Surg. 1986;78(1):122–3.
26. Coleman SR. Facial recontouring with lipostructure. Clin Plast Surg. 1997;24(2):347–67.
27. Tanna N, Broer PN, Roostaeian J, Bradley JP, Levine JP, Saadeh PB. Soft tissue correction of craniofacial microsomia and progressive hemifacial atrophy. J Craniofac Surg. 2012;23(7 Suppl 1):2024–7.
28. Denadai R, Raposo-Amaral CA, Buzzo CL, Raposo-Amaral CE. Isolated autologous free fat grafting for management of facial contour asymmetry in a subset of growing patients with craniofacial microsomia. Ann Plast Surg. 2016;76(3):288–94.
29. Tringale KR, Lance S, Schoenbrunner A, Gosman AA. Sustained overcorrection after autologous facial fat grafting in the pediatric population: a case series. Ann Plast Surg. 2017;78(5 Suppl 4):S217–21.
30. Nagata S. A new method of total reconstruction of the auricle for microtia. Plast Reconstr Surg. 1993;92(2):187–201.

31. Brent B. Auricular repair with autogenous rib cartilage grafts: two decades of experience with 600 cases. Plast Reconstr Surg. 1992;90(3):355–6.
32. Brent B, Upton J, Acland RD, Shaw WW, Finseth FJ, Rogers C, et al. Experience with the temporoparietal fascial free flap. Plast Reconstr Surg. 1985;76(2):177–88.
33. Brent B, Byrd HS. Secondary ear reconstruction with cartilage grafts covered by axial, random, and free flaps of temporoparietal fascia. Plast Reconstr Surg. 1983;72(2):141–52.

Chapter 13
Salvage of the Unsatisfactory Microtia Reconstruction

Daniel J. Gould, Youssef Tahiri, and John F. Reinisch

Introduction

Microtia reconstruction remains one of the most challenging operations in plastic and reconstructive surgery. It combines a difficult and often variable anatomy with a particularly challenging technical surgery all in the context of a rare disease [1]. Most microtia surgeons recognize that the rareness and variability of this condition present unique challenges to standardized outcomes. Unfortunately, those challenges also contribute to unsatisfactory outcomes for microtia patients. The etiology of unsatisfactory surgical outcomes includes poor preoperative planning, inadequate technical execution, postoperative trauma, infection or extrusion, and long-term physiologic and growth-related changes.

This chapter is devoted to secondary microtia reconstruction, including salvage procedures and advanced techniques.

D. J. Gould (✉)
University of Southern California, Plastic and Reconstructive Surgery, Los Angeles, CA, USA
e-mail: daniel.gould@med.usc.edu

Y. Tahiri
Plastic and Reconstructive Surgery, Cedars-Sinai Medical Center, Los Angeles, CA, USA
e-mail: Youssef.Tahiri@cshs.org

J. F. Reinisch
Keck School of Medicine, University of Souther California, Los Angeles, CA, USA

Craniofacial and Pediatric Plastic Surgery, Cedars Sinai Medical Center, Los Angeles, CA, USA

© Springer Nature Switzerland AG 2019
J. F. Reinisch, Y. Tahiri (eds.), *Modern Microtia Reconstruction*,
https://doi.org/10.1007/978-3-030-16387-7_13

Common Techniques for Microtia Reconstruction

The most common techniques for microtia reconstruction include prosthesis, costal cartilage, and porous high-density polyethylene (pHDPE) implant-based reconstruction [1]. Each of these techniques has been described in the literature at length, and satisfactory outcomes may be achieved with each depending on the surgeon's experience and patient's preference [2, 3]. No one technique can be ascribed in all situations, and anatomic and technical variations exist for each technique.

Prosthesis

Prosthesis can provide an excellent color match with aesthetically pleasing results. The results are durable, and the devices are replaceable; thus they can be revised and updated. They do not interfere with the ability to place bone-anchored hearing aids. Prosthesis can be designed to match the contralateral ear and may be more acceptable in adults, as they are more compliant.

A prosthesis can be glued to the mastoid skin or can be surgically anchored to the bone. Bone anchors exhibit excellent bio-integrative technology; however, they may be subject to infection, wound-healing issues, or implant loosening [4]. Native skin around the implant can atrophy from implant pressure, further contributing to wound complications. One advancement in osteointegrated prosthesis involves image-guided placement for precise positioning shown in cancer resection patients [5].

Challenges facing prosthesis include tissue feel, color match, fading, and replacement over time as well as the fact that the implant must be removed while bathing, swimming, or other social contexts [3]. The prohibitive social conditions, particularly swimming and other athletic activities, are often the trigger for secondary reconstruction.

Costal Cartilage

The most common surgical technique for microtia reconstruction is rib cartilage reconstruction. Costochondral cartilage is harvested, sculpted into the shape of an ear, and then implanted into the temporal area. Later this construct is elevated in a staged fashion, requiring a supportive base and skin grafting in a secondary procedure.

Common surgical methods include the Brent or Nagata techniques and variations with or without a temporoparietal flap. In the Brent and Nagata techniques, the patient undergoes rib harvest, ear carving, and construct implantation at the same first stage [6]. The cartilage construct is usually placed in a subcutaneous plane. Some surgeons utilize a TPF flap to cover the cartilaginous construct if the patient has a low hairline with an insufficient amount of native mastoid skin or significant scarring of the mastoid area. Later during the second stage, the construct is elevated to gain projection and is maintained with a block of supporting cartilage to keep the construct elevated, while the post-auricular area is skin grafted. One benefit of this surgical approach is that a TPF flap is not necessarily always needed for coverage as the cartilage is well tolerated under a skin flap.

Many perform the cartilage reconstruction in two stages; however, some do perform single stage-reconstruction. Most surgeons who perform cartilage reconstruction require a staged approach [7], including two surgeries and possibly additional operative procedures [8]. Potential risks and complications associated with costal cartilage harvest include pain at the harvest site, hypertrophic scar, pneumothorax, and pneumoperitoneum and complications. Surgeons typically place closed suction drains under the construct which they monitor them with a suction protocol, so generally this procedure requires an observational stay in the hospital. Limitations or disadvantages of this technique include low hairline; poor projection; resorbed, deformed, warped, or exposed cartilage; poor construct placement; or migration of the construct [3, 8].

PHDPE Ear Reconstruction

PHDPE ear reconstruction typically involves a single-stage surgery. The soft tissue coverage is very different than what a cartilage construct requires. The implant requires total coverage with a fascial flap to minimize the risk of implant exposure [8, 9]. Some of the benefits of pHDPE reconstruction include a single-stage procedure performed as an outpatient, minimal pain and discomfort, and it can be done as early as 3.5 years of age (before school age). Atresia repair can be done before or at the same time as the ear reconstruction [10, 11]. One important advantage is that pHDPE is biocompatible and resists deformational forces.

Complications associated with pHDPE reconstruction are rare in the hands of the experienced surgeon. They include exposure/extrusion, infection, implant fracture, implant migration, and unfavorable cosmetic result.

With each of these reconstructive options, patients can have unsatisfactory outcomes which may lead them to seek secondary reconstruction. The remaining portion of the chapter will discuss the secondary treatment of these outcomes.

Dichotomy of Expectations

Before addressing anatomic variations and pathophysiology associated with ear reconstruction failure, patient perception must be understood. It is important to understand the dichotomy of surgical expectations between surgeons and patients. Importantly, one must probe the patients' ideas about outcomes and surgical course first, as often patients will come with the expectation of a single-stage cosmetic procedure [12]. Surgeons' expectations on the other hand often involve a perception of these procedures as challenging reconstructive cases, involving complex anatomy, lack of soft tissue or poor soft tissue, and difficult surgical techniques. Surgeons may anticipate two or three surgeries to achieve the final satisfactory outcome in a secondary revision case. Usually both the surgeon and the patient wind up disappointed, as truthfully secondary salvage is neither perfectly aesthetic nor entirely reconstructive. Expectations are often the most critical to manage to ensure the surgeon and the patient can share a common vision for the goals of surgery.

Patients may present with preconceived notions and stories of several consultations after failed attempts – they may be very much psychologically affected by their condition. These patients are older than primary microtia patients, and as such, they often have more insight into their deformity. Also, they have essentially lived through much of the social stigma of having an unsatisfactory reconstruction which is noticeable as an ear deformity which in some ways is as visible as microtia. One must be mindful of the expectations and be forthcoming about failure and the options for management when informing patients about this surgery [12].

When complications or unsatisfactory outcomes arise, often patients and surgeons are extremely disappointed. Patients are disappointed because they invest in a long reconstructive journey and in the end wind up with an unsatisfactory outcome. In addition to being disappointed for the poor outcome, surgeons are then struggling to provide a secondary reconstruction in the context of scar and a poor soft tissue bed.

In efforts to better understand secondary reconstruction, surgeons must consider their own practice and identify patient and surgical factors that lead to better outcomes.

Salvage Following Prosthesis

Reasons for Dissatisfaction

Prosthesis patients offer a unique set of challenges for several reasons. They often present with issues related to the color match or the visibility of the implant. However, if a good anaplastologist or prosthetist is identified, these issues can be improved. The biggest issue for these patients is often the fact that certain social situations arise where they may have to remove the implant, and this can prove challenging. Patients may describe sports or pool parties where they were embarrassed by having to take off the prosthesis or situations like the gym or other physical activities where the prosthesis needs to be removed. These patients present a challenge due to their surgical and anatomical issues but also due to their complicated social dynamics. These factors all contribute to patients being unsatisfied with prosthetic reconstruction.

Reconstructive Considerations

Previous placement of a prosthesis could involve a bone anchor or simply skin glue [13]. As there is great variability in the options present for prosthesis, the secondary salvage options are diverse. Etiology of the defect is crucial, as trauma or burn patients may present more of a concern than congenital microtia or anotia patients

[4]. Similarly, oncological patients may present a unique problem if they have had radiation or other local therapies for their cancer treatment.

Prosthesis patients are often older and as such their cases may be complicated by scarring. The anatomy of the region should always be carefully studied, and the superficial temporal artery should be palpated or dopplered in clinic to ensure a robust supply to the TPF. If the TPF has not yet been harvested, then it provides an excellent soft tissue option for coverage which will allow for skin grafting and the use of pHDPE for reconstruction. On the other hand, if a TPF is not available, an occipital flap can be used for implant coverage.

Examples of Reconstruction

Figure 13.1a–e demonstrates two patients who presented with well-adapted prosthesis for reconstruction. The first patient (Fig. 13.1a–c) was born with microtia and craniofacial microsomia. The ear remnant and lobe were amputated and replaced with a skin graft. To camouflage the front of the prosthesis. a tissue expanded scalp flap was rotated to provide a robust sideburn. Reconstruction was done with a Pep implant covered with a radial forearm free fascia flap and skin graft. The patient sought out pHDPE reconstruction for durable and long-term reconstruction. The second patient presented (Fig. 13.1d, e) also was born with microtia treated with amputation and a prosthesis. This figure features the TPF flap used for soft tissue coverage of the pHDPE implant. These patients both had good long-term results as presented in Fig. 13.1c–e. Notably, both patients had spent a significant period with the prosthesis prior to seeking reconstruction

Salvage Following Autologous Ear Reconstruction

Reasons for Dissatisfaction

Autologous ear reconstruction is the most commonly practiced form of ear reconstruction. As such there are many more patients with autologous cartilage constructs, and this alone may account for the higher number of secondary revision patients from this group. Additionally, cartilage uniquely presents with loss of definition and shape over time leading to a deformed construct. Other issues surrounding secondary reconstruction of autologous constructs include a constricted pocket, scar tissue, and poor soft tissue envelope. These are secondary characteristics associated with wound healing that may lead to unsatisfactory outcomes. These patients may present after secondary elevation with loss of projection or loss of definition. Moreover, a low set hairline may complicate surgery, and in the case of cartilage, the surgeon may opt to place the construct under the hair-bearing scalp or at a level that is too low to avoid having to address a hairy construct at a later stage. Both anatomic issues create a situation where the anatomic placement is not ideal and contribute to unsatisfactory outcomes. Figure 13.2a, b demonstrates what constructs

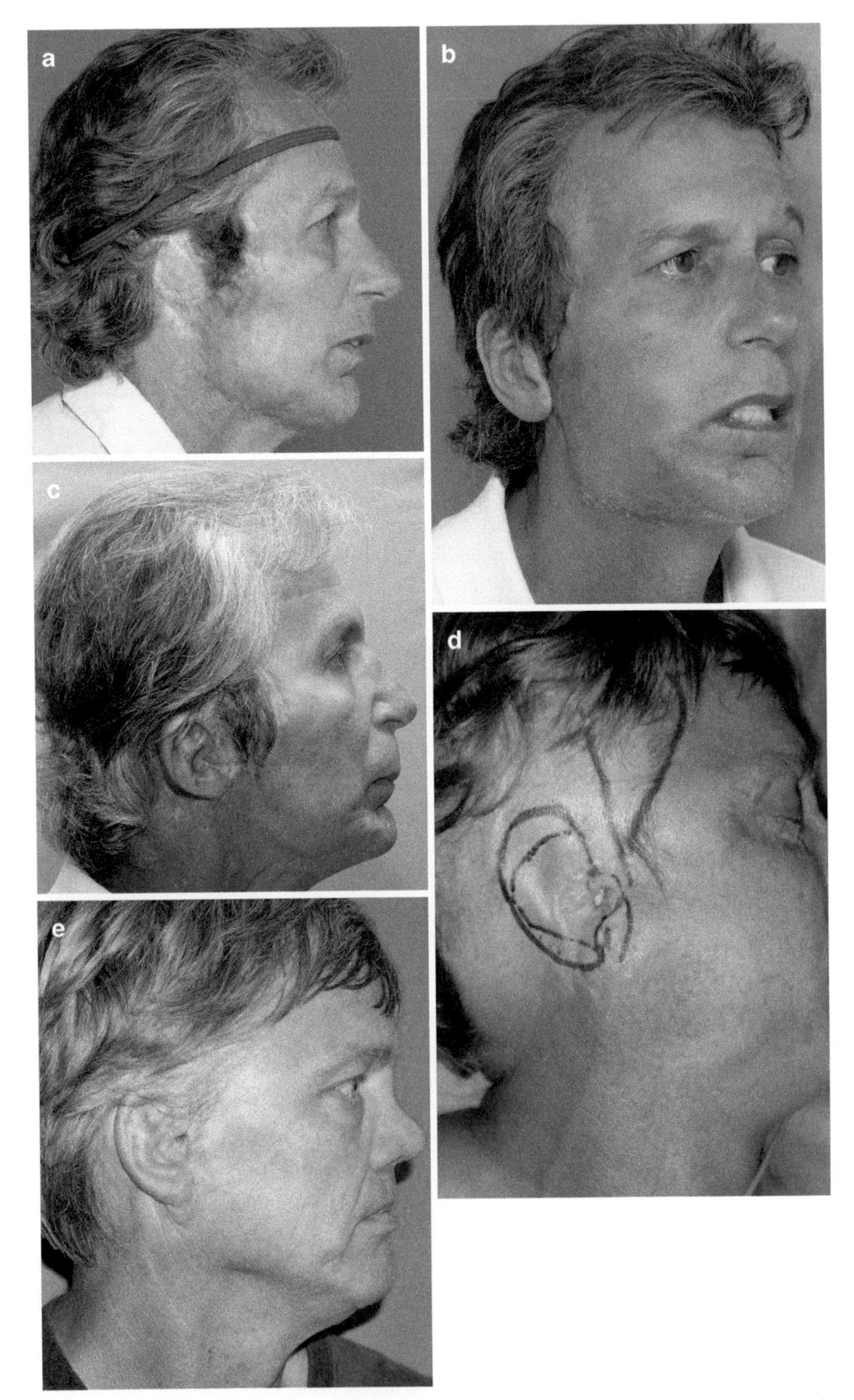

Fig. 13.1 (**a**–**e**) These two adult male patients were born with microtia treated with amputation and a prosthesis. Prosthesis patients often present as older patients who may have never been offered reconstruction. They both underwent successfully polyethylene ear reconstruction. The results are at 10-year postoperative (**c**) and 1-year postoperative (**e**)

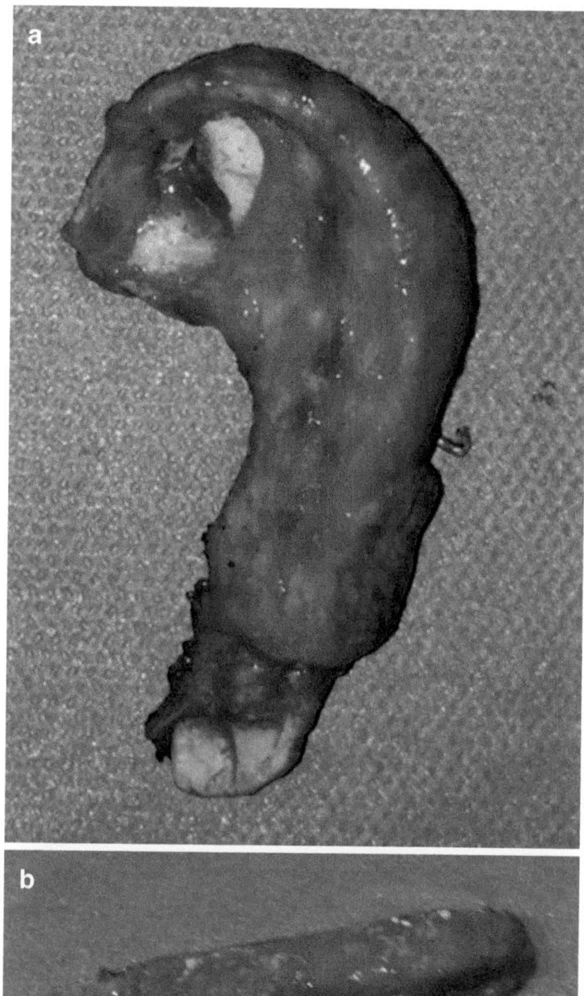

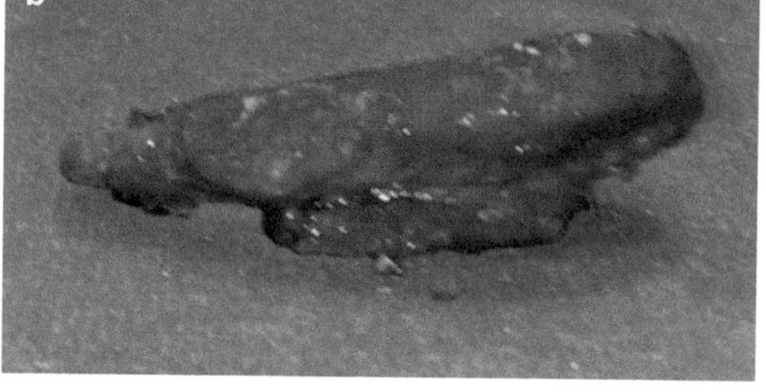

Fig. 13.2 (**a, b**) Representative example of autologous constructs at the time of explant when patients describe dissatisfaction with shape. The cartilage is often deformed and lacks anatomic definition

look like when explanted after this type of deformational process has occurred. Unfortunately, there is a high rate of this type of deformation in the cartilage construct reconstructions. Also, over time, warping, erosion, and ossification may further contribute to deformity of the construct. These issues all fall under the general problem of deformation of cartilage.

Reconstructive Considerations

The overall poor shape and definition as well as the lack of projection of the cartilaginous ear are the most common complaints of unsatisfied patients. The abnormal placement of the construct (often too low and anterior) is also a cause for dissatisfaction.

Prior to attempting reconstruction of cartilage ears, the surgeon must again survey for the presence of the STA and a TPF flap for soft tissue coverage. They must also identify the proper location of the ear based on a contralateral side or anatomic landmarks. If needed, they may have to significantly alter the location of the ear to reestablish normal anatomic relations.

Examples of Reconstruction

Figure 13.3a–e demonstrates an example of salvage secondary ear reconstruction with pHDPE constructs. This figure shows a young child who had an ear reconstruction with autologous cartilage and presented with concerns about projection, shape, and position (Fig. 13.3a, b). The cartilaginous ear was removed and a pHDPE ear reconstruction was performed. The result was improved projection, definition, and shape (Fig. 13.3c–e)

These outcomes can be replicated in different Fitzpatrick skin types and with different levels of deformity. Figure 13.4a–f shows several patients with satisfactory outcomes following secondary reconstruction. Importantly, when scar tissue is severe, the native skin may be difficult to utilize. Definition in the area may take time to develop if there is prolonged swelling and inflammation.

These types of outcomes can also be achieved in older patients with significant deformity, and the results are long lasting. In Fig. 13.5a–d, an older man with pHDPE salvage reconstruction is shown with excellent projection and definition. Figure 13.5e–h shows a further example which is a 20-year follow-up on a young girl who underwent secondary pHDPE ear reconstruction following failure of a cartilaginous ear reconstruction.

Physical examination and anatomic landmarks are keys in the salvage reconstruction process. Figure 13.6a–g shows several cases of extremely poor soft tissue pocket as well as poor implant position. In patients with low hairline, it is not uncommon to see patients with cartilage ears positioned too low to avoid the hairline.

Again, these results are long lasting. In Fig. 13.7a–c, a young girl is presented at 1 (Fig. 13.7b) and then 4 years (Fig. 13.7c) postoperatively. Note that over time, the swelling and edema subside, while the definition of the pHDPE ear reconstruction continues to improve.

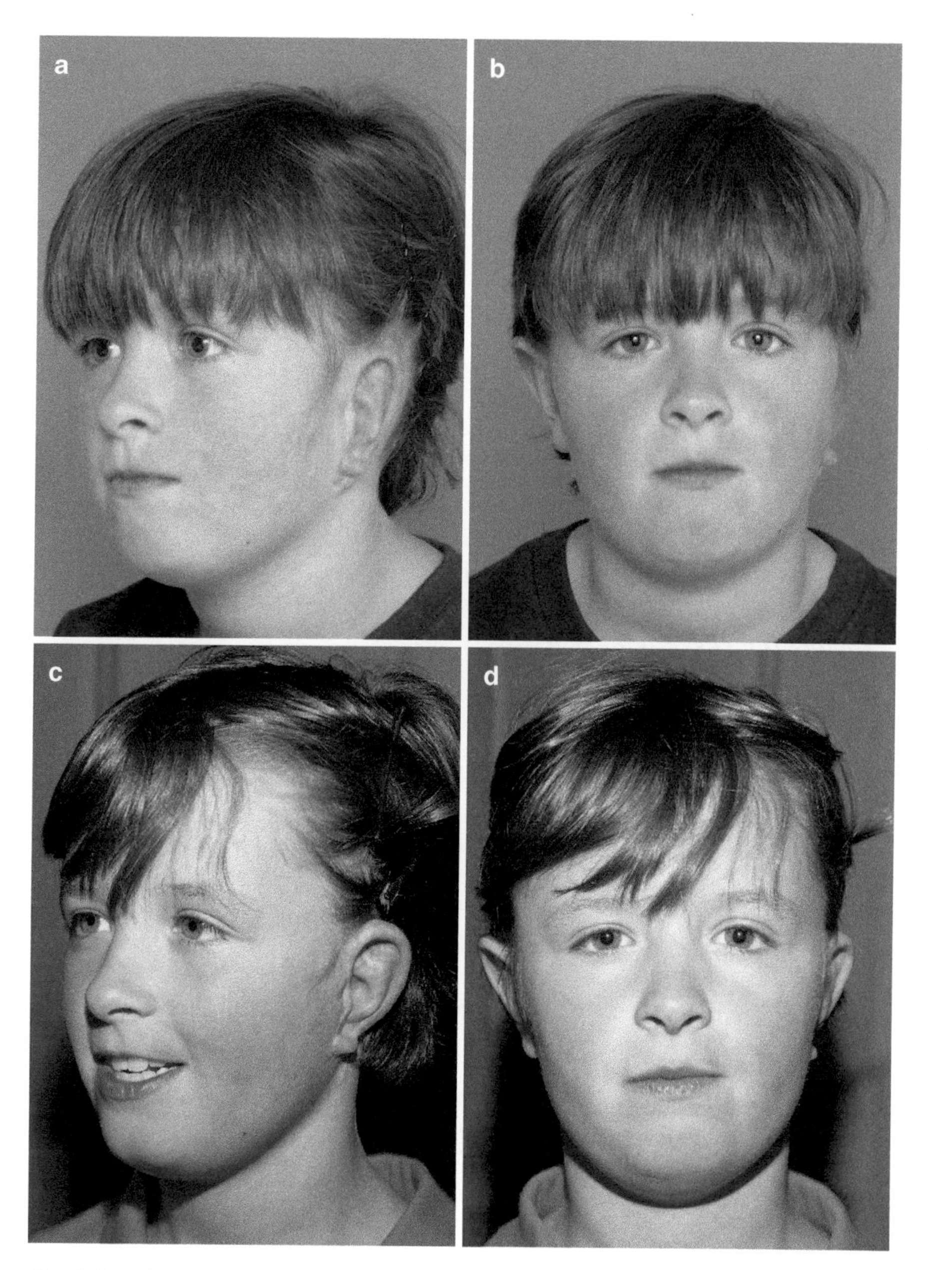

Fig. 13.3 This 9-year-old had microtia reconstruction with cartilage. The construct lacked projection and definition (**a**, **b**). The reconstructed polyethylene ear is presented at 14-month postoperative with excellent projection and form (**c**–**e**)

Fig. 13.3 (continued)

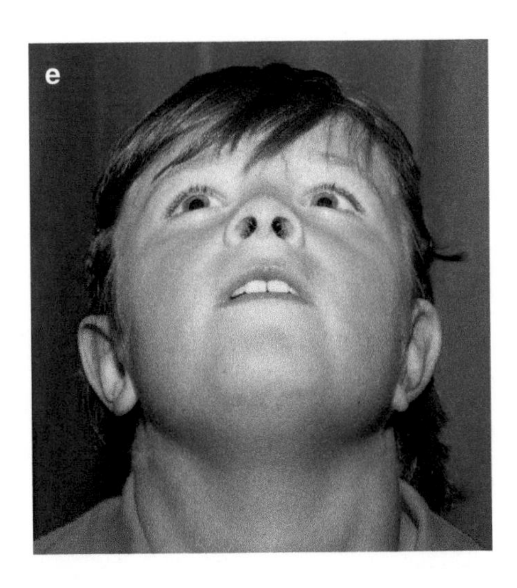

Salvage Following Alloplastic Ear Reconstruction

Reasons for Dissatisfaction

PHDPE constructs have their own set of drawbacks, including exposure and infection [3]. Porous polyethylene constructs have several advantages, including a porous network to allow ingrowth of tissue, relative biocompatibility, durability, and resistance to deformation and relatively easy manipulation and fabrication [14, 15]. Drawing upon parallels in plastic surgery, it is understood that micro texturing breast implants leads to less capsular contracture, which may occur due to the dramatic increase in surface area from texturing and changes in the fibrous capsule and its ability to constrict with this type of architecture. It is also known that these types of implants may be at greater risk of biofilm formation and resistance to antibiotic penetration. Care must be paid to the implants to avoid contamination and large or chronic exposures may necessitate complete salvage reconstruction [16].

Although large exposures, infections, and soft tissue loss are some of the most catastrophic reasons for dissatisfaction, other issues can present a challenge in pHDPE reconstruction such as fractured framework or malpositioning of the ear.

Reconstructive Considerations

Anatomic considerations are crucial in secondary pHDPE reconstruction. Rarely, surgeons will place the construct in a subcutaneous pocket which generally leads to skin loss and subsequent implant exposure. Conversely, if the patient has already had a TPF flap for coverage of the implant, other techniques are required for the

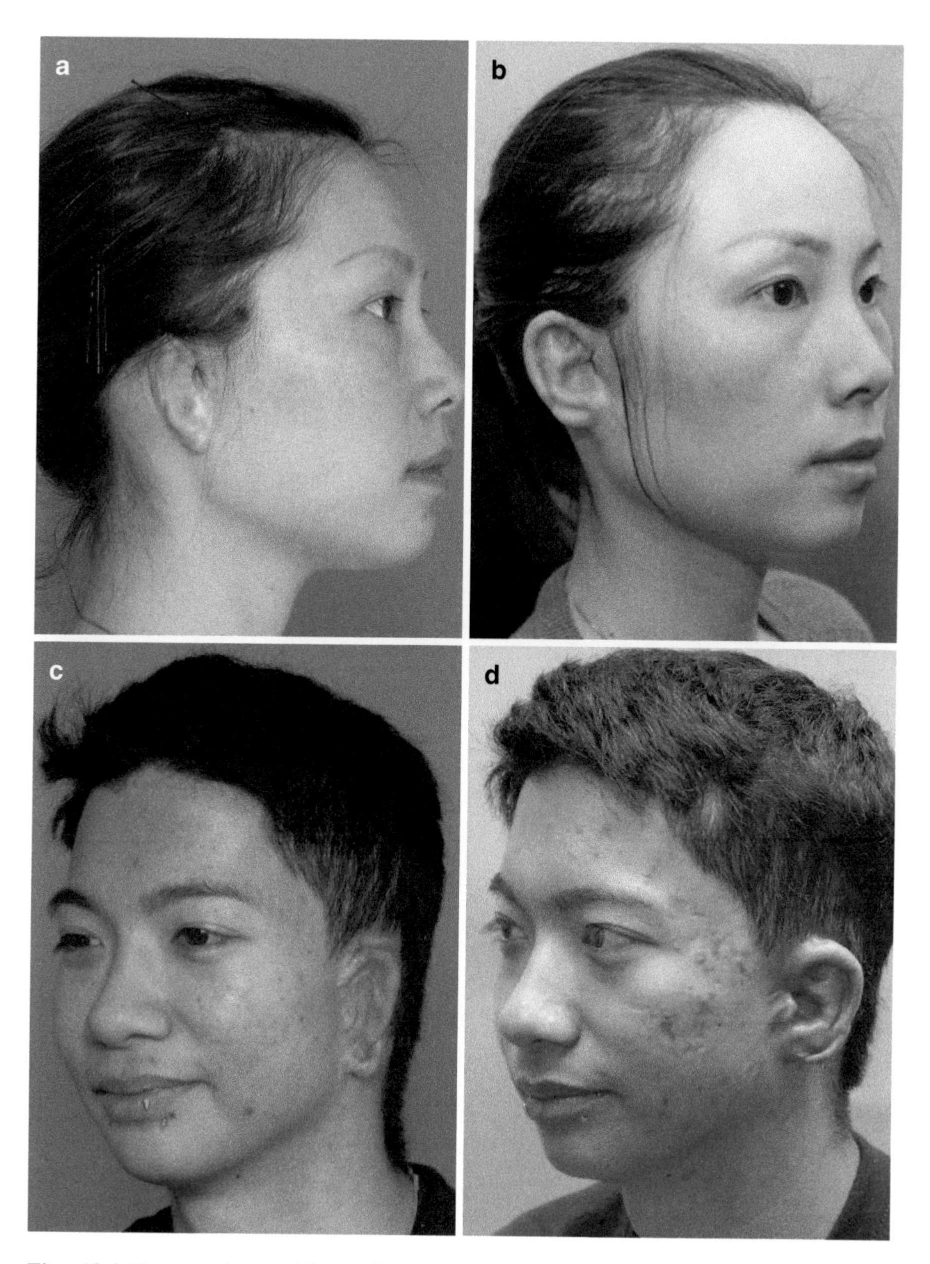

Fig. 13.4 Three patients with varying Fitzpatrick skin types with previous autologous reconstructions. (**a**, **b**) An Asian adult female preoperative and then 6 months postoperative. (**c**, **d**) A Filipino adult male with previous autologous rib and reconstruction at 1 year postoperative. (**e**, **f**) A Caucasian teenage girl with prior autologous rib and then 11 months postoperative with polyethylene reconstruction. All of these patients had improvements in projection, shape, and definition

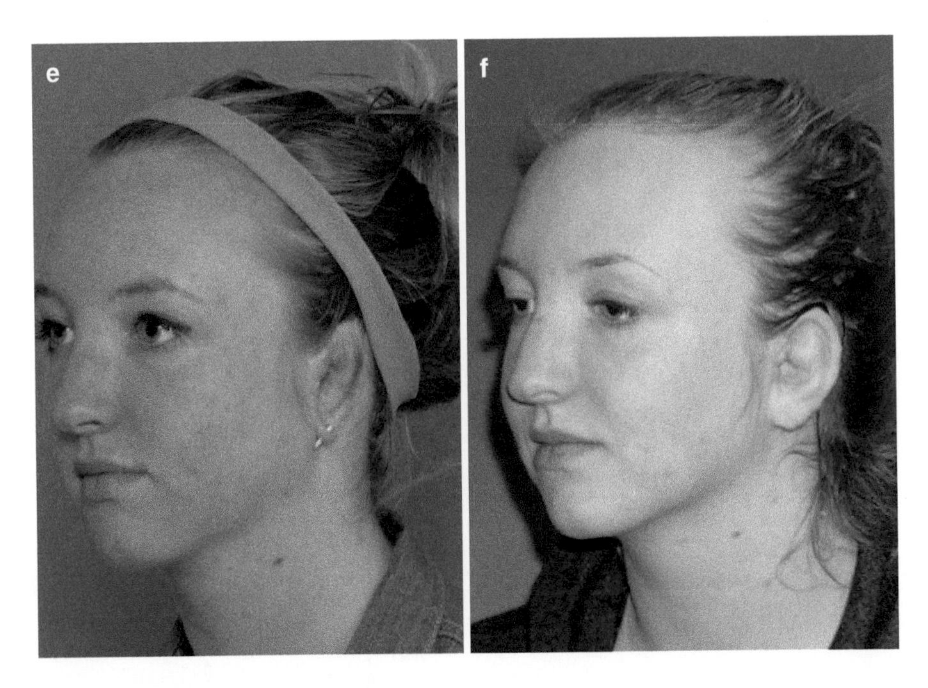

Fig. 13.4 (continued)

revision surgery. A pedicled occipital fascial flap, based on the occipital artery, is used for implant coverage when a TPF flap is not available.

Examples of Reconstruction

Figure 13.8a–e shows one patient who had a previous subcutaneous alloplastic reconstruction who presented with implant erosion and failure. The reconstruction was salvaged with an occipital flap, which is the preferred flap for secondary alloplastic reconstruction. The anatomy in this region is consistent, and a CT angiogram (CTA) in Fig. 13.9 demonstrates the typical course of this vessel. Note, the authors do not routinely obtain, nor do they recommend, CTA for vascular study of this region

Utilizing these techniques, even disastrous erosions and extrusions of alloplastic implants can be managed successfully as shown in Fig. 13.10a, b. This may require removal of the implant and staging for successful salvage as shown in Fig. 13.11a–f. In this case the child developed an implant extrusion after subcutaneous placement of the pHDPE implant at a different institution. Multiple attempts were tried to use pedicled flaps to improve coverage of the implant. Salvage required removal of the implant, antibiotics, and staging for definitive alloplastic reconstruction.

Figure 13.12a–c demonstrates another patient who presented with an exposure following subcutaneous placement of the pHDPE implant. Revision included the

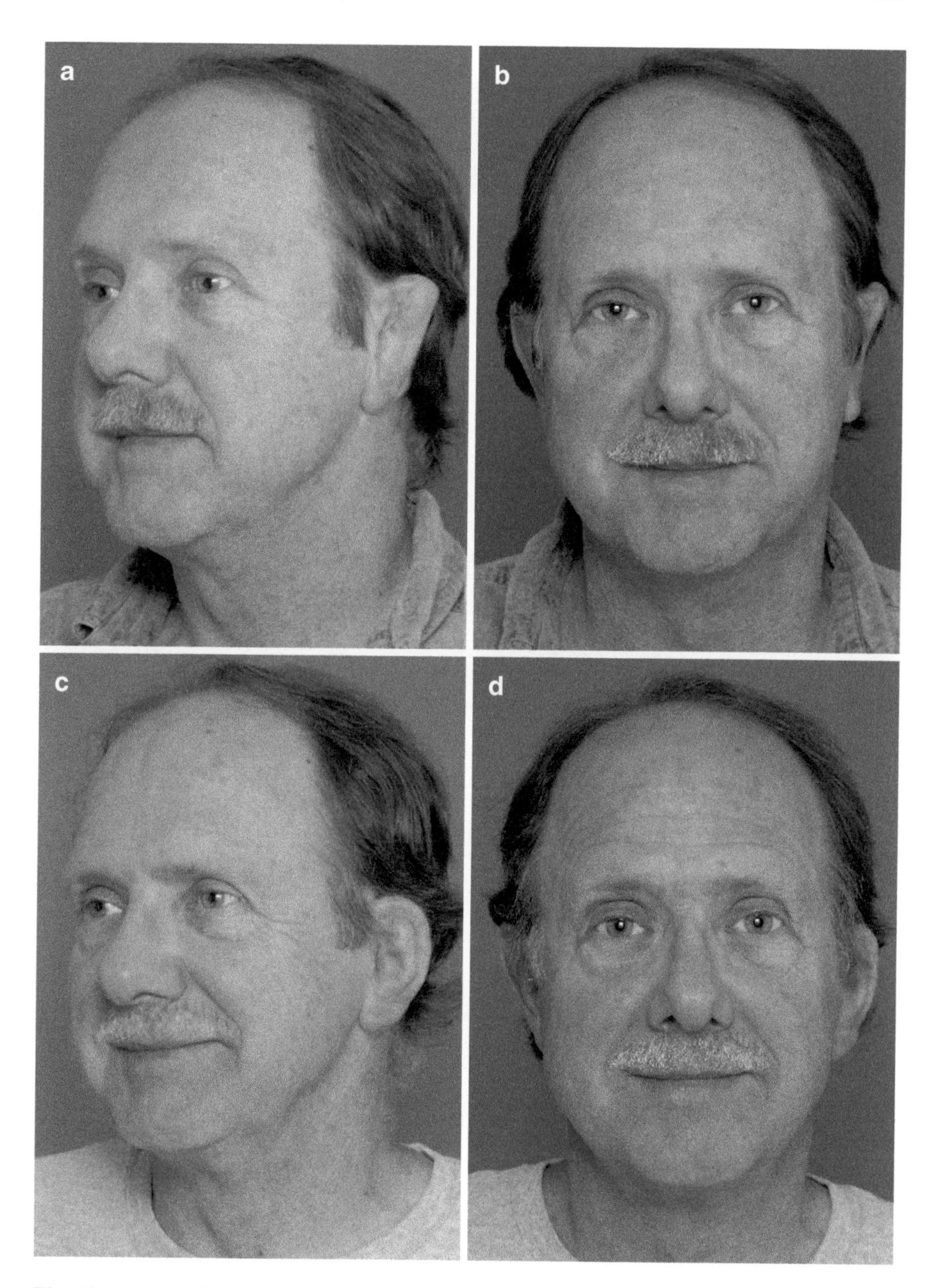

Fig. 13.5 (**a–d**) Older gentleman with severely deformed auricular cartilage with a good outcome following polyethylene ear reconstruction. (**e–h**) A young girl who presented after complete failure and scalp flap to cover the resultant defect at 10 years of age. She underwent a polyethylene ear reconstruction. (**g, h**) 17 years postoperative outcome in second patient

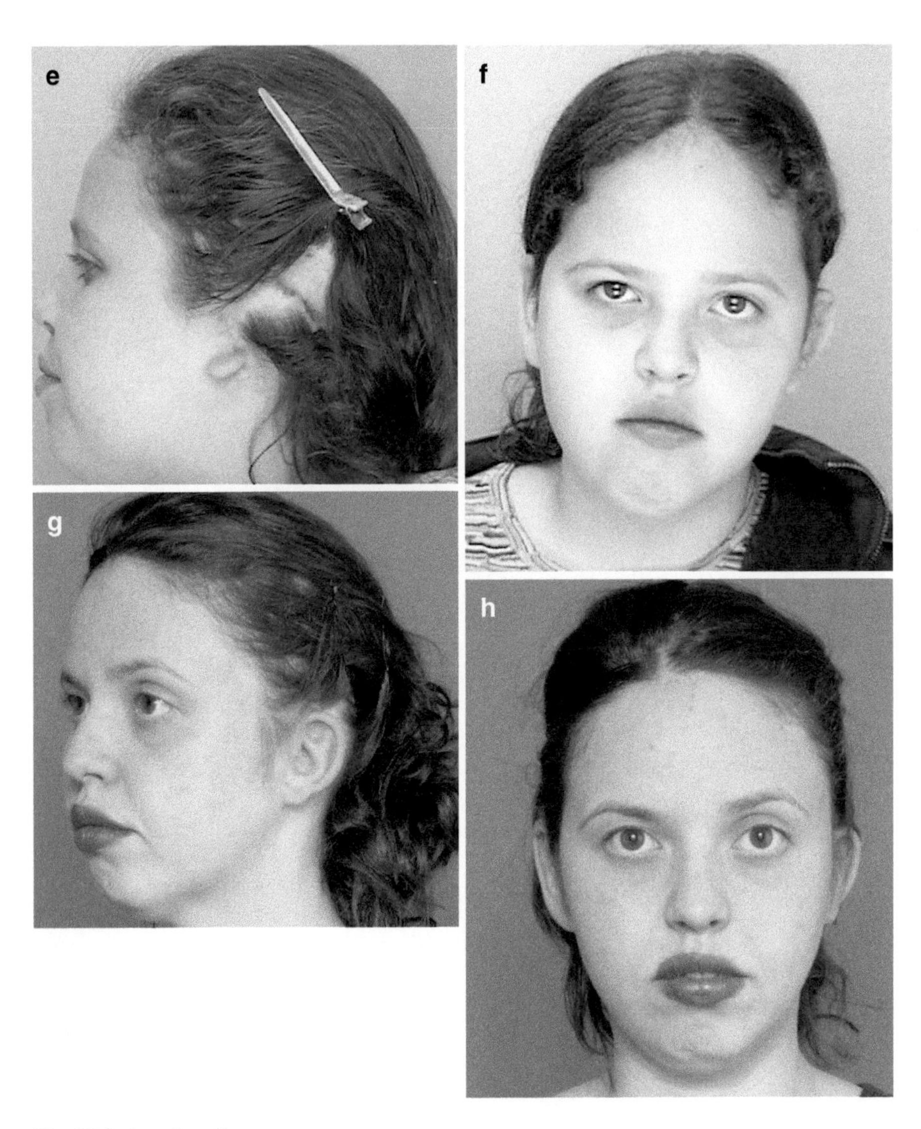

Fig. 13.5 (continued)

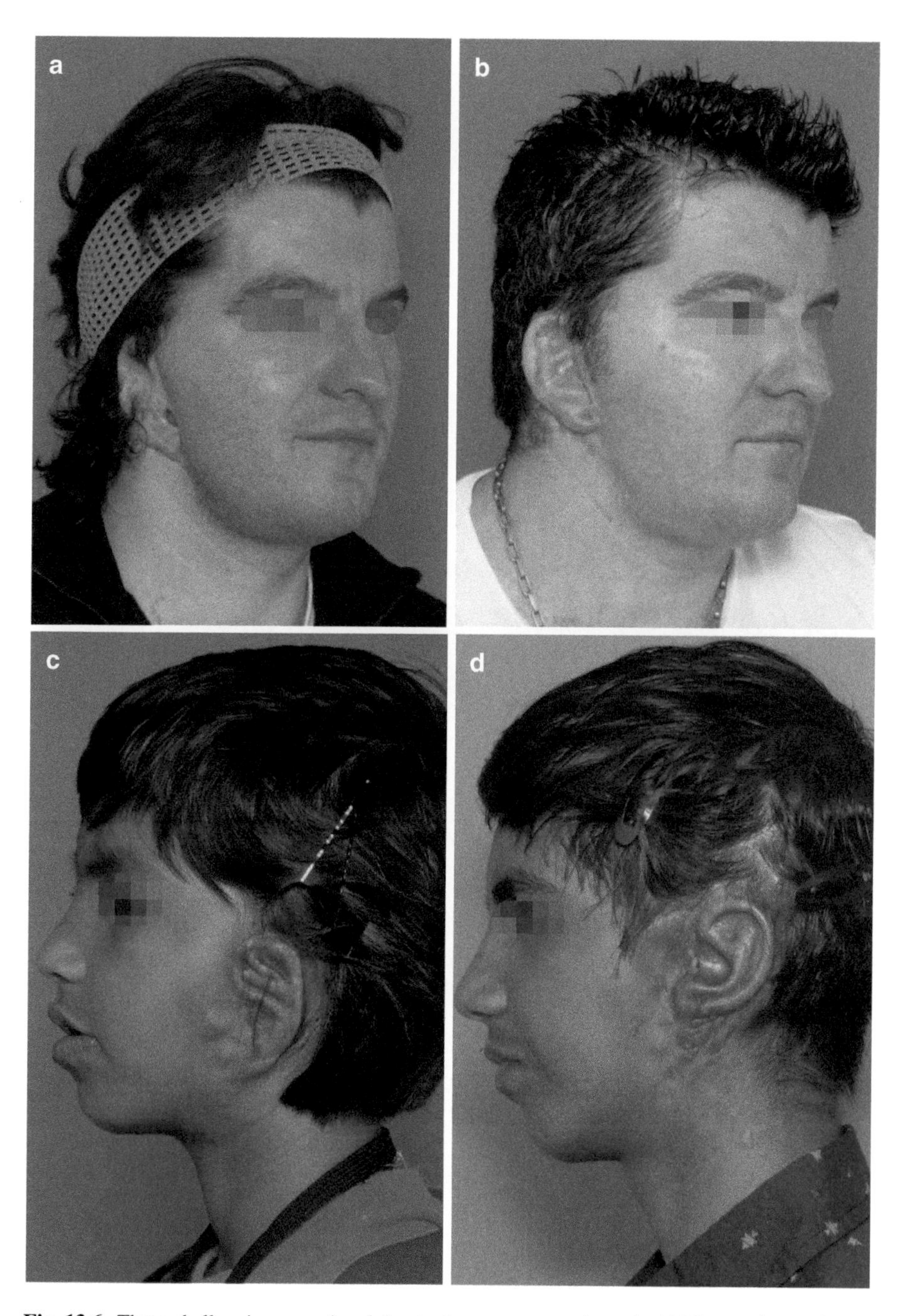

Fig. 13.6 Three challenging cases involving tertiary reconstructions. (**a, b**) The gentleman had at least three prior ear reconstruction attempts with rib cartilage and had extensive scarring. (**c–e**) The second patient had a poorly positioned rib construct, which was likely placed low to avoid the hairline. It was removed and a new construct was placed in the correct anatomic location and position as shown (**e**). (**f, g**) The last patient is a female who had multiple ear cartilage reconstruction attempts by several surgeons (**f**). She finally underwent a polyethylene ear reconstruction. Note the improved anatomic position and overall definition in the 3-month postoperative outcome (**g**)

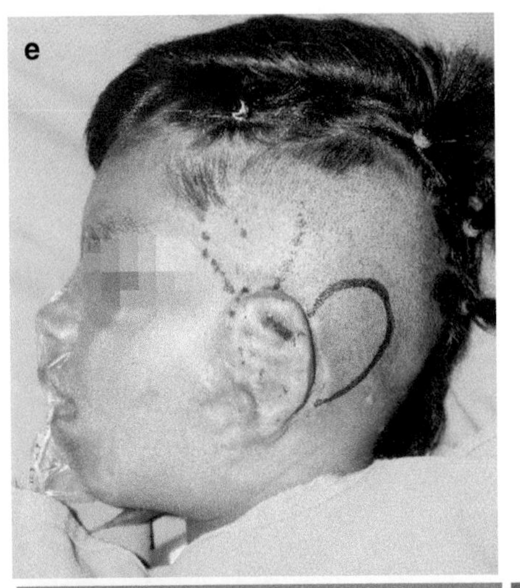

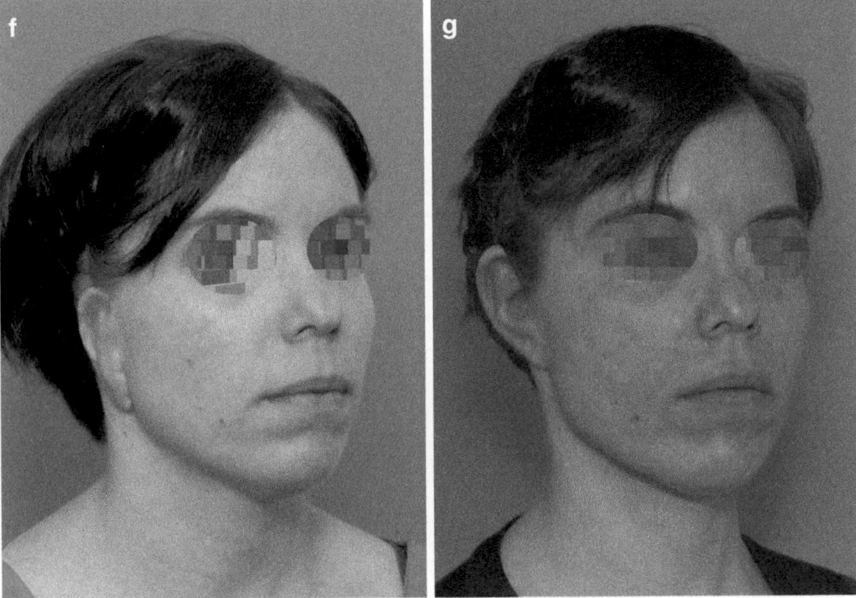

Fig. 13.6 (continued)

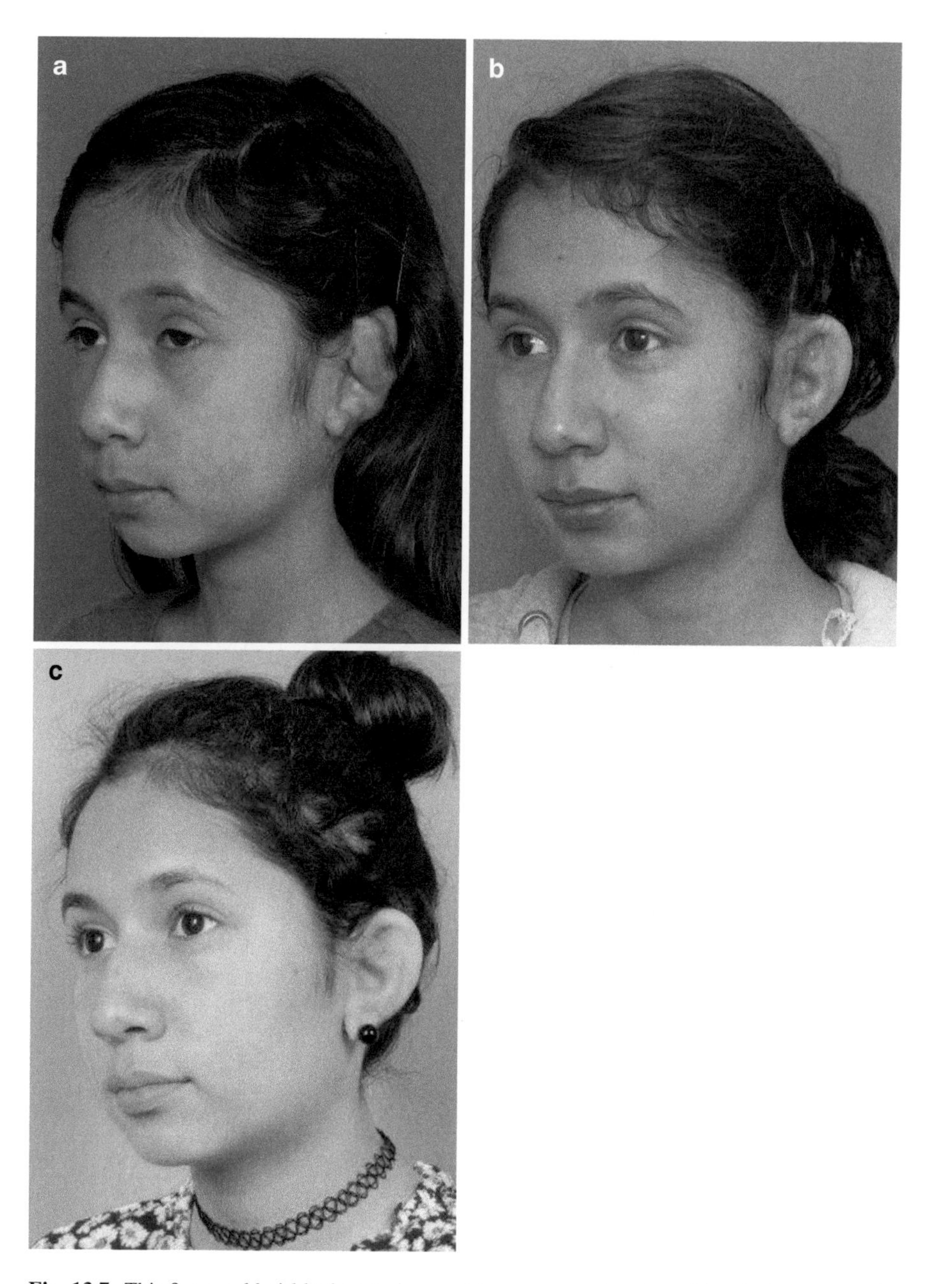

Fig. 13.7 This 9-year-old girl had a previous autologous reconstruction with soft tissue necrosis covered with a TPF flap. (**a**) She underwent polyethylene reconstruction using an inferiorly based occipital flap. (**b**, **c**) Outcomes at 1 year and 4 years postoperative, respectively

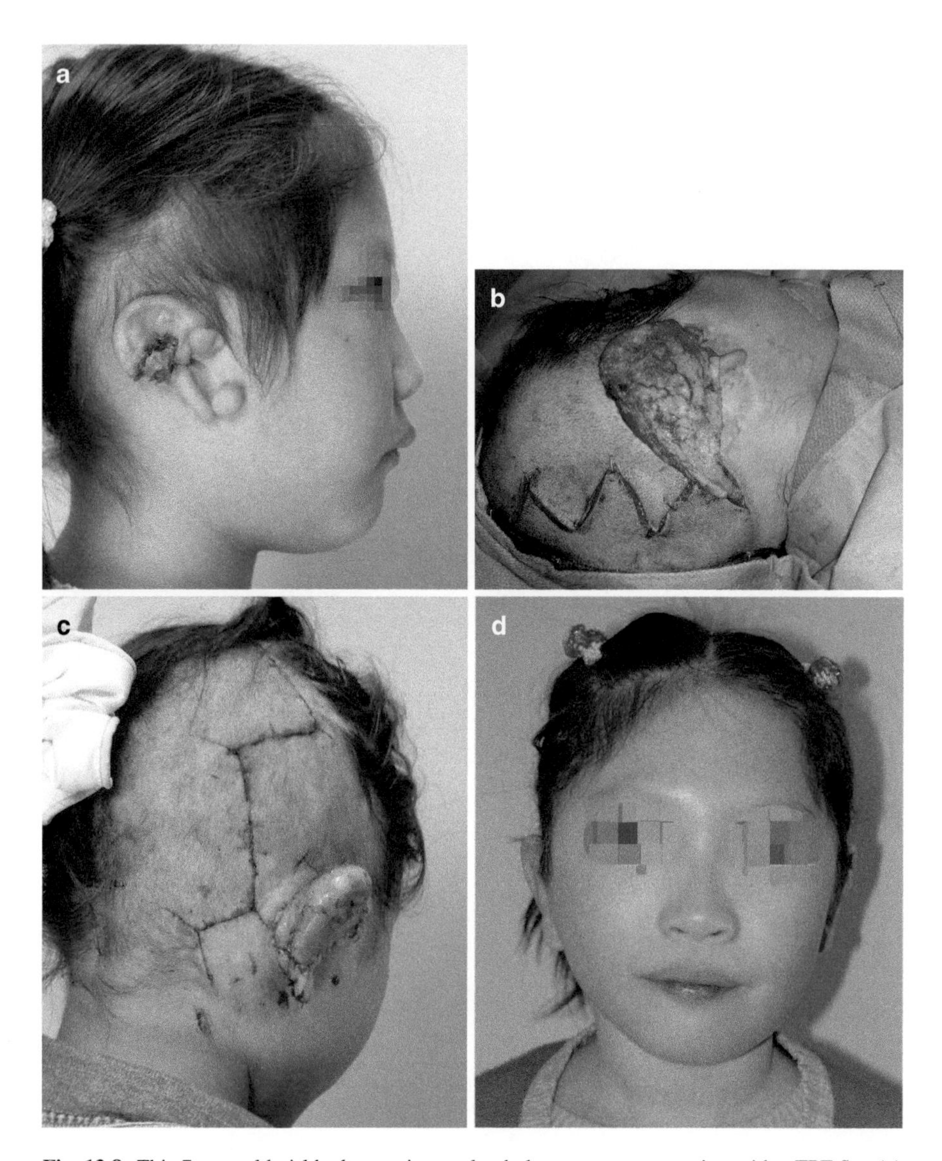

Fig. 13.8 This 7-year-old girl had a previous polyethylene ear reconstruction with a TPF flap (**a**) which failed. An occipital-based flap was utilized to complete a secondary reconstruction (**b–d**). The incision scar is well hidden in the occipital region (**e**)

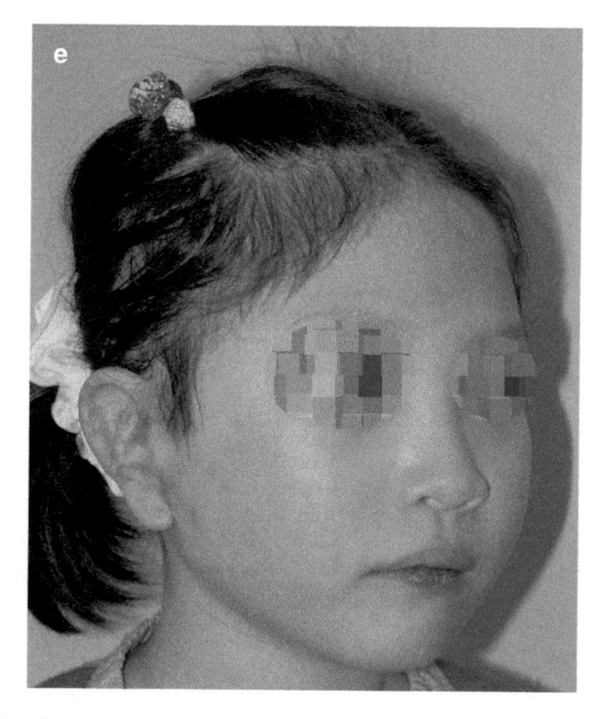

Fig. 13.8 (continued)

removal of the implant and new implant placement under a well-vascularized fascial flap. Exposures may be insidious and difficult to detect; in Fig. 13.13a–f, a small exposure in a reconstruction is highlighted. This patient required implant replacement with an occipital flap, and the outcome with several years of follow-up is shown

Conclusion

Secondary salvage of reconstructed patients offers a complex variety of challenges. Managing the patients' complicated anatomy, the surgical plan, and the social context is key to obtaining reasonable outcomes. Importantly, the patient and surgeon must carry out a thorough dialogue to discuss expectations prior to operating, as often there is a disconnection in expectations between the surgeon and patient.

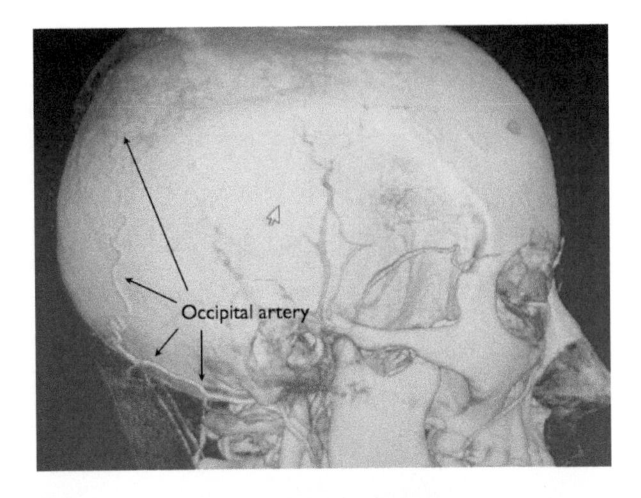

Fig. 13.9 CT angiogram demonstrating the course of the occipital artery

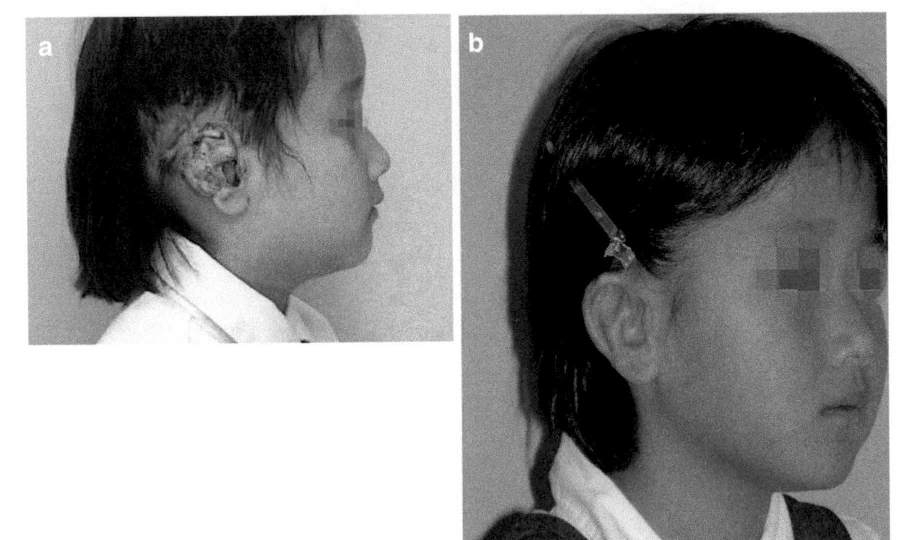

Fig. 13.10 (**a, b**) This 4-year old patient had a polyethylene implant placed by an inexperienced surgeon with necrosis and attempted secondary coverage with a local scalp flap. We removed the implant and reconstructed the ear 6 months later with a new PPE implant covered with an occipital fascia flap and skin graft

These patients may have had disappointing results previously, and this may lead to some hesitation to undergo secondary revision surgery. The pHDPE or alloplastic reconstruction is useful for secondary revision as it requires no secondary donor site, it is performed as a single-stage procedure in the outpatient setting, and it is less painful than rib. The outcomes from secondary revision are usually not as good as primary reconstruction, and patients again must be counseled that their results will not be the same as primary reconstruction patients, but generally patients have very good levels of satisfaction with these reconstructions.

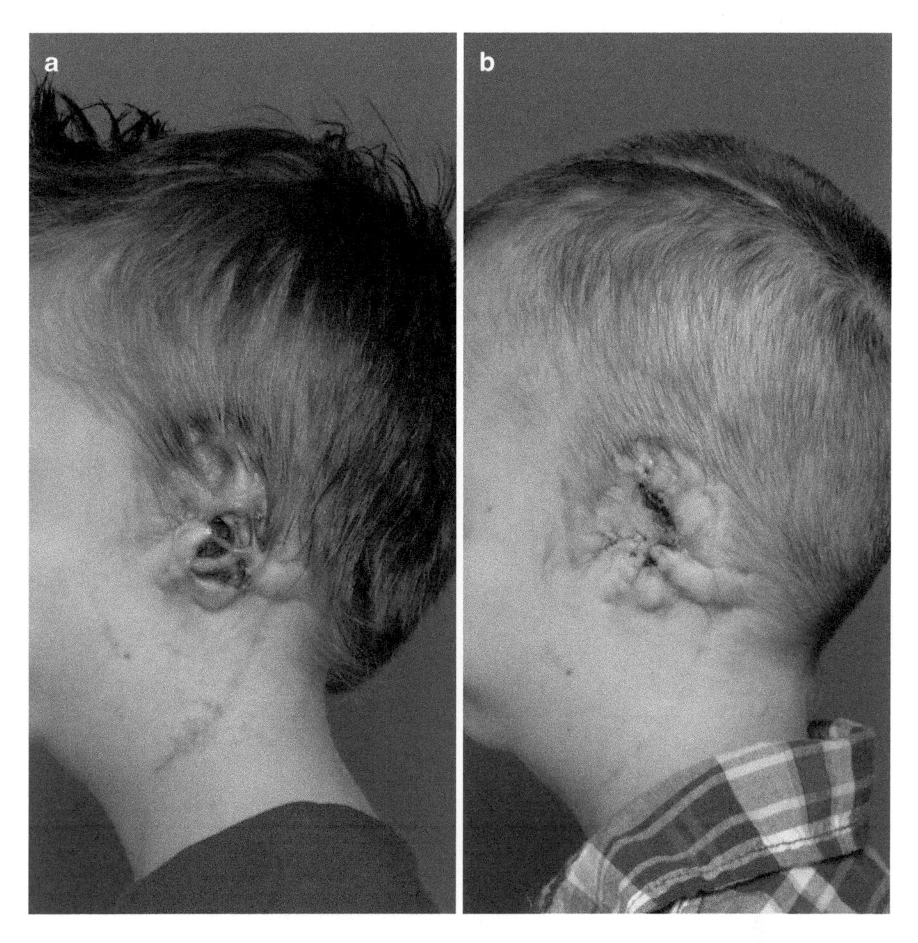

Fig. 13.11 Patient with bilateral microtia seen with PPE implant exposure secondary to TPF failure by an inexperienced surgeon. Multiple secondary attempts at coverage were made using local flaps (**a**). We removed the implant (**b**, **c**) at the time of the patient's right implant ear reconstruction (**e**, **f**). Six moths later, we performed a successful left polyethylene ear reconstruction (**d**) with an occipital flap

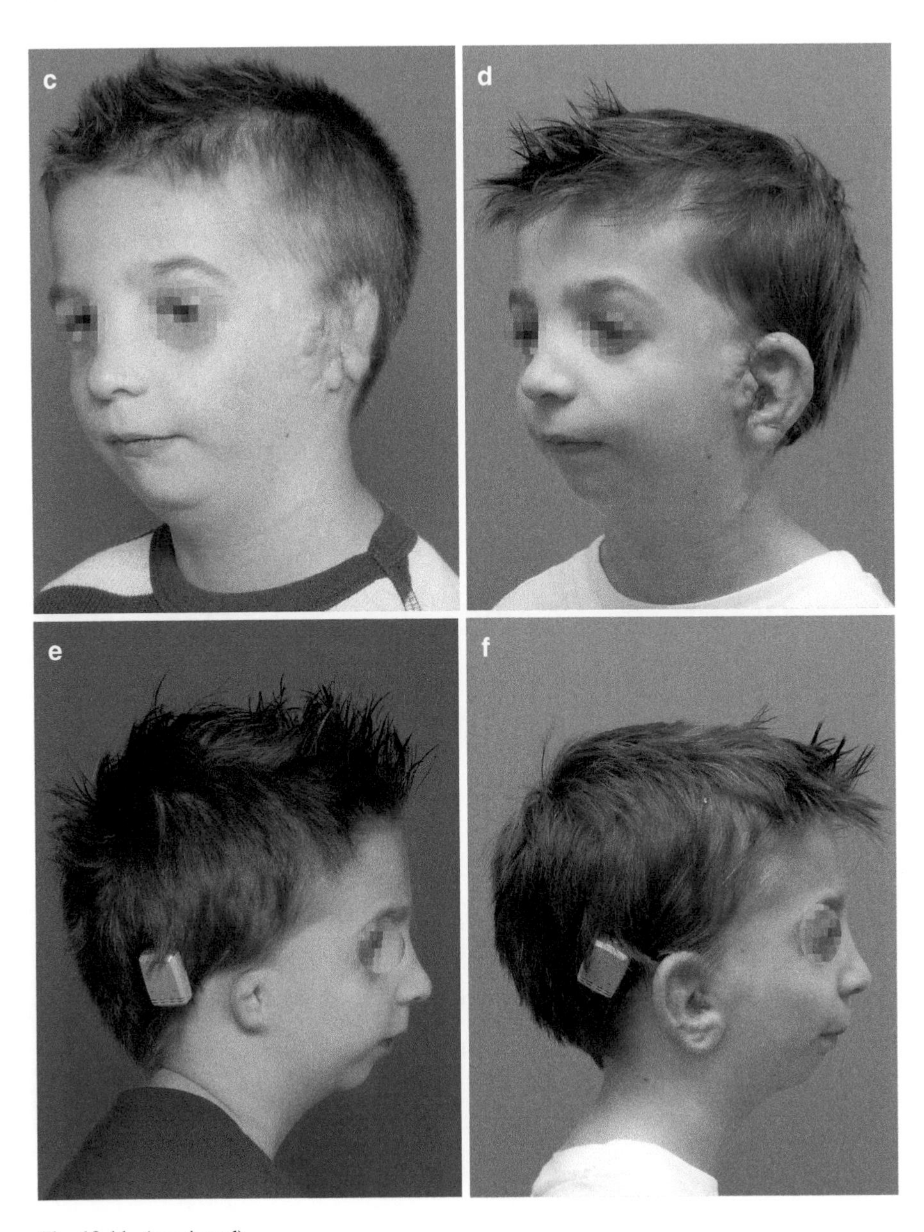

Fig. 13.11 (continued)

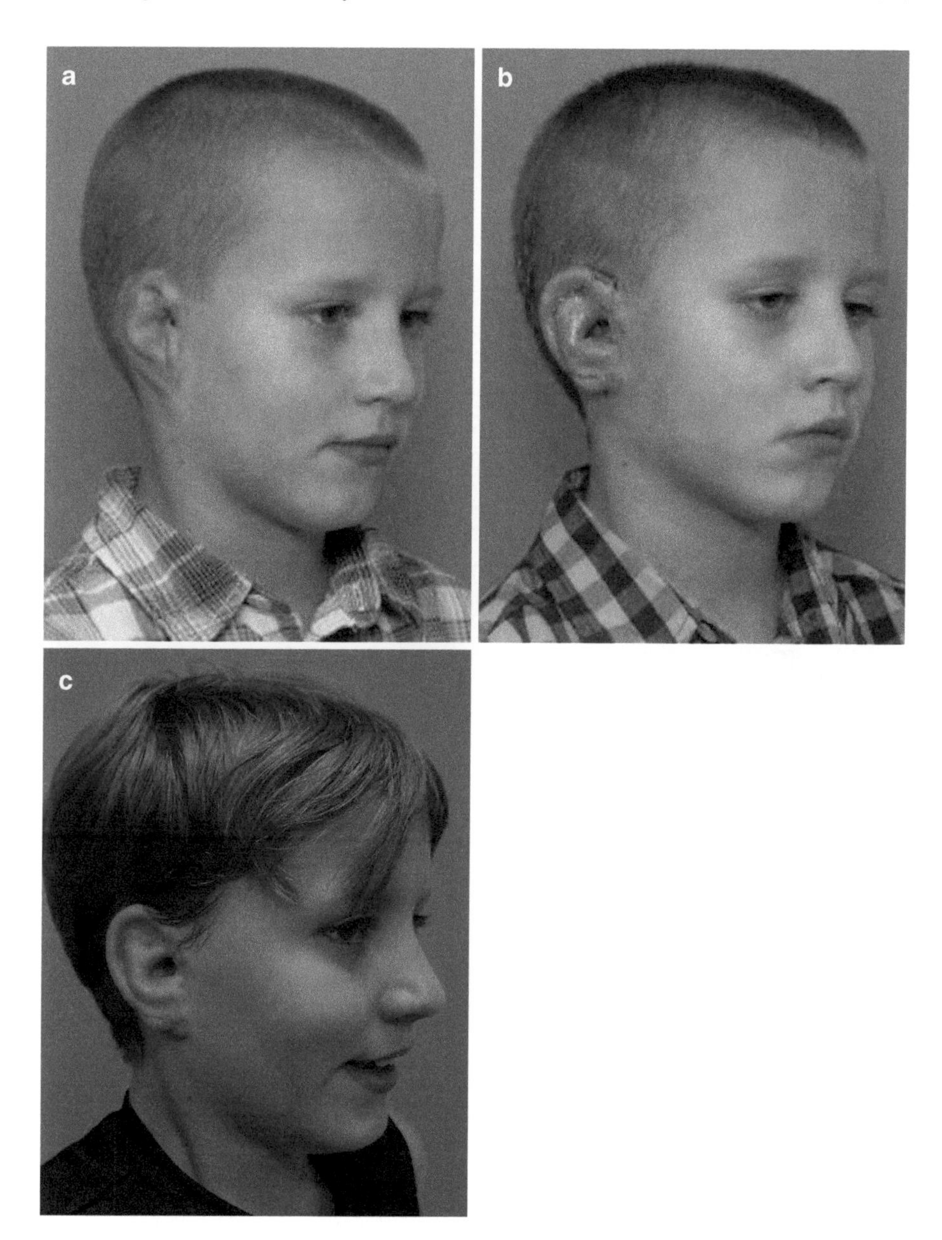

Fig. 13.12 This is an 8-year-old boy who underwent subcutaneous placement of a right polyethylene implant (**a**). We removed the implant and performed a full ear reconstruction with a new implant covered by a TPF flap (**b**). His 2-year follow-up is shown in (**c**)

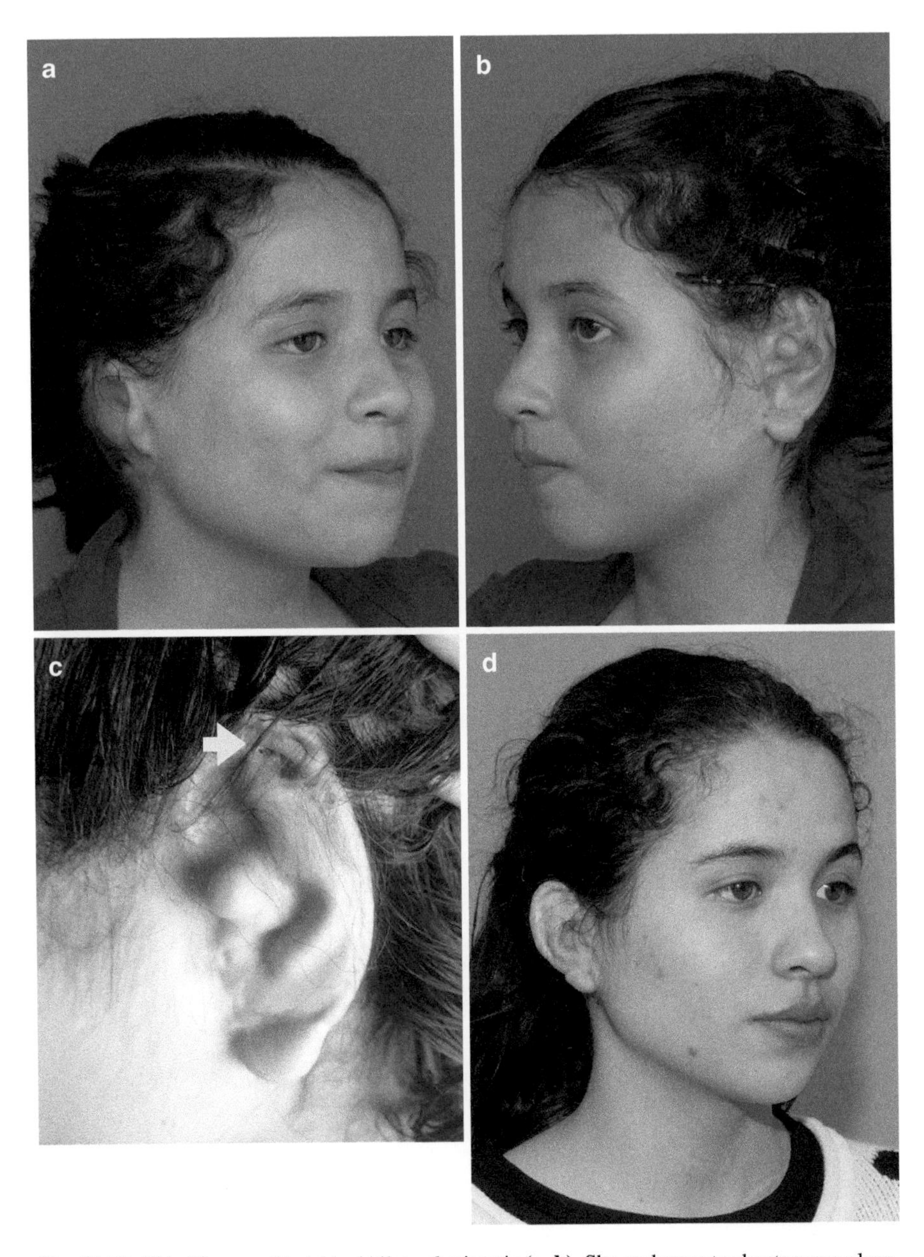

Fig. 13.13 This 13-year-old girl had bilateral microtia (**a**, **b**). She underwent subcutaneous placement of a left polyethylene implant following tissue expansion and had no surgery on the right side. Extrusion was noted on the left side (**c**). Similar to the patient in Fig. 13.12**a**–**c**, we performed a salvage ear reconstruction on the left side using a polyethylene implant and a TPF flap. She also underwent successfully primary ear reconstruction on the right side. Her 4-year follow-up is shown in (**d**–**f**)

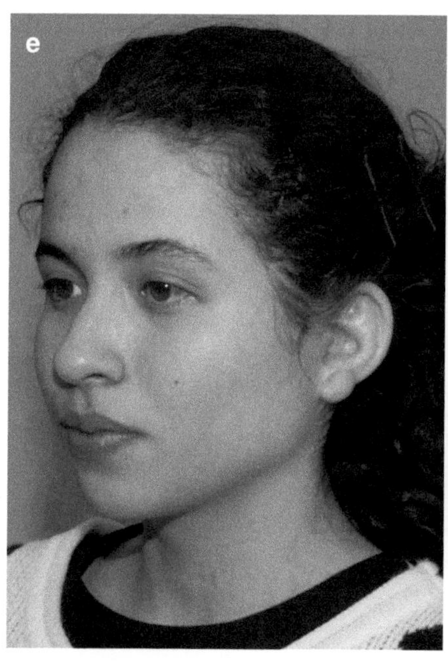

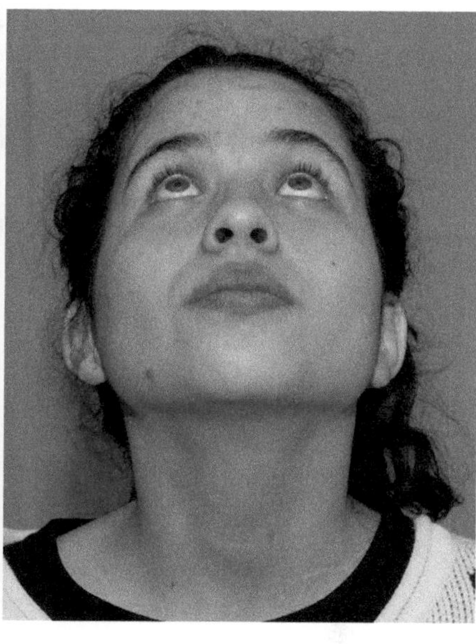

Fig. 13.13 (continued)

References

1. Im DD, Paskhover B, Staffenberg DA, Jarrahy R. Current management of microtia: a national survey. Aesthet Plast Surg. 2013;37:402–8.
2. Bly RA, Bhrany AD, Murakami CS, Sie KC. Microtia reconstruction. Facial Plast Surg Clin North Am. 2016;24:577–91.
3. Baluch N, Nagata S, Park C, Wilkes GH, Reinisch J, Kasrai L, et al. Auricular reconstruction for microtia: a review of available methods. Plast Surg (Oakville, Ont). 2014;22:39–43.
4. Giot JP, Labbe D, Soubeyrand E, Pacini R, Guillou-Jamard MR, Compère JF, et al. Prosthetic reconstruction of the auricle: indications, techniques, and results. Semin Plast Surg. 2011;25:265–72.
5. Choi KJ, Sajisevi MB, McClennen J, Kaylie DM. Image-guided placement of osseointegrated implants for challenging auricular, orbital, and rhinectomy defects. Ann Otol Rhinol Laryngol. 2016;125:801–7.
6. Nagata S. A new method of total reconstruction of the auricle for microtia. Plast Reconstr Surg. 1993;92:187–201.
7. Nagata S. Modification of the stages in total reconstruction of the auricle: part IV. Ear elevation for the constructed auricle. Plast Reconstr Surg. 1994;93:254–66; discussion 267–258.
8. Reinisch J. Ear reconstruction in young children. Facial Plast Surg FPS. 2015;31:600–3.
9. Reinisch JF, Lewin S. Ear reconstruction using a porous polyethylene framework and temporoparietal fascia flap. Facial Plast Surg: FPS. 2009;25:181–9.
10. Romo T III, Fozo MS, Sclafani AP. Microtia reconstruction using a porous polyethylene framework. Facial Plast Surg. 2000;16:15–22.
11. Romo T III, Morris LG, Reitzen SD, Ghossaini SN, Wazen JJ, Kohan D. Reconstruction of congenital microtia-atresia: outcomes with the medpor/bone-anchored hearing aid–approach. Ann Plast Surg. 2009;62:384–9.

12. Akter F, Mennie JC, Stewart K, Bulstrode N. Patient reported outcome measures in microtia surgery. J Plast Reconstr Aesthet Surg: JPRAS. 2017;70:416–24.
13. Federspil PA. Auricular prostheses. Adv Otorhinolaryngol. 2010;68:65–80.
14. Williams JD, Romo T 3rd, Sclafani AP, Cho H. Porous high-density polyethylene implants in auricular reconstruction. Arch Otolaryngol Head Neck Surg. 1997;123:578–83.
15. Wellisz T. Reconstruction of the burned external ear using a Medpor porous polyethylene pivoting helix framework. Plast Reconstr Surg. 1993;91:811–8.
16. Wilkes GH, Wong J, Guilfoyle R. Microtia reconstruction. Plast Reconstr Surg. 2014;134:464e–79e.

Chapter 14
Non-microtia Ear Reconstruction

Youssef Tahiri and John F. Reinisch

Introduction

Although this book focuses on microtia, we have included this chapter on reconstruction of the non-microtia ear because the method used to restore a large acquired loss of an ear can be similar to those used for microtia.

Patients with an acquired absence of their ear differ from patients with congenital microtia in several ways.

The first difference is that most patients with a traumatic or postsurgical loss of their ear usually have normal hearing so that the functional aspect of auricular reconstruction does not need to be addressed.

A second difference relates to the quality of the available skin and underlying fascia. With microtia, there is supple, unscarred, color-matched mastoid skin that can be used for cutaneous coverage of the reconstructed ear. The temporoparietal fascia beneath the scalp is intact. In the non-microtic situation, there is scarring and less local skin available. The TPF fascia may not be present or its blood supply may have been disrupted [1, 2].

Finally, microtia patient are younger and are both male and female. They never had a normal ear. Patients with an acquired absence are older and usually male. They have sustained the loss of what was a normal structure. The resulting deformity not only causes an external asymmetry but also serves as an internal reminder of what is usually a psychologically traumatic event [3]. Moreover, acquired defects

Y. Tahiri (✉)
Plastic and Reconstructive Surgery, Cedars-Sinai Medical Center, Los Angeles, CA, USA
e-mail: Youssef.Tahiri@cshs.org

J. F. Reinisch (✉)
Keck School of Medicine, University of Souther California, Los Angeles, CA, USA

Craniofacial and Pediatric Plastic Surgery, Cedars Sinai Medical Center, Los Angeles, CA, USA

© Springer Nature Switzerland AG 2019

J. F. Reinisch, Y. Tahiri (eds.), *Modern Microtia Reconstruction*,
https://doi.org/10.1007/978-3-030-16387-7_14

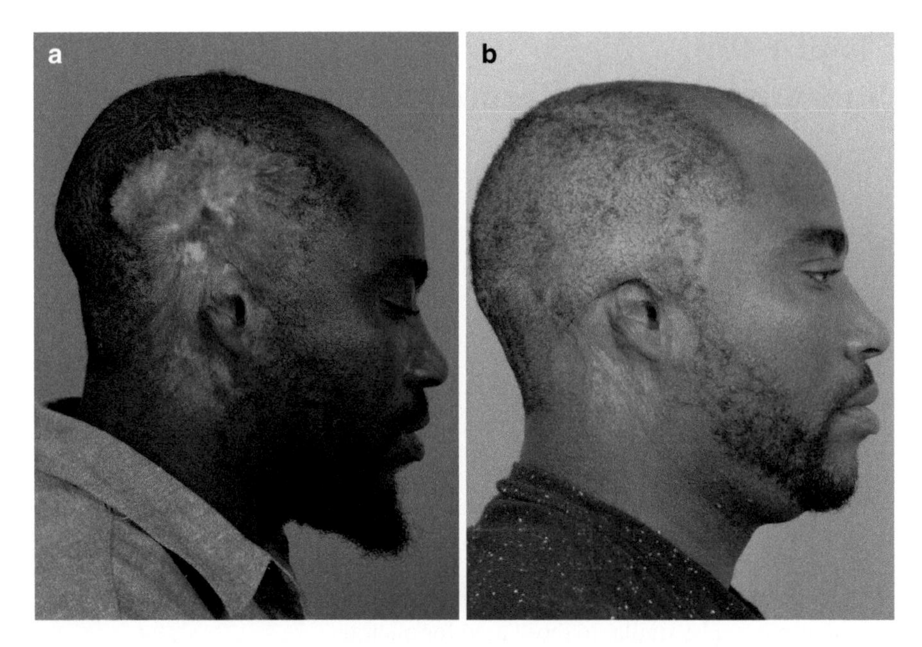

Fig. 14.1 A 33-year-old man who sustained a burn as a child to the right scalp and ear (**a**). He cannot hide his acquired ear deformity because of his surrounding alopecia. We performed a scalp reconstruction using staged expansion and adjacent tissue rearrangement (**b**)

generally occur in patients who, because of employment or alopecia, are often less able to cover their deformity with their hair. See Fig. 14.1a, b.

Causes of Acquired Ear Loss

Acquired auricular defects can present with partial or total loss of the ear structures. In this chapter, we will focus mostly on large acquired auricular defects requiring total ear reconstruction.

The most common causes of large acquired ear defects requiring a full ear reconstruction include sharp traumas/amputations, burns, and defects following tumor resections. In the following sections, we will discuss the challenges associated with auricular reconstruction in each setting.

Sharp Trauma/Amputation

Traumatic amputations most often occur following car accidents or cuts with sharp objects. Car accidents are often associated with avulsion-type injuries of the ear and surrounding scalp. Partial or total amputation of the ear can also happen due to a sharp instrument in the setting of accidents and physical fights.

Ear replantations are notoriously challenging, and most attempts to replant an amputated ear will fail. Some authors report excellent results of ear replantation; however, failure is very common, and thus any attempt at replantation must consider that success is unlikely and may result in scars that limit later reconstructive attempts. Replantation failures are often due to lack of finding necessary veins for drainage [4]. Unfortunately, an attempt at ear replantation can cause additional incisions/scars, while some important fascial and/or vascular structures that could be useful for secondary reconstruction may be sacrificed [5].

When the amputated ear is available, it is difficult to convince a patient to discard the part without an attempt at replacement. It is a challenging dilemma, since the use of the superficial temporal artery to revascularize the replanted ear precludes the use of this pedicle and a well-vascularized TPF flap for secondary reconstruction.

Reattaching the amputated ear as a composite graft is extremely unlikely to work. However, it does not disrupt the surrounding soft tissues and vessels; thus, it does not compromise a secondary ear reconstruction. It may also have a positive psychological impact on the patient.

An alternative to composite grafting or replantation include burying the cartilaginous framework under skin flaps or even covering it with a TPF flap. Some authors suggest removing the entire skin from the amputated ear and inserting the cartilaginous framework under postauricular skin flaps [6, 7] (Fig. 14.2a–i). In our experience, this does not work well since the thin and pliable cartilaginous framework does not maintain its structure against the contracting scars. The same applies for the proponents of inserting an cartilaginous framework (from the amputated ear) under a TPF flap. We feel this does not provide an adequate reconstruction and aesthetic outcome, while the important TPF flap that could be useful for secondary reconstruction is sacrificed.

Some authors reported successful ear salvage with removal of the posteromedial skin of the amputated ear and fenestration of the cartilage. The retroauricular skin is excised, and the fenestrated portion of the ear is applied on the retroauricular bed. This technique depends on the cartilage and anterior ear skin being revascularized as a graft from the posterior bed via the fenestrations.

As far as we are concerned, when faced with an amputated ear, our preferred approach would be a replantation without additional scarring or additional incisions and using a vessel different from the superficial temporal artery. This has been also encouraged in some reports [8]. In the event of failed ear replantation, we recommend a total ear reconstruction using a porous high-density polyethylene implant covered by a vascularized temporal parietal fascia flap and FTSG (Fig. 14.3a–d).

Burns

Ears can also be severely damaged by burn trauma. Burns cause ear damage via one of two processes: (1) a suppurative chondritis due to a severe secondary infection following the burn that causes destruction of the cartilage (2) an

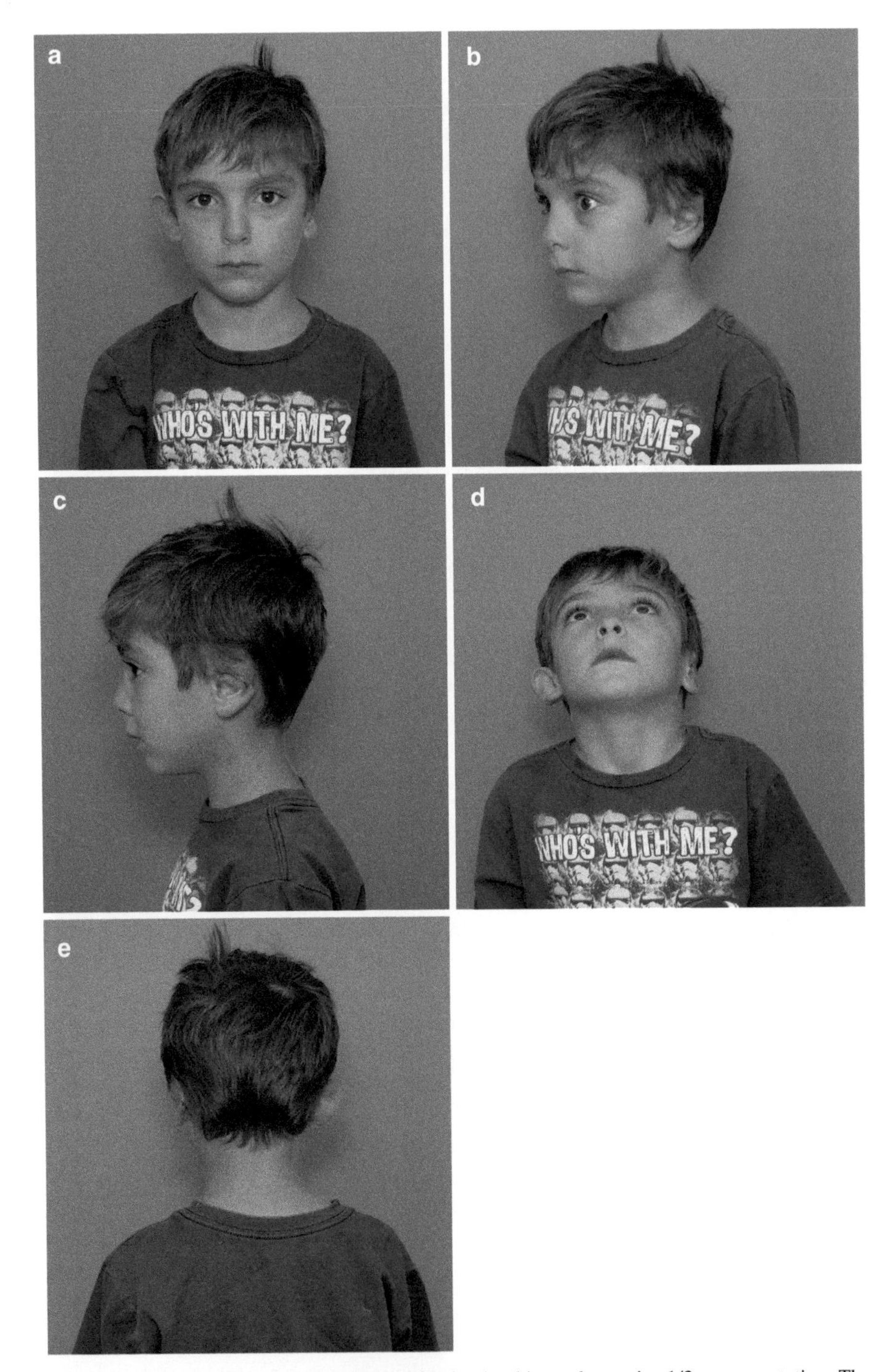

Fig. 14.2 (**a–i**) A 6-year-old boy who sustained a dog bite and superior 1/3 ear amputation. The amputated part was denuded from the skin. The cartilage was then attached to the remaining ear placed under a postauricular scalp flap. The cartilage and the flap were then elevated as one unit. The post mastoid/parietal scalp was advanced to close the donor site, and a groin full-thickness skin graft was used to cover the posterior aspect of the ear

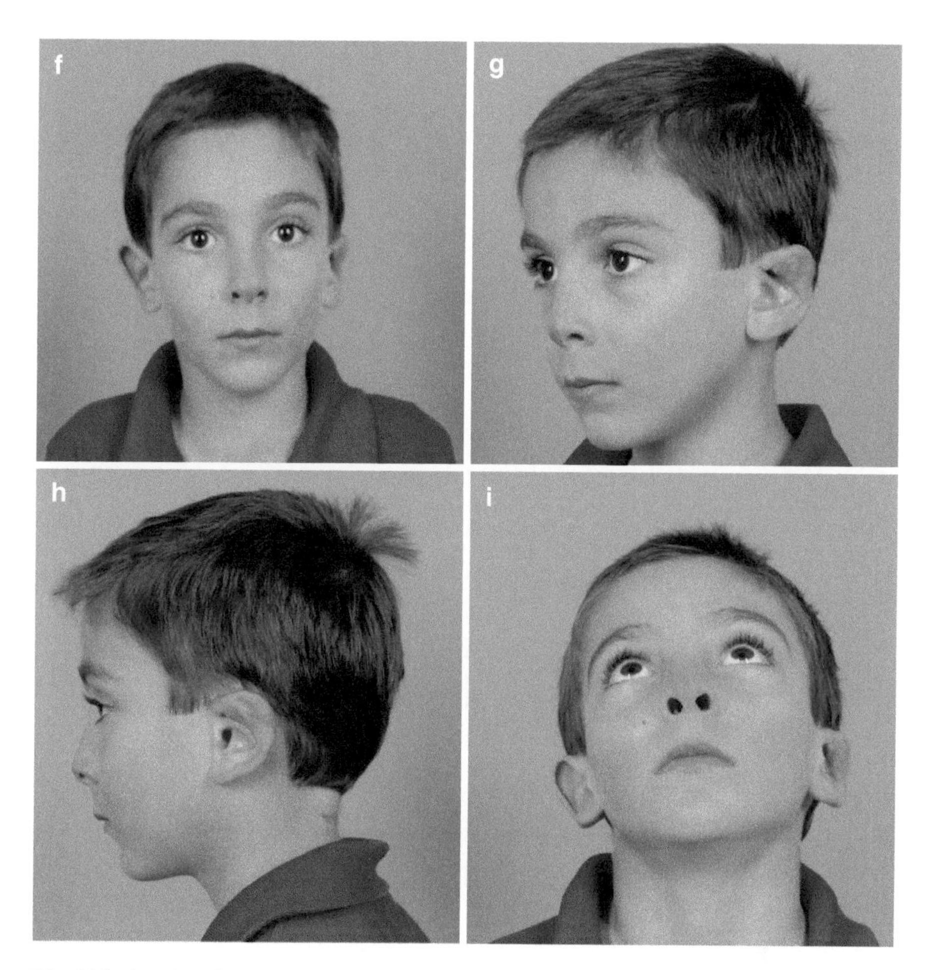

Fig. 14.2 (continued

auto-chondrectomy due to the full-thickness burn associated with the direct thermal injury [9]. Most common causes of burn include fire, hot liquids, chemical liquids, and frostbite.

Patients with burned ears often seek reconstruction once they are healed and they are unsatisfied by their ear. The ear is often distorted and severely scared, with a significant loss of definition, domain, and skin quality.

In the instances where the superficial skin is burned but not the cartilage, the ear can be salvaged by simply debriding the necrotic skin and applying a skin graft on the healthy cartilage [10]. We focus here on more severe burn causing significant auricular damage.

Figure 14.4a–h illustrates a 3-year-old boy who sustained an electrical burn to his left ear causing significant damage and leading a near total loss of his ear. We performed on him a total ear reconstruction using a pHDPE implant covered with a TPF flap. The remaining cartilage was discarded, while the skin was harvested as a FTSG to cover part of the reconstructed ear.

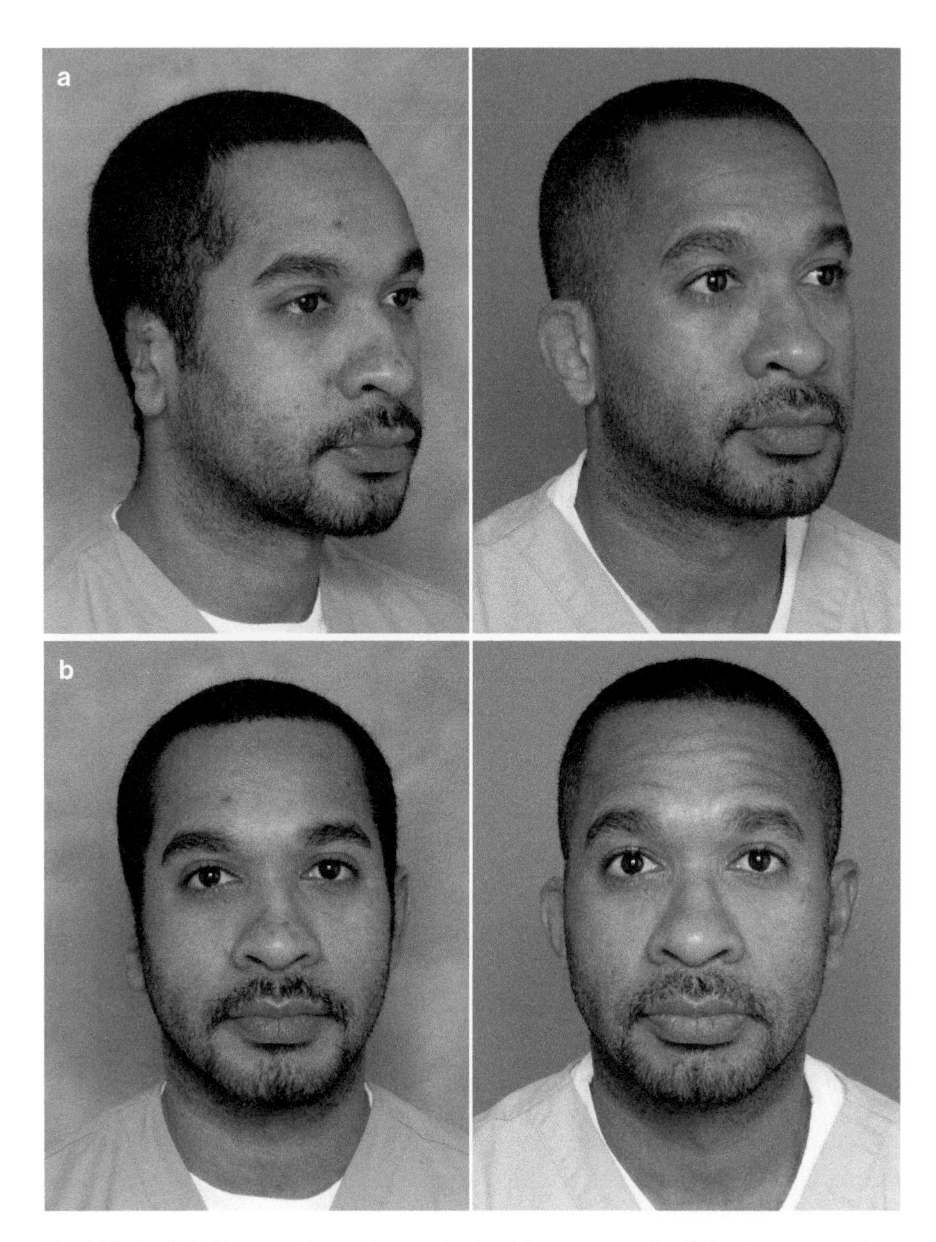

Fig. 14.3 (**a–d**) A 36-year-old man who sustained a right ear amputation following a car accident. We performed a right ear reconstruction using a porous high-density polyethylene (pHDPE) implant covered with a vascularized temporoparietal fascia (TPF) flap and full-thickness skin grafts

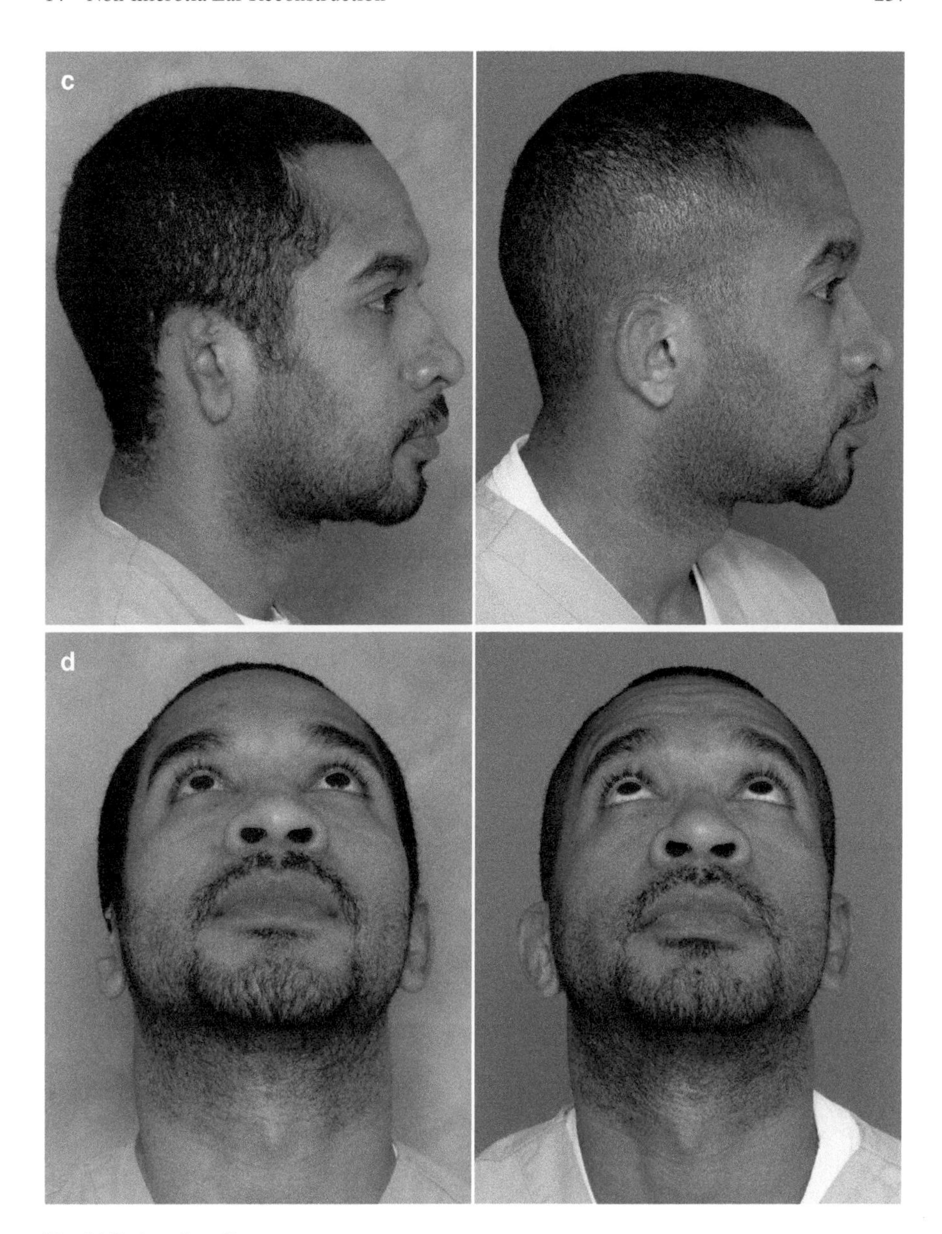

Fig. 14.3 (continued)

Tumors

Ablative surgery for benign and malignant tumors is a common cause of near total auricular defects. The most common skin cancers involving the ear include basal cell carcinoma, squamous cell carcinoma, and melanoma.

Basal cell carcinoma is the most common skin cancer involving the ear. In fact, 90% of all malignant cutaneous lesions in the head and neck region are basal cell carcinomas. It makes up one fifth of neoplasms that involve the ear and the temporal bone [11]. The vast majority of those basal cell carcinomas are located on the auricular helix and periauricular area which are especially susceptible as they are exposed to the most UV light. Moreover, 15% arise in the external auditory canal. Basal cell carcinomas are classified in five different clinical forms: nodular-ulcerative (most common), pigmented, cystic, superficial multicentric, and morphealike.

Squamous cell carcinoma is the second most common skin cancer involving the ear. It originates on the helix and antihelix margins where the skin receives the greatest actinic exposure; but it can arise anywhere on the outer ear and potentially involves the middle ear and the lateral skull base. Diagnosis is usually made on patients in their fifth to sixth decade of life, whereas lesions originating primarily from the external auditory canal generally present 10–15 years earlier. Sun exposure, fair complexion, cold injury, radiation exposure, and chronic infection as well as an association with HPV-induced viral carcinogenesis are among the predisposing factor [11–13].

Approximately 20% of all primary melanomas are located at the head and neck, of which 7–14% are located at the ear's helix and antihelix. Peripheral parts of the ear are more frequently affected. Interestingly, the left ear is more often affected than the right ear. The most accepted theory for this phenomenon is the asymmetric UV dosage in Anglo-Saxon countries with left-hand driven cars. Furthermore, a male predisposition of 61.5–90.5% is reported in the literature with a predisposition for fair-skinned individuals. It can be explained with different hairstyles which correlate with UV exposition [14–19].

In Fig. 14.5a–k, we present a 58-year-old female who was diagnosed with a BCC at the level of her right ear and underwent an amputation of the lower half of her ear and a reconstruction with a radial forearm free flap. Similar to the patient presented in Fig. 14.3a–d, we performed on her a total ear reconstruction using a pHDPE implant covered with a TPF flap. The remaining cartilage was discarded, while the skin was harvested as a FTSG to cover part of the reconstructed ear.

Other Causes

Other less common causes of large acquired defects include human and animal bites, infections from piercing, vascular malformations, chronic trauma from martial arts, and specific diseases such as Hansen's disease (Leprosy), Winkler disease, and lymphocytoma.

In Fig. 14.6a–n, we present a patient that was born with PHACES syndrome. She was born 3 months prematurely. She presented to our office with bilateral ear ulcerations

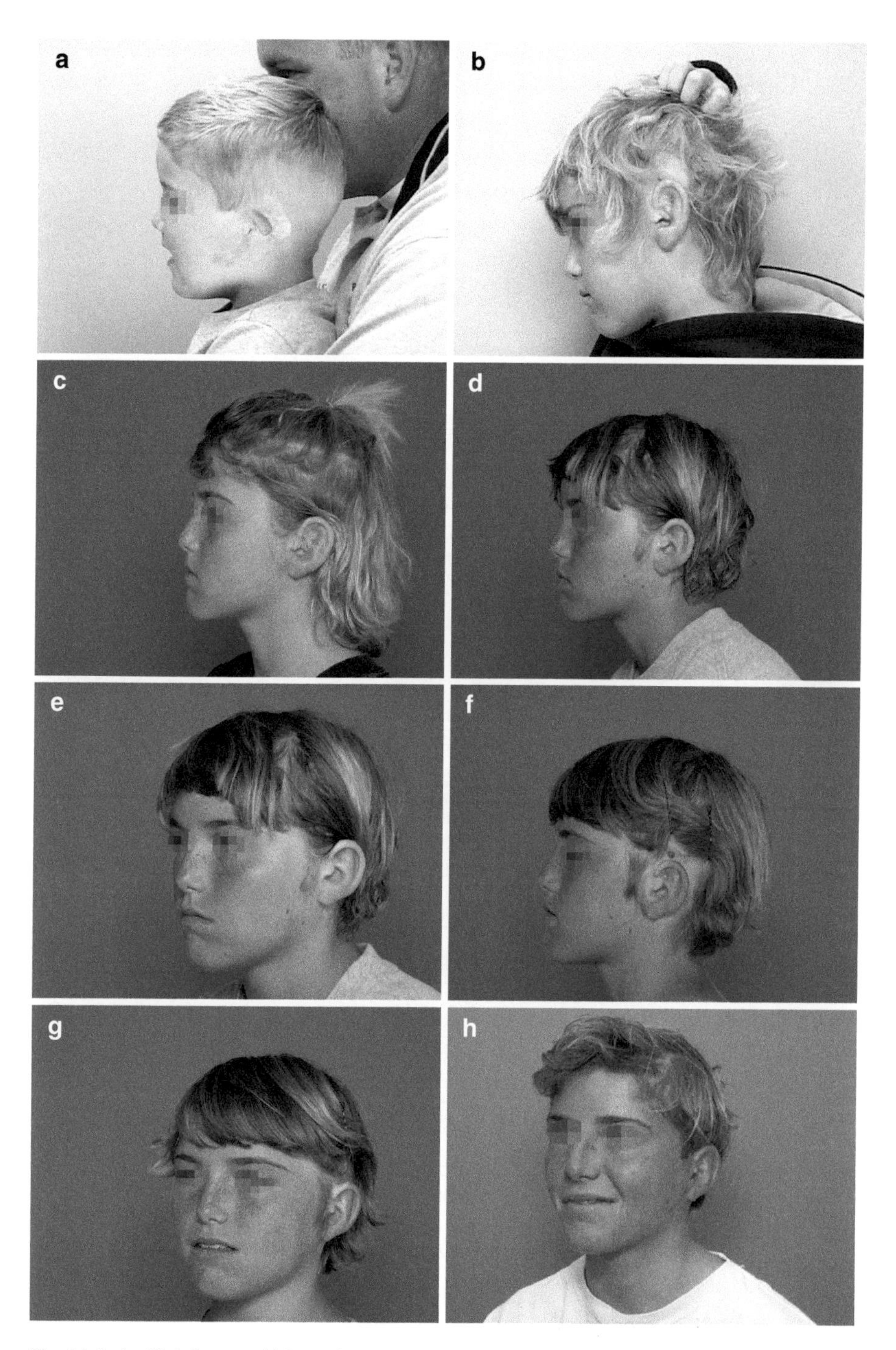

Fig. 14.4 (**a–h**) A 3-year-old boy who sustained an electrical burn to his left ear causing significant damage and leading a near total loss of his ear. We performed on him a total ear reconstruction using a pHDPE implant covered with a TPF flap. The remaining cartilage was discarded, while the skin was harvested as a FTSG to cover part of the reconstructed ear

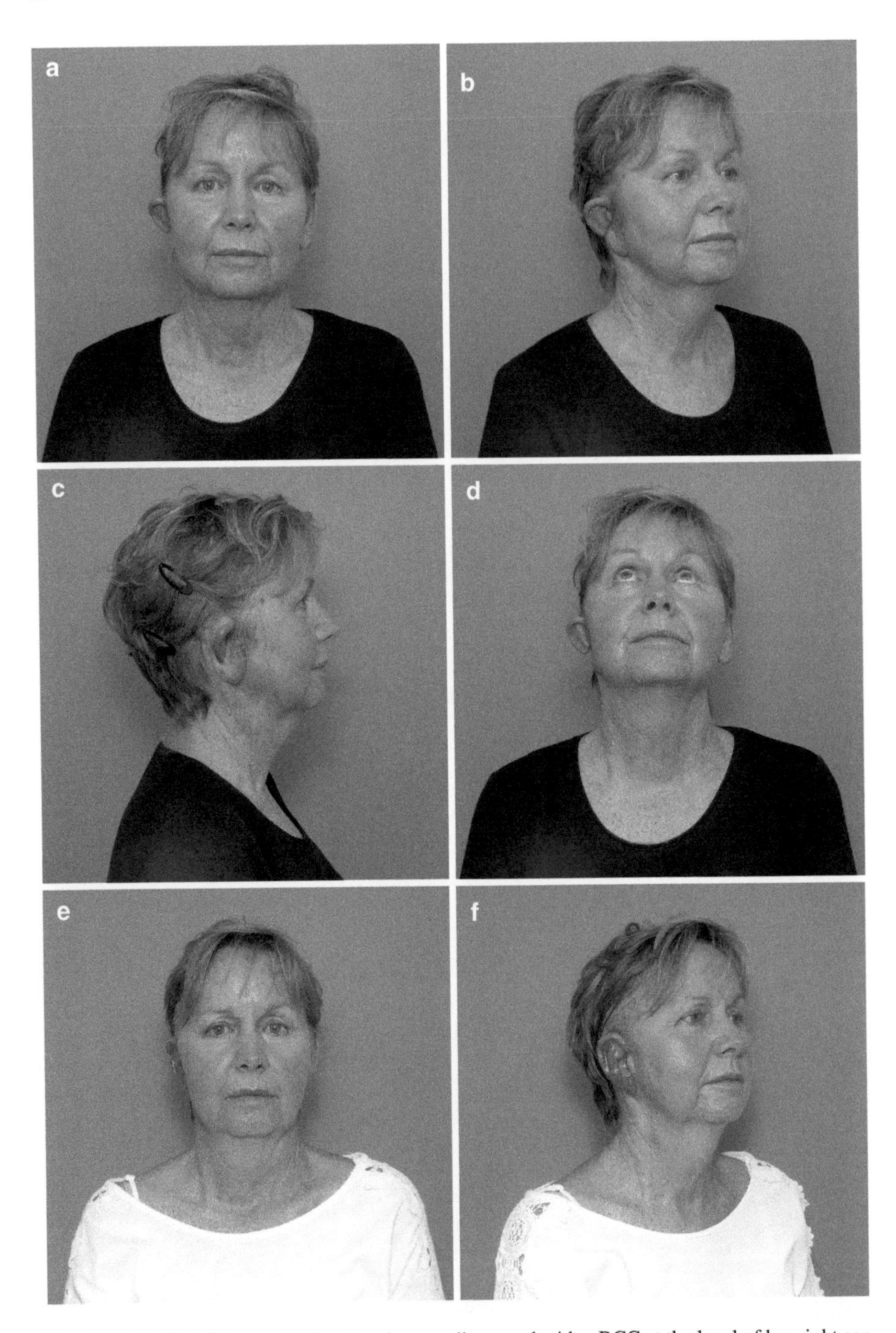

Fig. 14.5 (**a–k**) A 58-year-old female who was diagnosed with a BCC at the level of her right ear and underwent an amputation of the lower half of her ear and a reconstruction with a radial forearm free flap. We performed on her a total ear reconstruction using a pHDPE implant covered with a TPF flap. The remaining cartilage was discarded, while the skin was harvested as a FTSG to cover part of the reconstructed ear

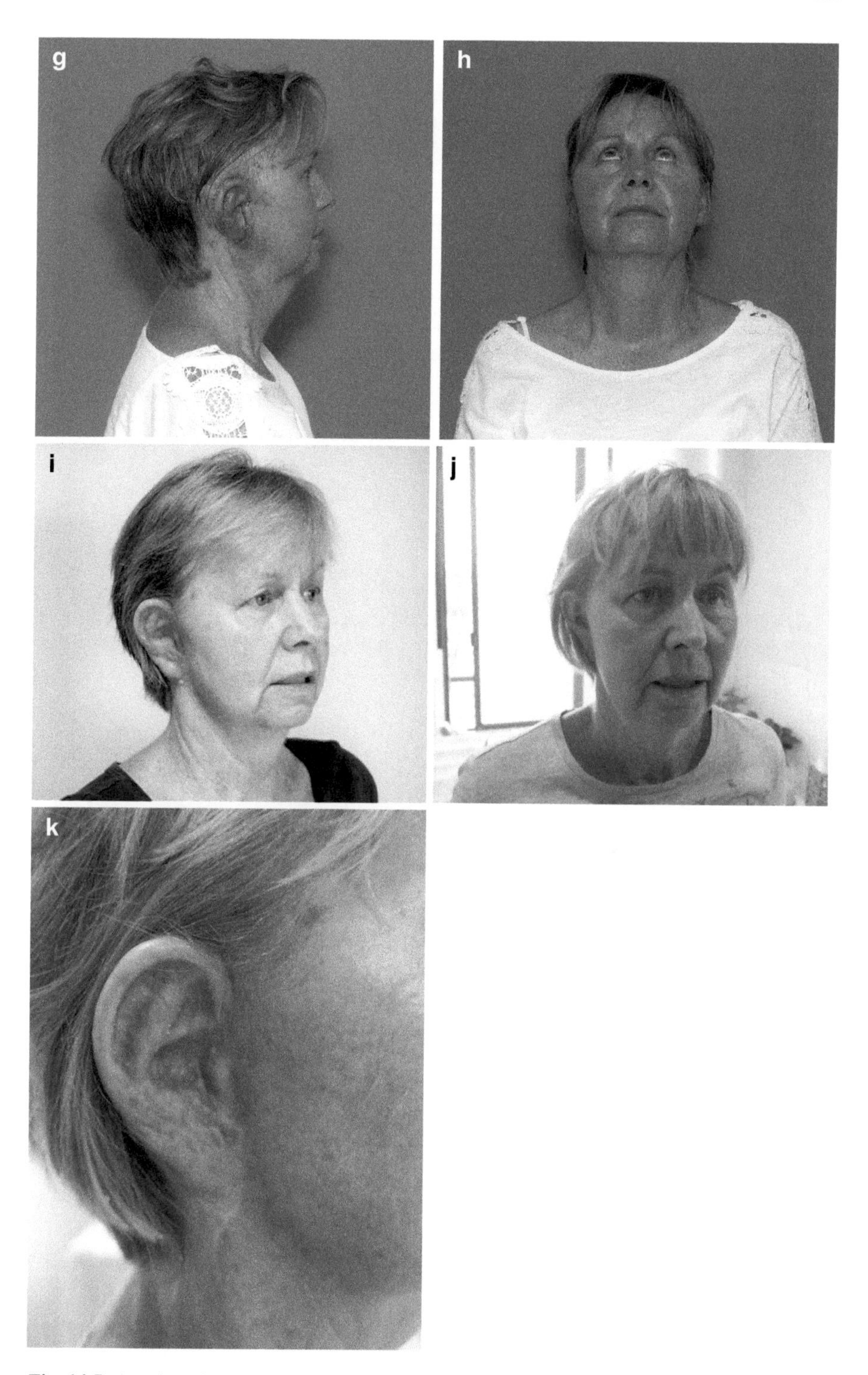

Fig. 14.5 (continued)

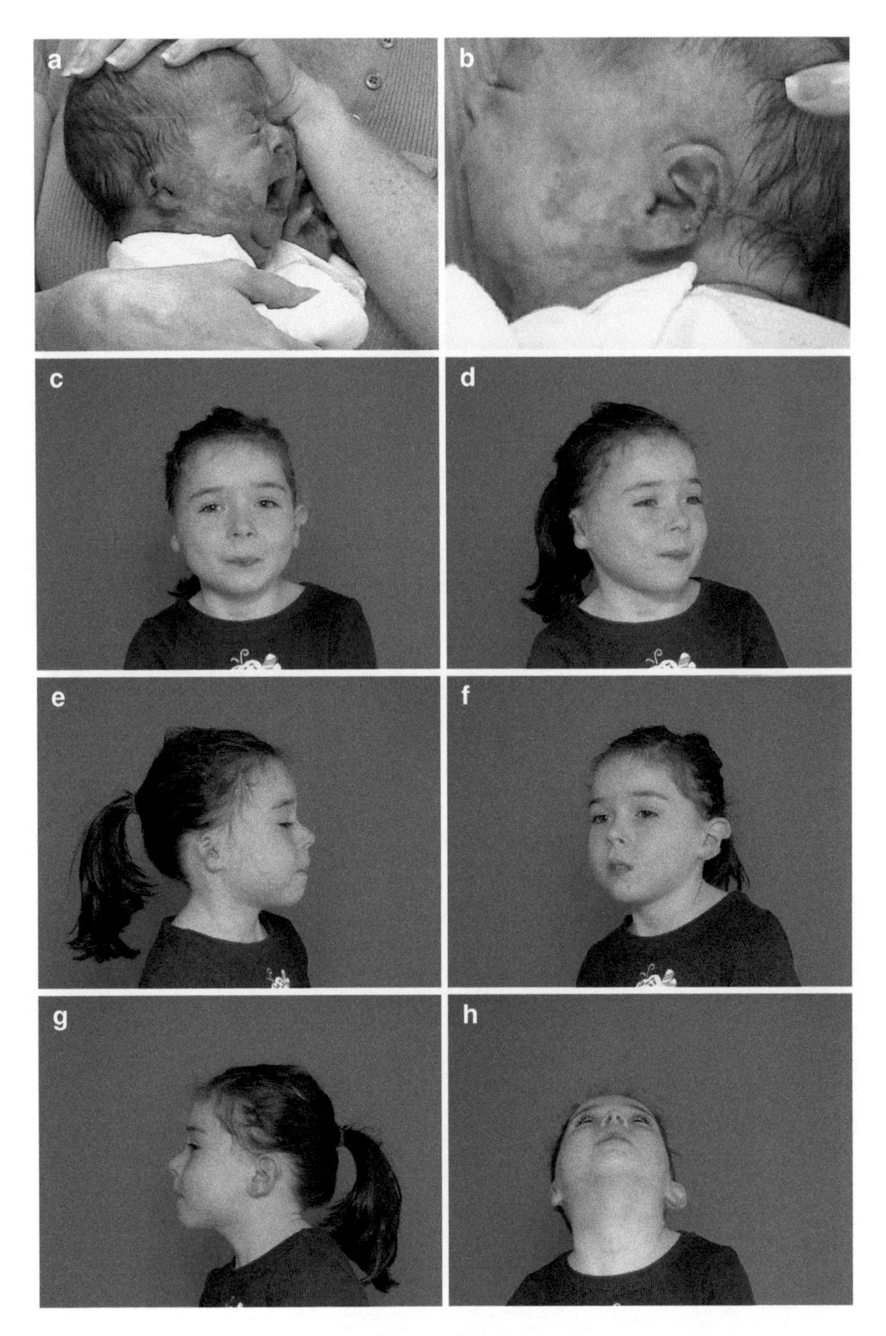

Fig. 14.6 (**a–n**) This patient was born with PHACES syndrome. She presented to our office with bilateral ear ulcerations due to the ulcerated hemangiomas. The right ear was more severely affected than the left ear. The left ear was reconstructed using a left conchal cartilage (2 × 1.5 cm) graft and postauricular flap. The postauricular flap was released at the time of the right ear pHDPE reconstruction 6 months later. The right ear was completely reconstructed using a pHDPE implant covered with a well-vascularized TPF flap and FTSG

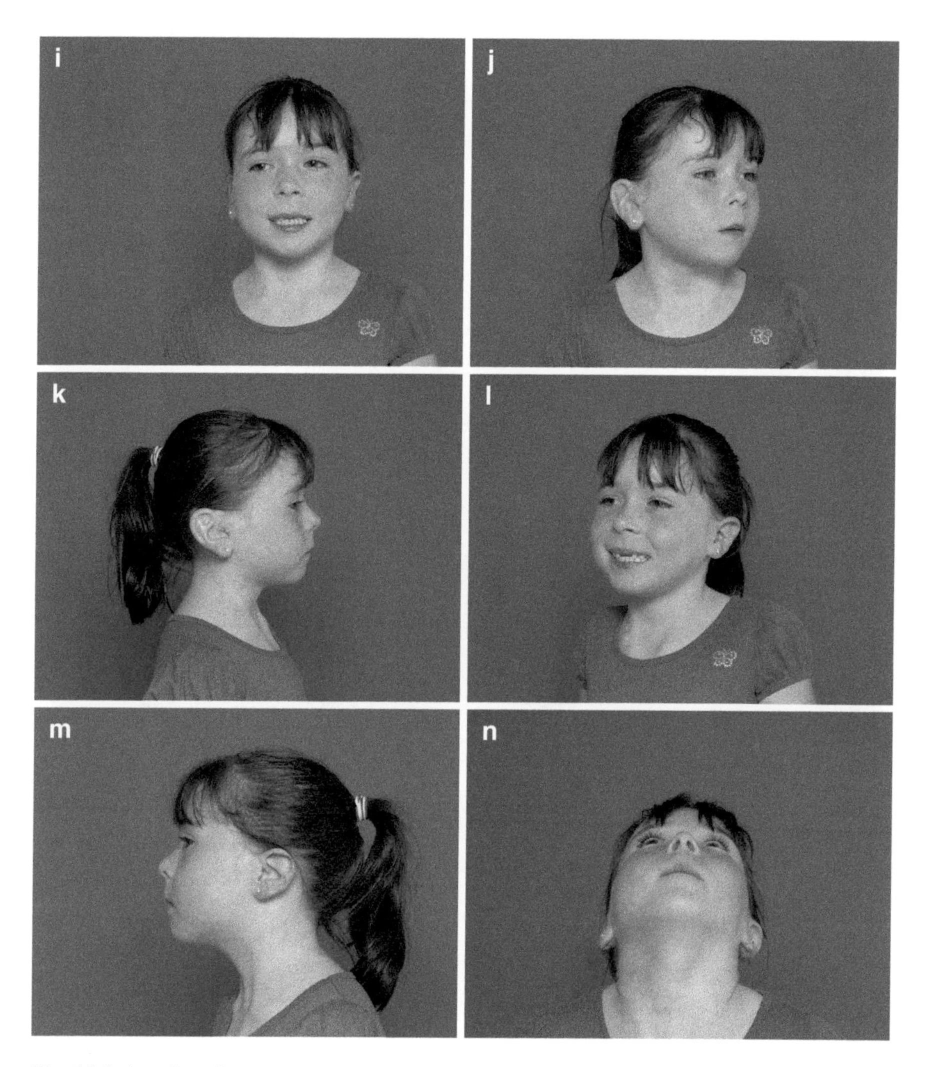

Fig. 14.6 (continued)

due to the ulcerated hemangiomas. The right ear was more severely affected than the left ear. The left ear was reconstructed using a left conchal cartilage (2 × 1.5 cm) graft and postauricular flap (Fig. 14.7a–d). The postauricular flap was released at the time of the right ear pHDPE reconstruction 6 months later. The right ear was completely reconstructed using a pHDPE implant covered with a well-vascularized TPF flap and FTSG.

Surgical Planning

As mentioned earlier in this chapter, ear reconstruction in patients with post-traumatic or ablative ear defects is different than ear reconstruction for congenital microtia. It differs in various aspects, including:

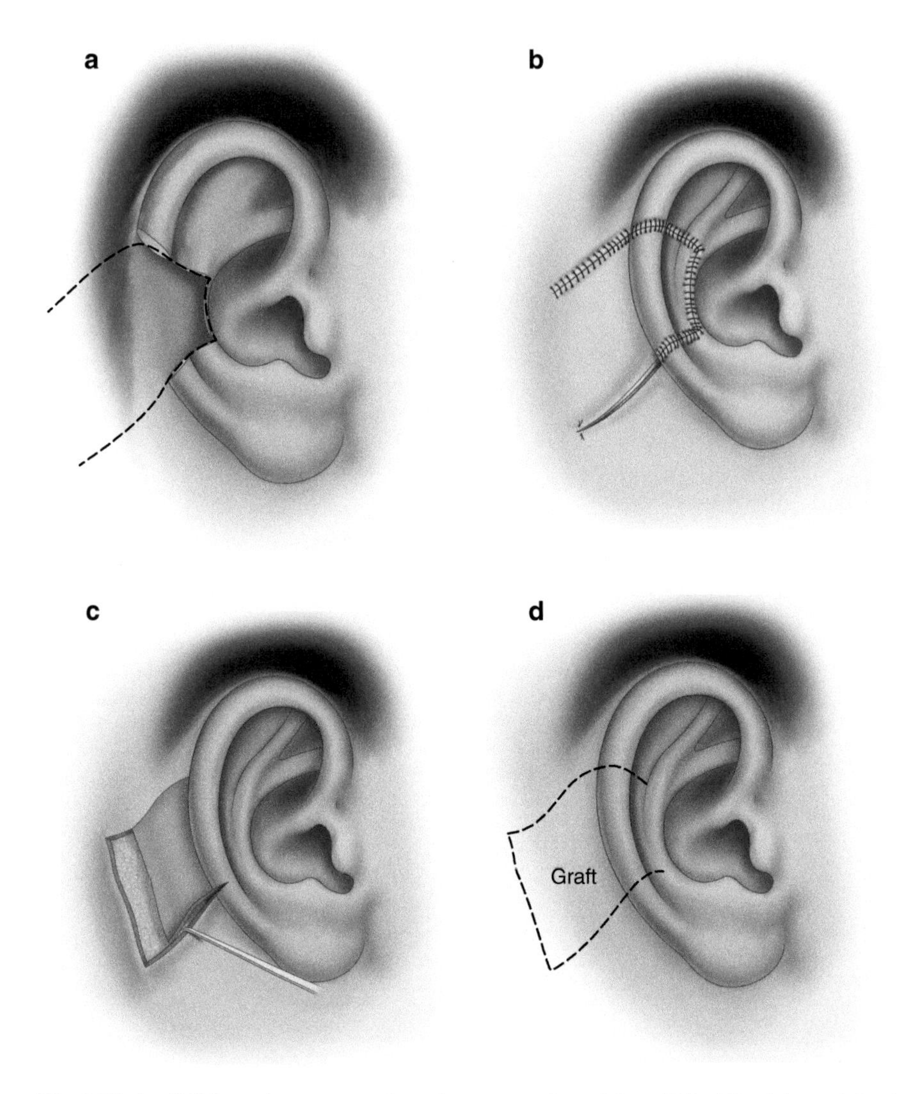

Fig. 14.7 (**a–d**) Schematic representation of reconstruction of the middle 1/3 of the auricle. A cartilage graft is covered with a mastoid flap. In a second stage, the flap is divided at the base and folded posteriorly. The donor side can be closed primarily by advancing the mastoid scalp or can be covered with a skin graft if necessary

- Available skin/scar: Patients with traumatic or ablative ear defects have usually less skin and more scars than patients with a congenital ear defect.
- Tragal reconstruction: The tragus is often maintained in the traumatic/ablative ear defect patient, while it almost always requires reconstruction in congenital microtia.
- External auditory canal (EAC): As for the tragus, the AEC is often maintained in the traumatic/ablative ear defect patient, while it is absent in congenital microtia.
- Psychological: Microtia patient are younger and never had a normal ear. Patients with an acquired absence are older and have sustained the loss of what was a nor-

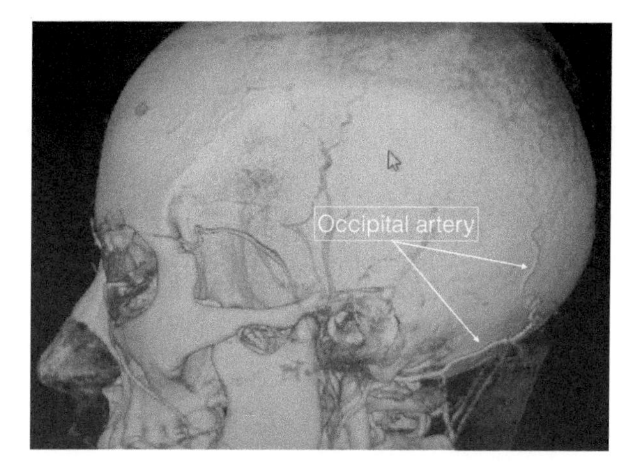

Fig. 14.8 CT angiogram demonstrating the course of the occipital artery

mal structure. The resulting deformity not only causes an external asymmetry but also serves as an internal reminder of what is usually a psychologically traumatic event.

Surgical concepts in auricular reconstruction remain somewhat similar. However, due to these differences, the operative planning differs slightly when treating patients with large traumatic or ablative ear defects not amenable to local reconstruction.

In all cases of large acquired ear defects, it is first recommended to wait an adequate amount of time (at least 6 months to 1 year) to allow the scar tissue to mature.

Since our preferred method of ear reconstruction is using a pHDPE implant covered by a TPF flap and FTSG, we first evaluate the integrity of the superficial temporal vessels as well as integrity of the TPF flap. Large penetrating injuries to the temporal scalp may prevent the use of a TPF flap. The superficial temporal artery along with its anterior and posterior branches is evaluated using a Doppler.

In the unfortunate case where a TPF flap cannot be used, our second choice is the use of an occipital fascia flap, based on the occipital artery, as illustrated in Fig. 14.8.

Alternatively, if a TPF flap and an occipital fascia flap are not available, our third option is to perform a free radial forearm fascia flap. The vascular bundle is anastomosed to one of the branches of the external carotid artery (most often the facial artery).

The main advantage of using a porous high-density polyethylene implant is that the ear reconstruction does not rely on surrounding skin for being intact. The implant is covered with a well-vascularized fascia flap and full-thickness skin grafts.

High-Density Porous Polyethylene Ear Reconstruction

The authors prefer to use a porous polyethylene ear reconstruction because, in their experiences, it addresses comprehensibly the cosmetic, the functional, and the psychological issues associated with microtia.

Patients are already recovering from the trauma associated with the loss of their ear. Undergoing a complex ear reconstruction with multiple stages can be difficult for them. The use of an implant covered with a TPF flap allows a single-stage reconstruction. Furthermore, by eliminating the discomfort of the costal cartilage harvest, an alloplastic implant reconstruction can be done as an outpatient with its obvious psychological and economic advantages.

As discussed extensively in previous chapters, polyethylene framework requires a different type of soft tissue coverage to avoid exposures. Covering the entire alloplastic material with a well-vascularized temporoparietal or occipitoparietal fascia flap reduces exposures to a very low rate.

Figure 14.9a–f demonstrates a 54-year-old healthy male who sustained a left ear amputation with loss of skin following a surf injury. Immediately after the injury, the defect was covered with a full-thickness skin graft at a local hospital. Seven months later we performed a left ear reconstruction using the technique described above.

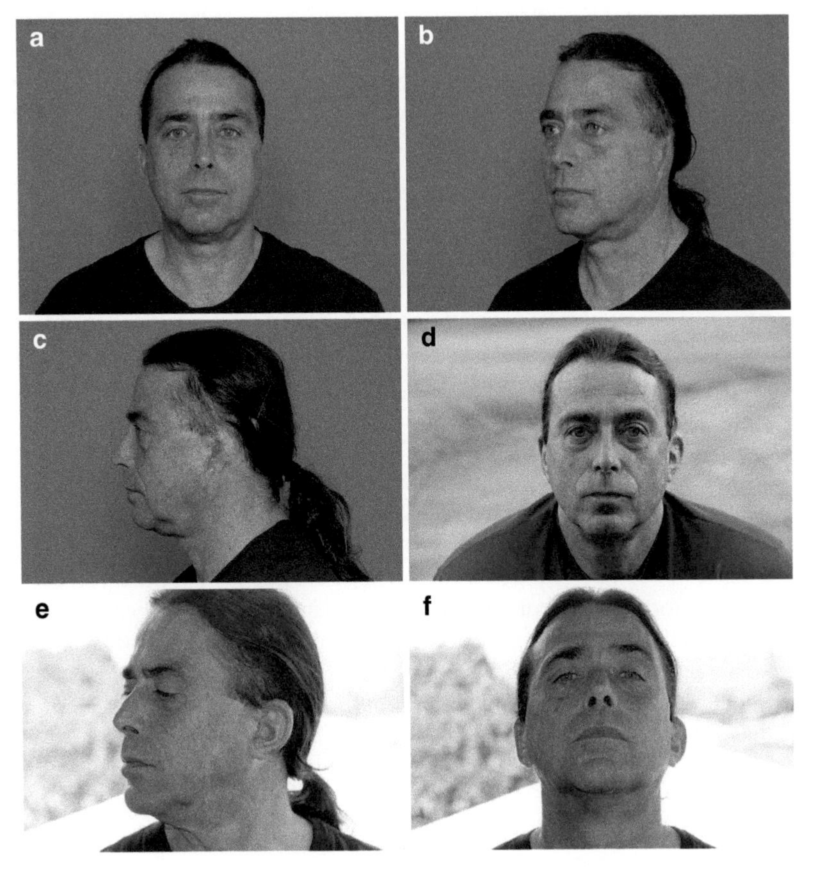

Fig. 14.9 **(a–f)** A 54-year-old healthy male who sustained a left ear amputation with loss of skin following a surf injury. Immediately after the injury, the defect was covered with a full-thickness skin graft at a local hospital. Seven months later we performed a left ear reconstruction with pHDPE

Reconstruction of Partial Defects

Partial ear defects with loss of skin with or without cartilaginous loss would first be addressed using local reconstruction techniques including composite grafts, skin grafts, and local or regional flaps.

Skin grafts can be used if there is skin loss with intact perichondrium. Skin grafts can also be used if a segment of skin and cartilage have been excised as long as there is an intact posterior skin to lay the graft on and an intact cartilage at the helical margin to prevent late collapse.

For some helical margins or anti-helical defects, primary closure can be attained. In order to obtain a tension-free closure, one may have to discard adjacent cartilage, advance posterior skin, and possibly excise accessory triangles [20]. The main disadvantage of this technique is the reduction of the auricular circumference/size (Fig. 14.10a–f).

Chondrocutaneous advancement flaps [21, 22] (Fig. 14.11a–e) can be used to reconstruct defects less than 3 × 3cm of the helical rim, middle 1/3, and earlobe. This technique involves advancement of the local skin and cartilage along the

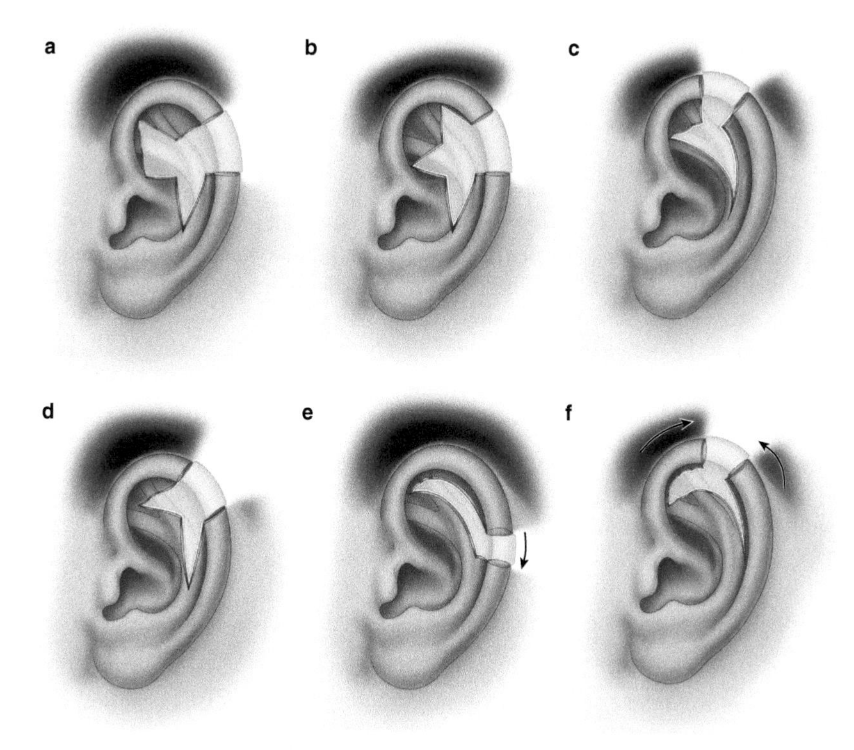

Fig. 14.10 **(a–f)** Techniques used to close primarily some helical defects. Triangular excisions are designed to reduce tension at suture lines. These techniques inherently reduce the ear circumference

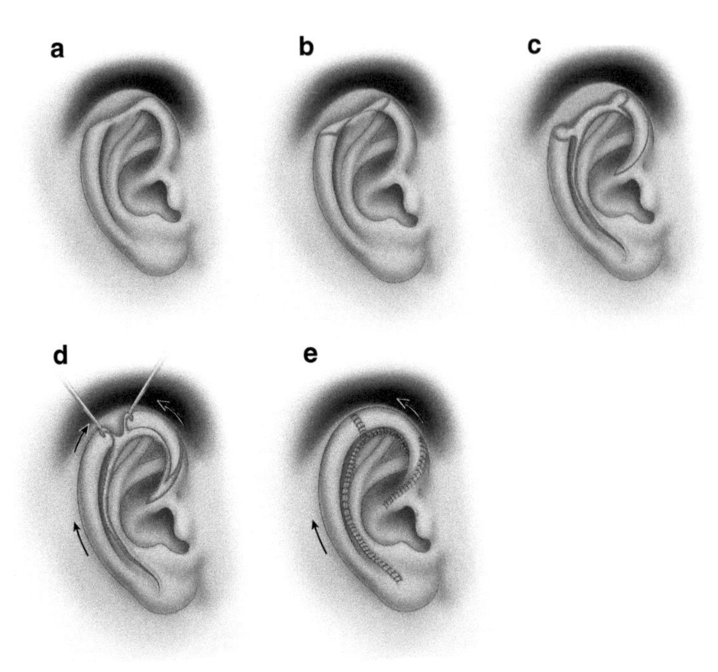

Fig. 14.11 (**a**–**e**) Helical defect reconstructed with advancement of auricular skin and cartilage. Note the extension into the earlobe

helical rim. The entire helix is freed from the scapha via an incision in helical sulcus through the anterior skin and cartilage, while the posteromedial auricular skin is undermined until the entire helix is freed as a chondrocutaneous component based on a wide postauricular pedicle. More length can be gained by performing a V-Y advancement of the helical crus. The main disadvantage of this technique is a reduction in the ear height (particularly at the lobe but less than with wedge excisions).

Other local procedures include:

- The mastoid flap (cephaloauricular flap) where a postauricular skin flap is raised to cover a defect. A second stage is sometimes necessary. It can be used along with a cartilage graft and is indicated for long shallow defects.
- The tunnel procedure: indicated for moderate-sized defects of the middle third (Fig. 14.12a–g).
- Dieffenbach's technique: also indicated for moderate-sized defects of the middle third (Fig. 14.7a–d).

We present in Fig. 14.13a–f a 50-year-old male who had a BCC excised on his left ear. He presented with a middle 1/3 helical defect of the left ear. Instead of proceeding to a larger ear reconstruction (with mastoid flap and cartilage graft), we offered him a primary closure of the defect under local anesthesia in the office. This offered an immediate aesthetic improvement in exchange for a slightly smaller ear. The option of later reconstruction was still available.

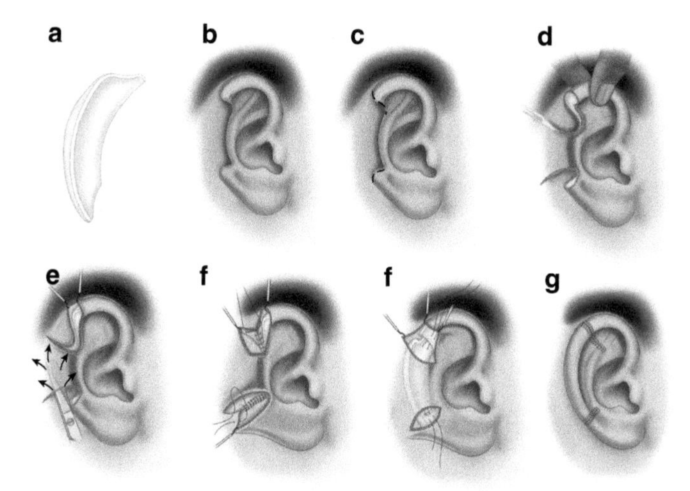

Fig. 14.12 (**a–g**) The tunnel procedure is used to repair large middle third defects. Two incisions at each edge of the defect are made, and the mastoid skin is undermined. A carved costal cartilage graft is inserted into a mastoid pocket. The costal cartilage is anchored to the remaining cartilage on each side. Incisions are closed as illustrated

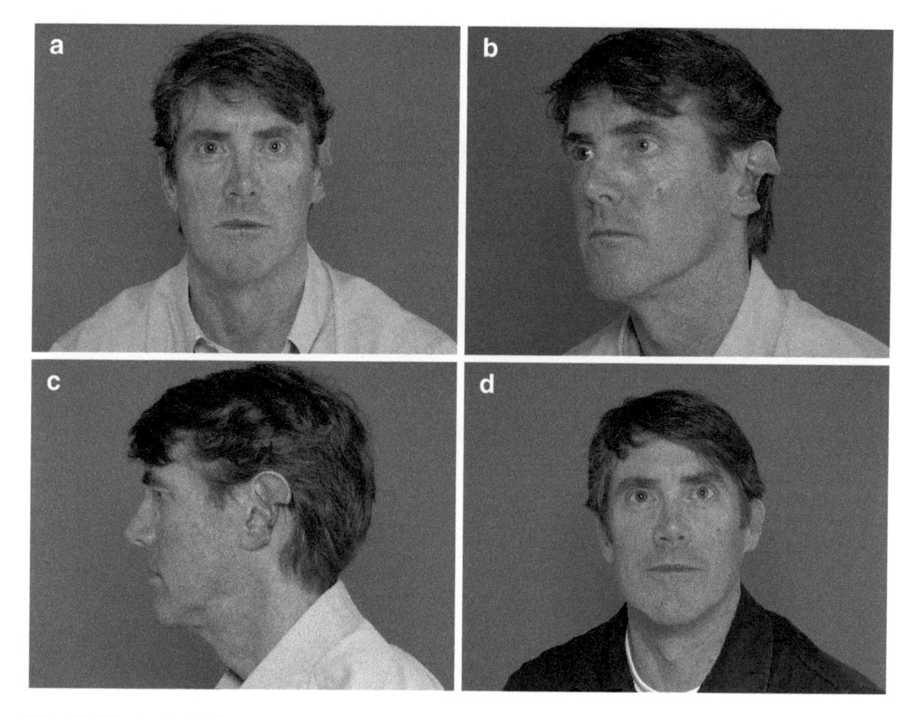

Fig. 14.13 (**a–f**) A 50-year-old male who had a BCC excised on his left ear. He presented with a middle 1/3 helical defect of the left ear. Instead of proceeding to a larger ear reconstruction (with mastoid flap and cartilage graft), we offered him a primary closure of the defect under local anesthesia in the office. This offered an immediate aesthetic improvement in exchange for a slightly smaller ear

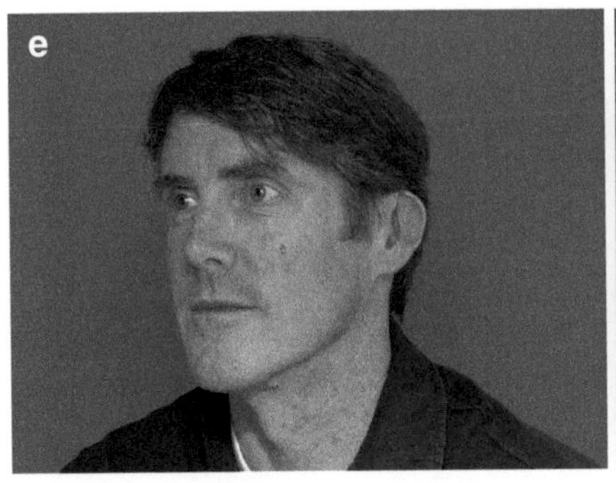

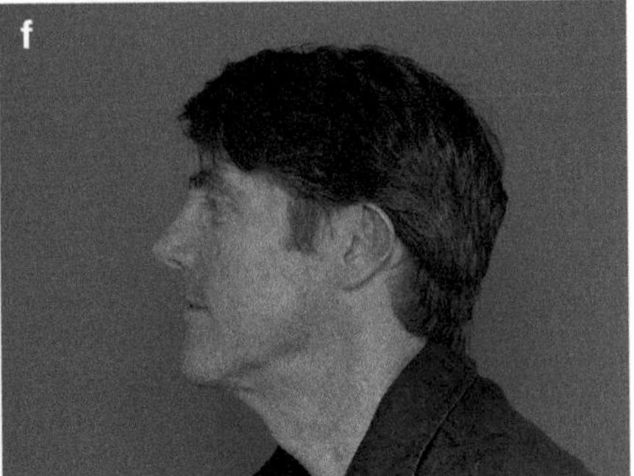

Fig. 14.13 (continued)

Conclusion

Reconstruction of acquired total ear defects is a very challenging task to undergo given the complex three-dimensional architecture and cosmetic expectations of patients.

Auricular reconstruction following trauma or ablative surgery can be performed using a porous high-density polyethylene implant covered by a healthy well-vascularized thin fascia flaps and color-matched full-thickness skin grafts.

References

1. Avelar JM. A new technique for reconstruction of the auricle in acquired deformities. Ann Plast Surg. 1987;18(5):454–64.
2. Pearl RA, Sabbagh W. Reconstruction following traumatic partial amputation of the ear. Plast Reconstr Surg. 2011;127:621–9.
3. Steffen A, Klaiber S, Katzbach R, Nitsch S, König IR, Frenzel H. The psychosocial consequences of reconstruction of severe ear defects or third-degree microtia with rib cartilage. Aesthet Surg J. 2008;28:404–11.
4. Bada AM, Pope GH. Use of hyperbaric oxygen as adjunct in salvage of near-complete ear amputation. Plast Reconstr Surg Glob Open. 2013;1:e1–5.
5. Kalus R. Successful bilateral composite ear reattachment. Plast Reconstr Surg Glob Open. 2014;2:e174–9.
6. Mladick RA, Carraway JH. Ear reattachment by the modified pocket principle: case report. Plast Reconstr Surg. 1973;51:584–7.
7. Park C, Lee CH, Shin KS. An improved burying method for salvaging an amputated auricular cartilage. Plast Reconstr Surg. 1995;96:207–10.
8. Steffen A, Katzbach R, Klaiber S. A comparison of ear reattachment methods: a review of 25 years since Pennington. Plast Reconstr Surg. 2006;118:1358–64.
9. Dowling JA, Foley ED, Monerief JA. Chrondritis in the burned ear. Plast Reconstr Surg. 1968;42:115–22.
10. Avelar JM. Artigo expefical; Reconstrucao da orella pos—quiemadura. Revista Brasileira De Queimaduras. 2009;8(2):42–50.

11. Hyams VJ, Batsakis JG, Michaels L. Tumors of the upper respiratory tract and ear. In: Hartmann WH, Sobin LH, editors. Atlas of tumour pathology, vol. 25. Washington, DC: Armed Forces Institute of Pathology; 1988. p. 343.
12. Nindl I, Gottschling M, Stockfleth E. Human papillomaviruses and non-melanoma skin cancer: basic virology and clinical manifestations. Dis Markers. 2007;23:247–59.
13. Molho-Pessach V, Lotem M. Viral carcinogenesis in skin cancer. Curr Probl Dermatol. 2007;35:39–51.
14. Byers RM, Smith JL, Russell N, Rosenberg V. Malignant melanoma of the external ear. Review of 102 cases. Am J Surg. 1980;140:518–21.
15. Davidsson A, Hellquist HB, Villman K, Westman G. Malignant melanoma of the ear. J Laryngol Otol. 1993;107:798–802.
16. Arons MS, Savin RC. Auricular cancer. Some surgical and pathologic considerations. Am J Surg. 1971;122:770–6.
17. Pockaj BA, Jaroszewski DE, Dicaudo DJ, Hentz JG, Buchel EW, Gray RJ, et al. Changing surgical therapy for melanoma of the external ear. Ann Surg Oncol. 2003;10:689–96.
18. Narayan D, Ariyan S. Surgical considerations in the management of malignant melanoma of the ear. Plast Reconstr Surg. 2001;107:20–4.
19. Dost P, Lehnerdt G, Kling R, Wagner SN. Surgical therapy of malignant melanoma of the external ear. HNO. 2004;52:33–7.
20. Tanzer RC. Congenital deformities of the Auricle. Ch 35. In: Converse JM, editor. Reconstructive plastic surgery, vol. 3. 2nd ed. Philadelphia: WB Saunders; 1977. p. 1671–719.
21. Antia NH, Buch VI. Chondrocutaneous advancement flap for the marginal defect of the ear. Plast Reconstr Surg. 1967;39:472.
22. Antia NH. Repair of the segmental defects of the auricle in mechanical trauma. In: Tranzer RC, Edgerton MT, editors. Symposium on reconstruction of the auricle. St. Louis: Mosby. p. 218.

Chapter 15
Treacher Collins-Franceschetti Syndrome

Patricia Cecchi and Darina Krastinova

Introduction

Treacher Collins-Franceschetti syndrome (TCFS) is a congenital syndrome with bilateral microtia as well as other anomalies affecting the hard and soft tissues of the face. The most noticeable feature of the syndrome are the bilateral down-slanting lids, due to the missing support of the underlying skeleton and specifically the zygomatic-malar bone.

TCFS is a rare autosomal dominant disorder, with an incidence of one in 50,000 live births. Forty percent of cases have a positive family history although often the affected parent has very slight features of the syndrome and the diagnosis is made when the child is born. The rest of the cases (60%) appear from de novo mutations. In most cases it is caused by a mutation of the TCOF1 gene named Treacle, a nucleolar phosphoprotein essential for the development of the first and second brachial arches [1]. Phenotypic expression of the syndrome is, however, variable in affected subjects.

The characteristic phenotypic features of TCFS involve absence or hypoplasia of the malar bones and orbito-palpebral region with the typical antimongoloid slant of the palpebral fissures, which constitutes the "hallmark" of the malformation. Maxillary and severe mandibular hypoplasia with an anterior open bite completes the clinical picture and is responsible for the typical birdlike profile. Bilateral microtia with absent or malformed ears is associated to varying degrees of middle ear hypoplasia and hearing loss.

Treatment for these complex patients requires a multidisciplinary approach which may begin at birth, when airway and feeding problems are the main focus and may require a tracheostomy [2]. Conductive hearing loss should be addressed very

P. Cecchi (✉)
Bambino Gesu Hospital, Plastic Surgery Unit, Rome, Italy

D. Krastinova
Clinique Chateaux de la Maye, Paris, France

© Springer Nature Switzerland AG 2019

J. F. Reinisch, Y. Tahiri (eds.), *Modern Microtia Reconstruction*,
https://doi.org/10.1007/978-3-030-16387-7_15

early with a banded hearing aid until a bone-anchored aid can be inserted [3]. There is a 23% estimated incidence of cleft palate which also requires early surgery.

Once the initial functional issues have been treated adequately, the more "cosmetic" deformities can be addressed. There is a strong demand on behalf of the family to "normalize" the face, especially the down-slanting lids, when the full phenotypic expression of the syndrome is present. Although optimal timing and treatment of eyelid deformities has not been fully established, problems such as corneal abrasion due to eyelid ectropion may require early treatment [4]. See Fig. 15.1a–c.

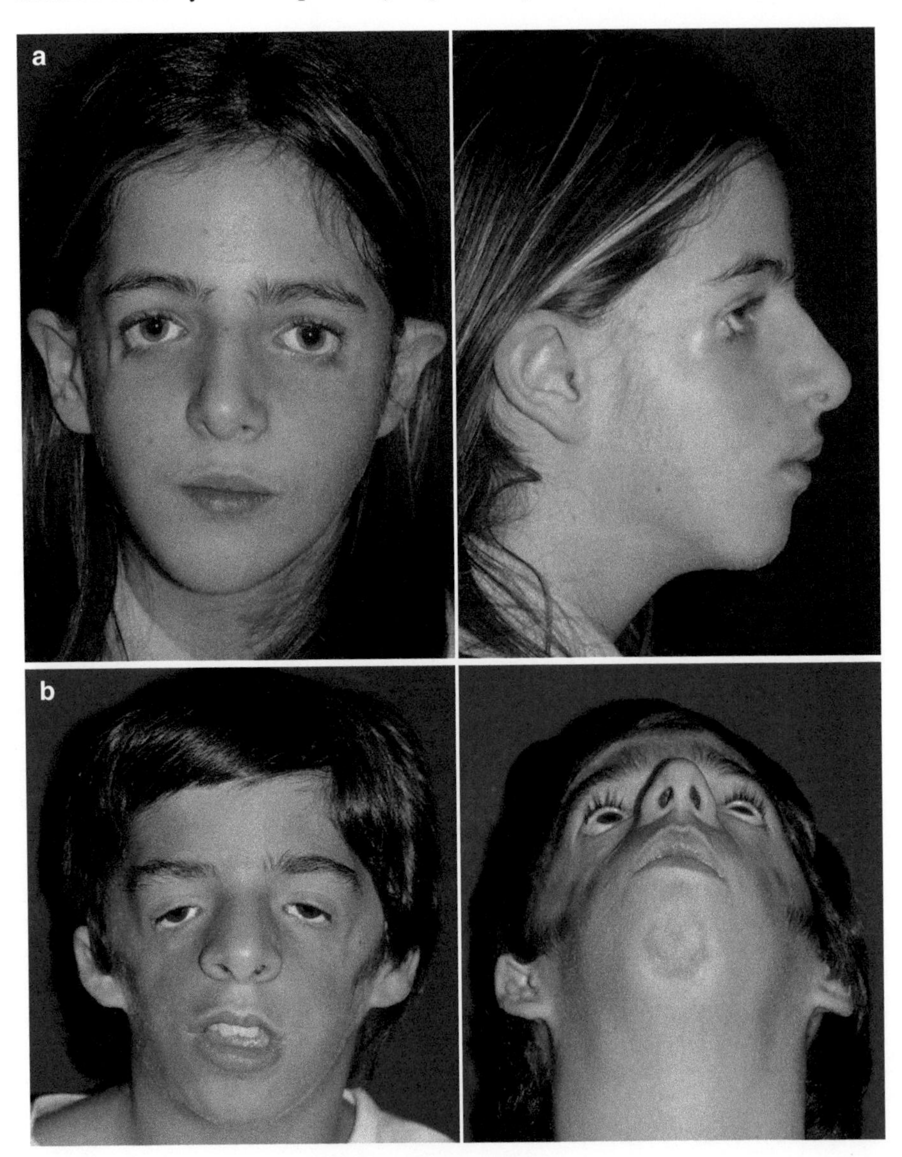

Fig. 15.1 Treacher Collins-Franceschetti syndrome. (**a**) Mild form. (**b**) Moderate form. (**c**) Severe form with asymmetry of lids and orbits

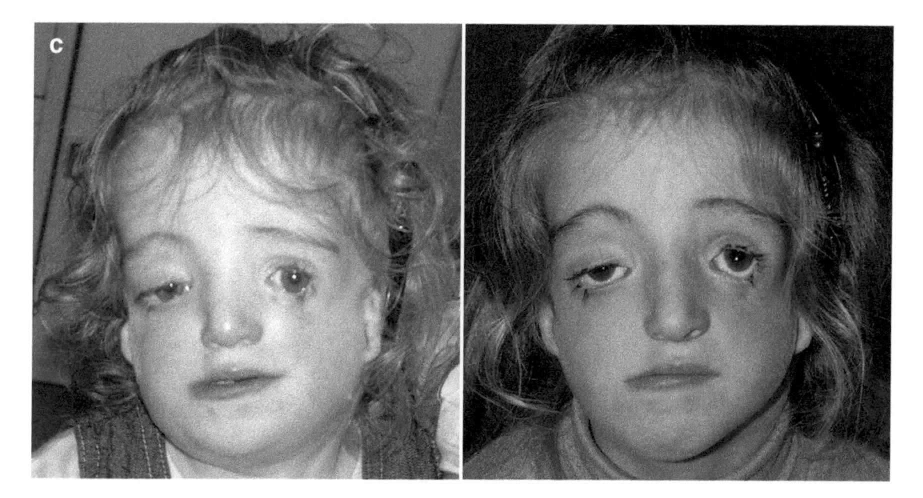

Fig. 15.1 (continued)

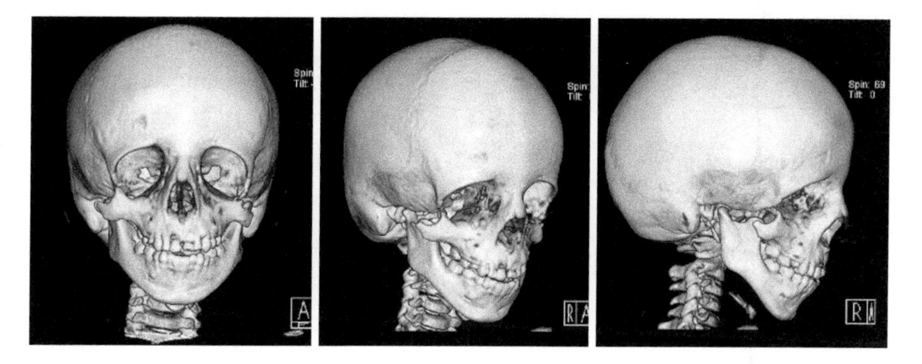

Fig. 15.2 Preoperative CT scan

Treatment Algorithm

The first reconstructive procedure is usually performed at age 6 or 7 and is aimed at correcting the antimongoloid slant of the palpebral fissures (typical stigmata of the syndrome). It involves simultaneous correction of the bony defect as well as the lower lid hypoplasia. A coronal approach associated with a short lower eyelid incision allows for complete dissection of the malformed orbit and the zygomatic-malar defect. These two approaches will also enable dissection of the periorbita in the inferolateral and inferior cleft and allow freeing of the retracted soft tissues causing the typical hollow on the lateral aspect of the cheek. Preoperative evaluation of the bony defect is carried out with computed tomography (Fig. 15.2).

Malar and Eyelid Reconstruction

The procedure we describe for correction of the hard and soft tissue deficiency of the orbito-malar and palpebral region is the result of more than 40 years of cranio-facial surgery of the senior author Dr. Darina Krastinova. She assisted Paul Tessier for 12 years during his most productive period at Foch Hospital in Paris. This experience has permitted the mastering of techniques such as the coronal approach, subperiosteal dissection of the facial skeleton, osteotomies, cranial bone grafts as well as medial and lateral canthopexy [5–7]. Personal variations in applying these procedures over the years have led to the establishment of a stepwise approach required for an optimal reconstruction of the missing and malformed elements in the orbito-palpebral area [8].

Split calvarial bone grafts are harvested from the outer cortex of parietal skull, and care is taken to preserve the integrity of the contralateral parietal bone, for a second reconstructive procedure. The grafts are positioned to reconstruct the lateral orbital wall, malar bone, and zygomatic arch. Important aspects for graft survival are preparation of the recipient bony bed by light burring, followed by adequate fixation with small plates and screws (Fig. 15.3a, b).

Further remodeling of the orbital contour is achieved by burring the superolateral orbital rims with a rotary drill, thus correcting its oblique vector. In the reconstructed

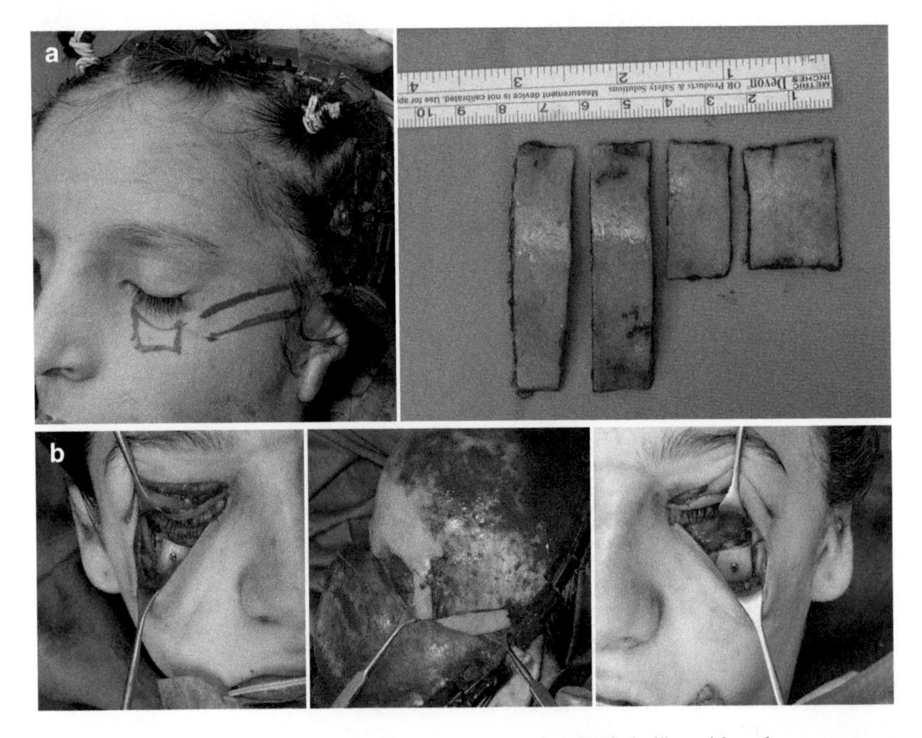

Fig. 15.3 Bone grafts (harvested from the outer cortex of parietal skull) positioned to reconstruct the lateral orbital wall, malar bone, and zygomatic arch. (**a**) Cranial bone grafts. (**b**) Intraoperative view of the orbito-malar reconstruction

lateral orbital wall, a groove has to be created to correctly place the new position of the lateral canthus.

When the bony reconstruction is completed, the facial flap is repositioned, and the antimongoloid slant of the palpebral fissure is corrected via a lateral canthopexy. This maneuver brings into light the lack of tissue in the lower lid, which will be corrected by the transposition of an upper eyelid flap.

Since patients with TCFS often have distended upper eyelids, this facilitates harvesting and dissection of large myocutaneous flaps, taking care to leave at least 25 mm of residual upper lid, with the fold located at 6–8 mm from the eyelid margin. This pedicled flap is based right above the lateral canthus and extends to the medial canthus along the entire length of the upper eyelid. The lower eyelid incision is at this point extended to the upper lid incision (Fig. 15.4a, b).

To avoid shortening of the palpebral fissure when the flap is transposed, it is mandatory to fix the lateral extremity of the palpebral fissure and the base of the flap to the temporal fascia. The distal part of the flap will then be anchored to the medial canthus creating a hammock (Fig. 15.4c).

The postoperative dressing will require suspension of the reconstructed lower lid to the forehead. To obtain better positioning of the lower lids, it is best to place a tarsorrhaphy stitch for 4–5 days.

This procedure addresses the reconstruction of the external lamella of the lower lid, but most cases also require reconstruction of the inner lamella. This can be done with chondromucosal grafts from the nose or fibromucosal grafts from

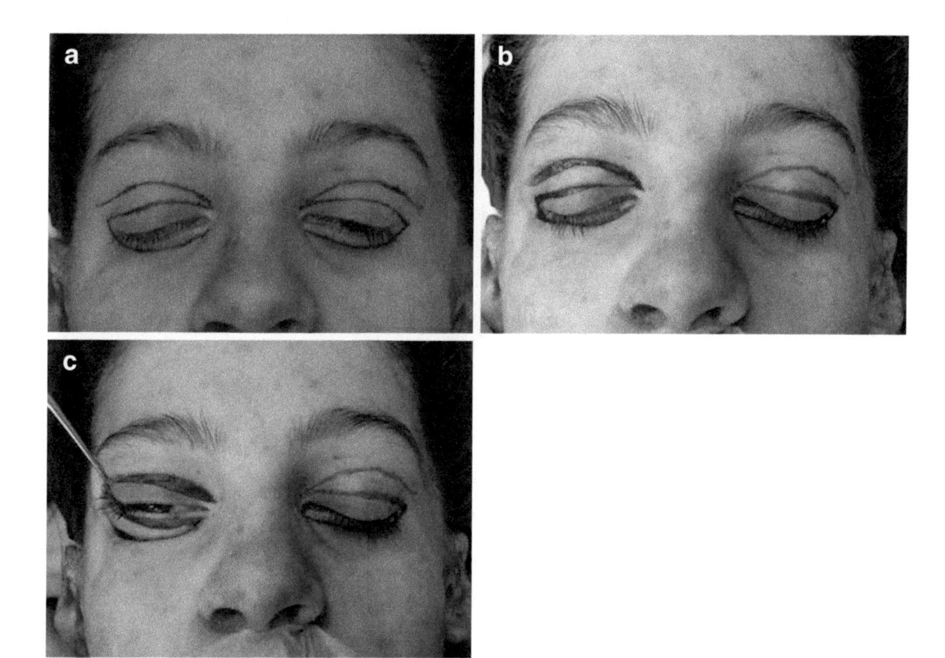

Fig. 15.4 Myocutaneous upper eyelid flap. (**a**) Design. (**b**) Myocutaneous flap incised. (**c**) Flap anchored to the medial canthus

the hard palate (Fig. 15.5a–c). Reconstruction of the inner lamella can be challenging in cases of severe ectropion in which the lower lid is practically absent (Figs. 15.6a–c and 15.7).

The aim of this first procedure is to correct the missing or hypoplastic elements of the malar region and the surrounding soft tissues. According to Dr. Krastinova's algorithm, a second set of bone grafts, harvested from the other parietal bone, is used to reinforce, stabilize, and complete the reconstructed bony skeleton. This second procedure is carried out 1 year later. The approach is via the previous coronal scar which also allows harvesting of the necessary split calvarial bone grafts.

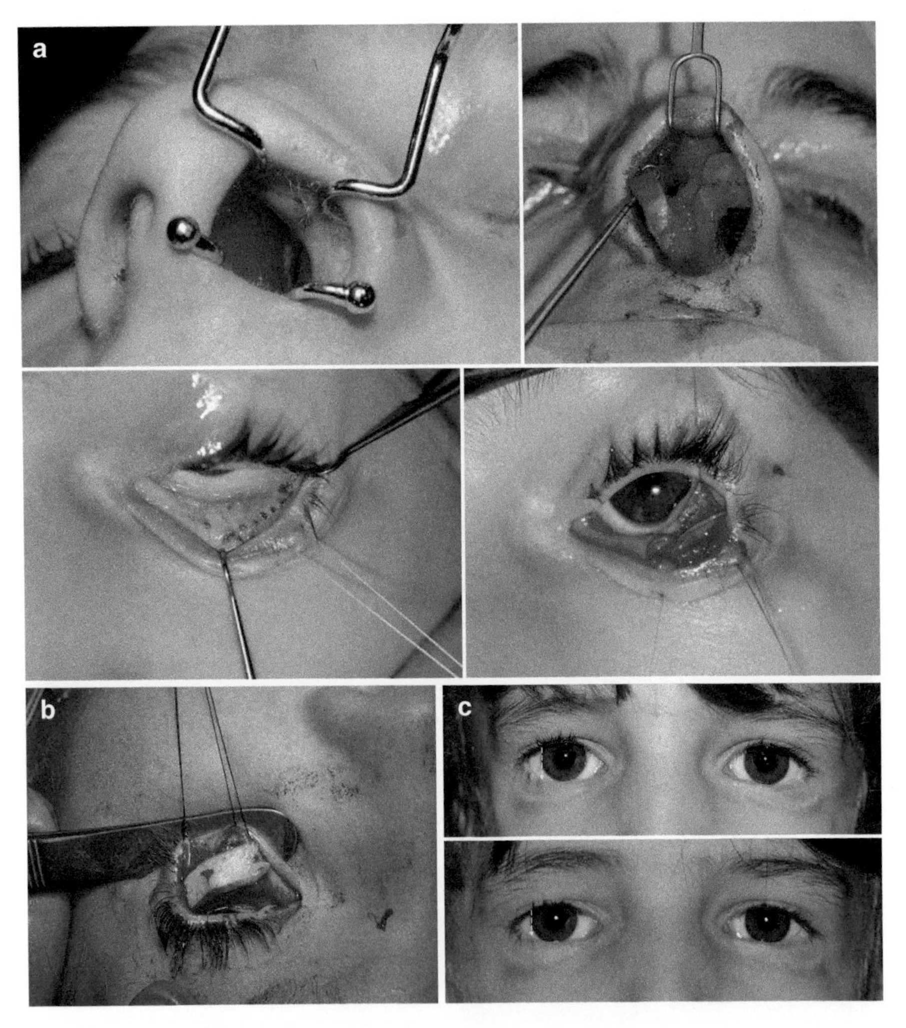

Fig. 15.5 Reconstruction of the inner lamella. (**a**) Condromucosal grafts from the nose. (**b**) Fibromucosal grafts from the hard palate. (**c**) After correction of inner lamella

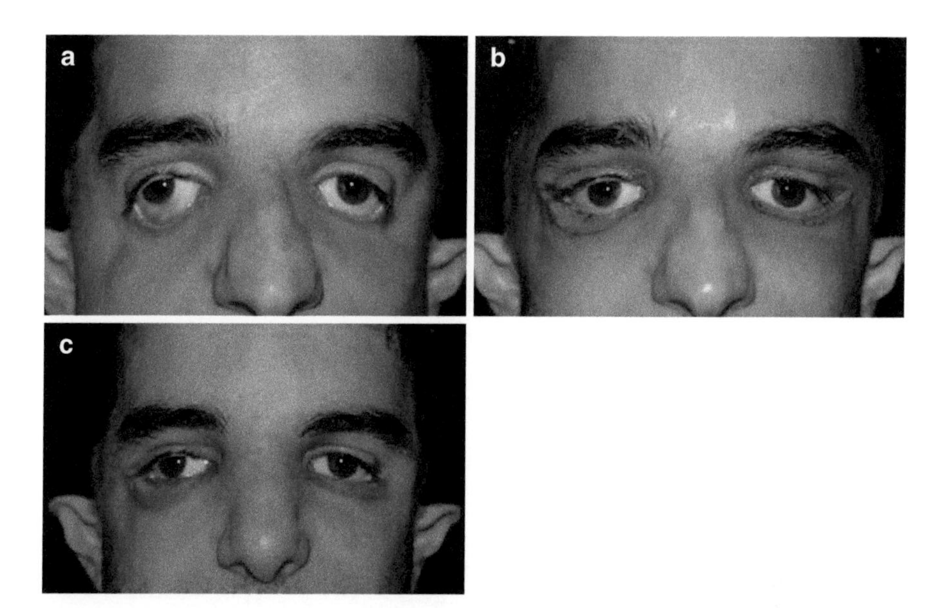

Fig. 15.6 Reconstruction of the inner lamella. (**a**) Severe lower lid ectropion. (**b**) One month after bone grafts and upper lid flap with canthopexy, residual important lower lid insufficiency requiring a prompt solution. (**c**) After reconstruction of the inner lamella with alar condromucosal cartilage grafts and contemporary rhinoplasty

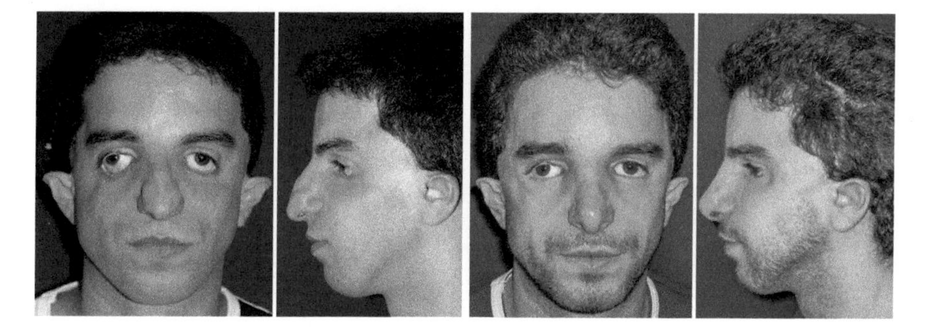

Fig. 15.7 Same patient as in Fig. 15.6. Long-term result after 10 years

The grafts are stacked on top of the bone placed in the first stage, especially the malar prominence (Fig. 15.8a–c).

In the personal experience of the first author, not all the patients required a second bone grafting procedure, for various reasons: some patients were satisfied with the initial result, some did not want to repeat the operation, and others have decided to wait (Fig. 15.9a, b).

Lipofilling has proved very useful as a primary procedure in cases with severe soft tissue hypoplasia. In all other cases, it has been used as a final procedure to

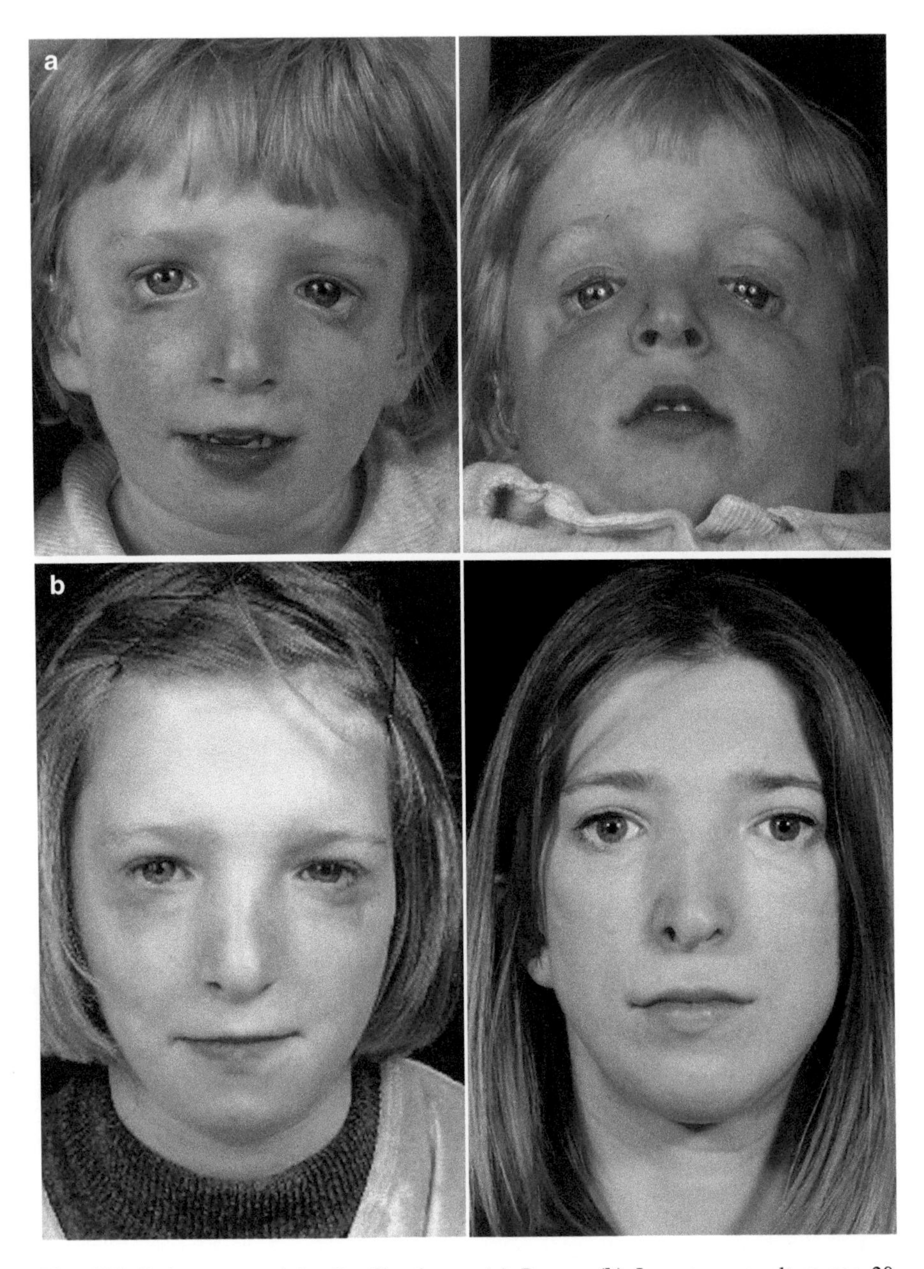

Fig. 15.8 Patient operated by Dr. Krastinova. (**a**) Pre-op. (**b**) Long-term result at age 20. (**c**) Post-op CT scan at age 20

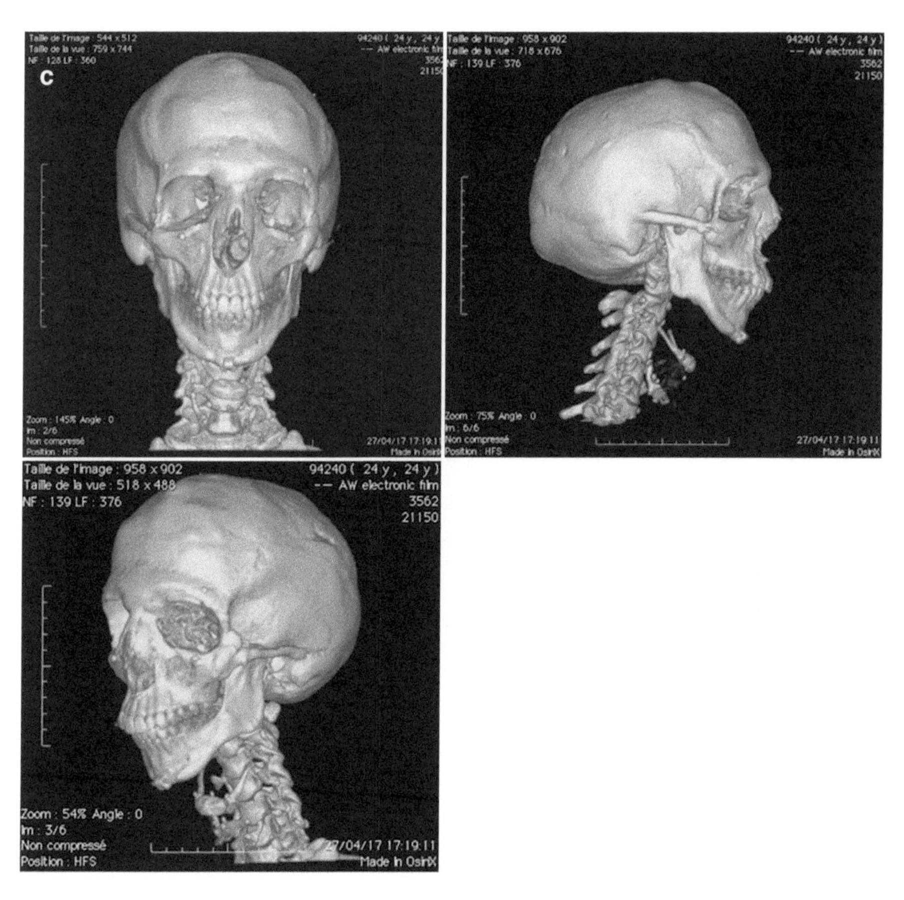

Fig. 15.8 (continued)

harmonize, obtain symmetry, and soften contours. The procedure should be executed with great care in this area where the soft tissues are hypotrophic, injecting small aliquots at a time, in various planes using the Coleman technique. Unpleasant surprises may appear years later such as fat tissue cysts, or if the patient gains weight, the fat in this area seems to increase twofold [9].

Treatment of maxillary and mandibular deformities is usually undertaken as late as possible toward skeletal maturity and according to different requirements. Occasionally, a severe mandibular hypoplasia may require a tracheostomy to safely approach surgery (Fig. 15.10a, b). Figure 15.11a–d illustrates a patient with severe open bite who had presurgical orthodontics, tracheostomy, and bimaxillary osteot-

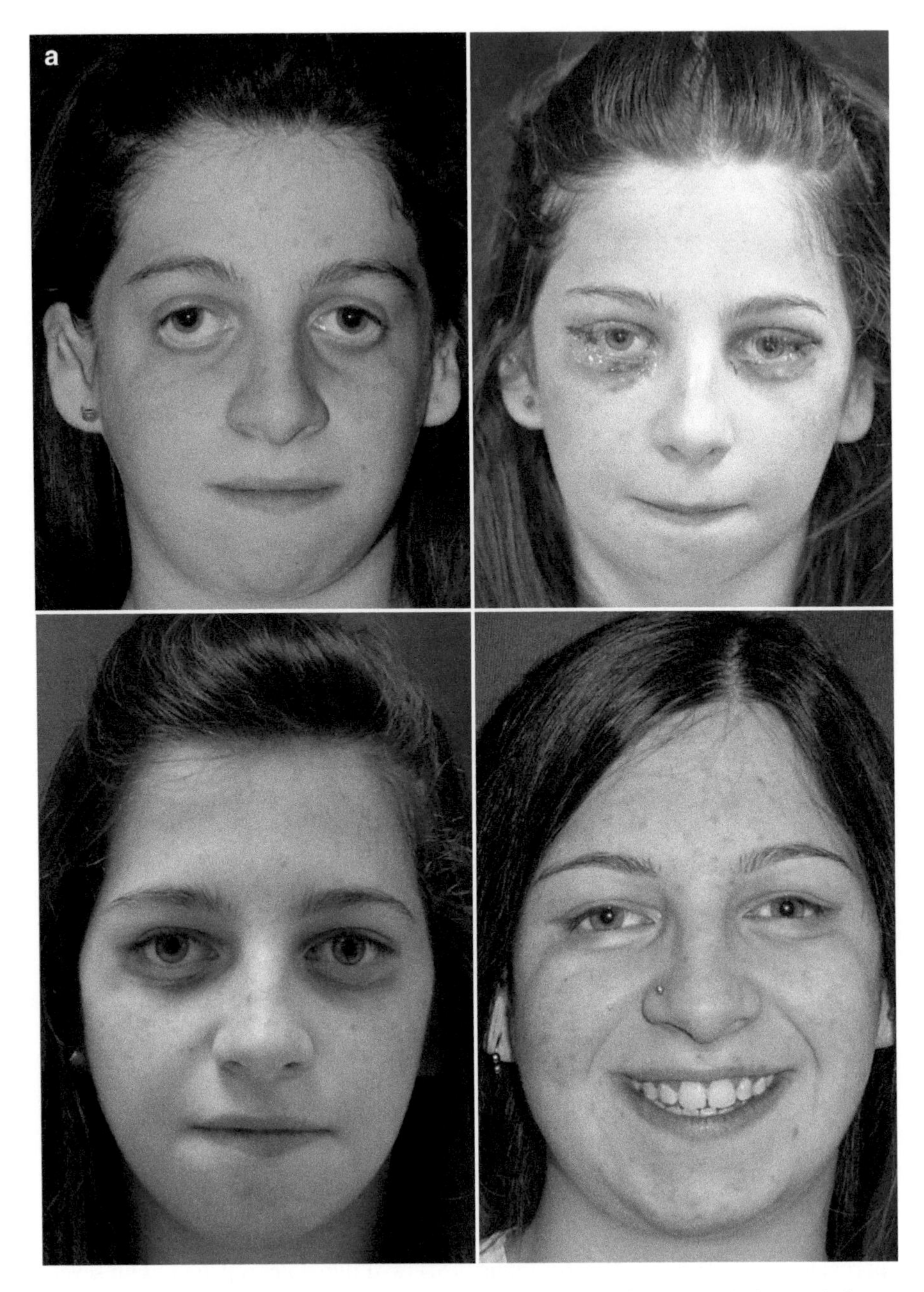

Fig. 15.9 (**a**) A 12-year-old patient pre- and postoperative result. (**b**) CT scan before and after

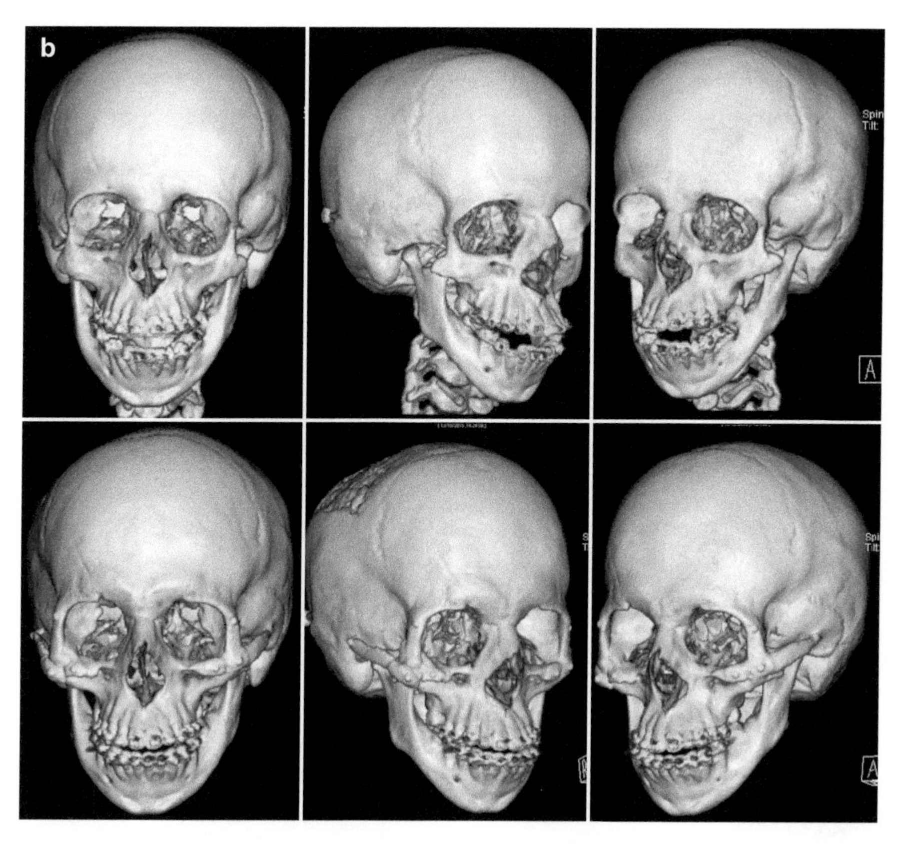

Fig. 15.9 (continued)

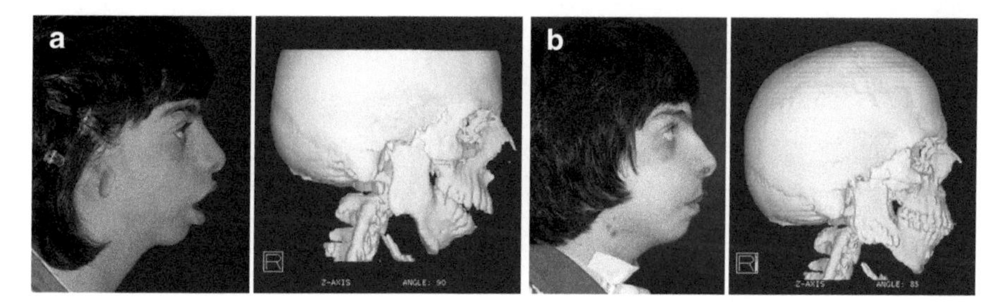

Fig. 15.10 Pre- (**a**) and post-op (**b**) profile view of the bimaxillary osteotomy

omy. With the tracheostomy in place, 6 months later, orbito-palpebral reconstruction with bone grafts was carried out.

Genioplasty is certainly a fundamental procedure for these patients with retruded chins and may be either repeated or enhanced with onlay bone grafts. Rhinoplasty, when required is usually the final procedure performed, when all other craniofacial surgeries are completed [10–15].

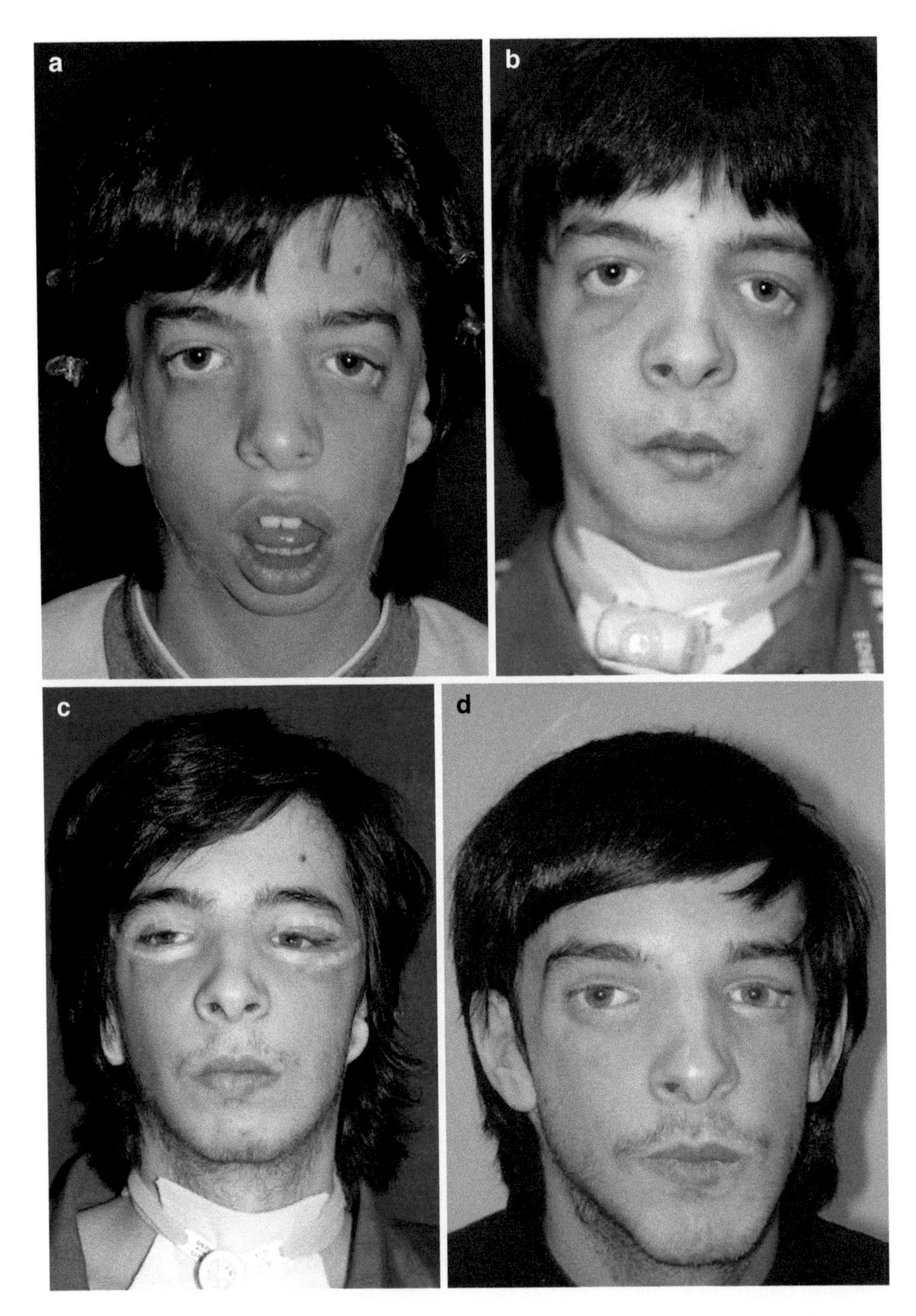

Fig. 15.11 Pre-op front view (**a**), after the bimaxillary osteotomy (**b**), after malar and lid reconstruction with cranial bone grafts (**c**), and long-term result with bilateral epithesis (**d**)

Some patients present small colobomas on the lateral aspect of the lower eyelid which should be treated in separate procedures. Usually a small pentagonal excision (Kuhnt-Szymanowski-type procedure) is sufficient to correct the defect.

Ear Reconstruction

Patients with TCFS often present with bilateral microtia as well as bilateral conductive hearing loss. Primary concern is for adequate and early correction with a banded hearing aid.

Pinna reconstruction is approached later and the first requests are usually before school age.

Most patients will by this time be equipped with bone-aided hearing appliances.

There are two main ways of reconstructing the outer ear. One involves an alloplastic reconstruction using a porous polyethylene implant covered by a vascularized thin temporoparietal fascia flap. As discussed in the previous chapters, this procedure can be performed as an outpatient procedure, at an early age (as early as 3.5 years of age). The second technique involves an autologous ear reconstruction using costal cartilage and is usually performed at a much later age [16–19].

Our personal experience in ear reconstruction is based on an apprenticeship with Françoise Firmin in Paris, which translates into waiting until age 10 for the possibility of obtaining an adequate cartilage harvest. A second stage is necessary to create a retroauricular sulcus, and this procedure requires the use of a fascia to cover the cartilage wedge that gives projection to the ear (Fig. 15.12). Initially a temporoparietal fascia flap was used, but this did not avoid the frequent contraction of the sulcus so a mastoid fascia with a local flap is preferred [20].

TCF patients often present a very low hairline in the mastoid region and also a very low set ear remnant, often located at the level of the mandibular angle. In some patients, a preliminary procedure is planned for repositioning of the earlobe and surgical epilation of a skin flap if an autologous reconstruction is planned (Fig. 15.13). An alloplastic reconstruction does not rely on the position of the hairline of the mastoid skin, thus surgical epilation is not necessary.

The reconstruction is then carried out according to the Nagata/Firmin two-stage procedure with a cartilage harvest (Fig. 15.14a–c). The procedure has then to be repeated on the contralateral side. Results may be sub-optimal in this region due to previous scarring and the low hairline. Lobe repositioning is, however, a procedure which is particularly appreciated (Fig. 15.15).

Most patients have a coronal scar due to the previous craniofacial reconstruction and scars in the mastoid region due to a BAHA positioning. This scarring and possible damage during the surgical procedures may alter the vascular integrity of the underlying temporoparietal fascia anteriorly and the occipital fascia posteriorly (Fig. 15.16). This condition would certainly influence the possibility of using the porous polyethylene implant with a temporoparietal fascia flap or an occipital flap.

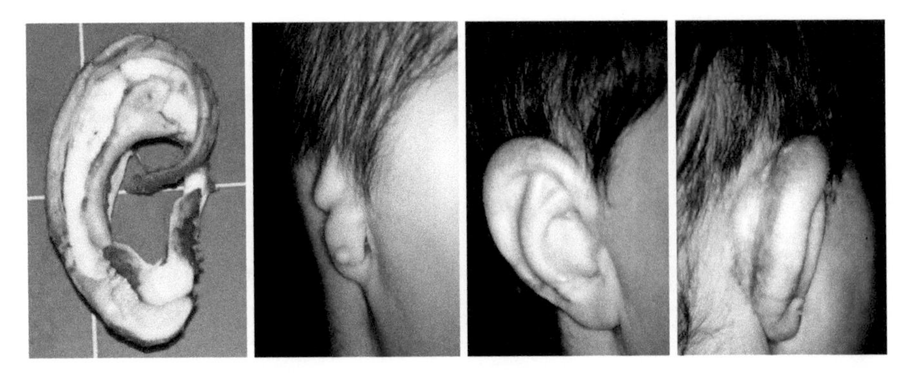

Fig. 15.12 Cartilage framework. Result in a classical microtia case

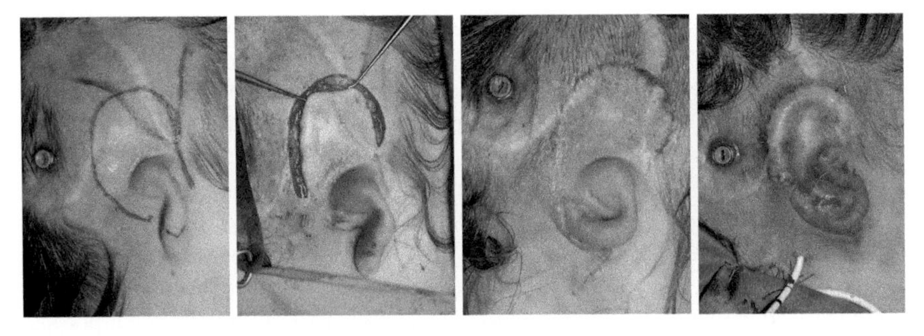

Fig. 15.13 Preliminary procedure for repositioning of the earlobe and surgical epilation of a skin flap

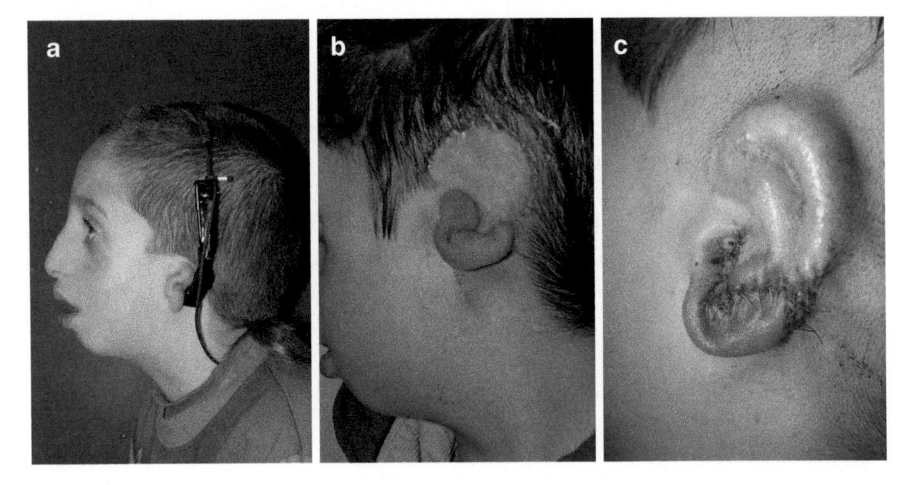

Fig. 15.14 (**a**) Low set ear remnant. (**b**) After repositioning and epilation of the flap. (**c**) After positioning of the cartilage framework

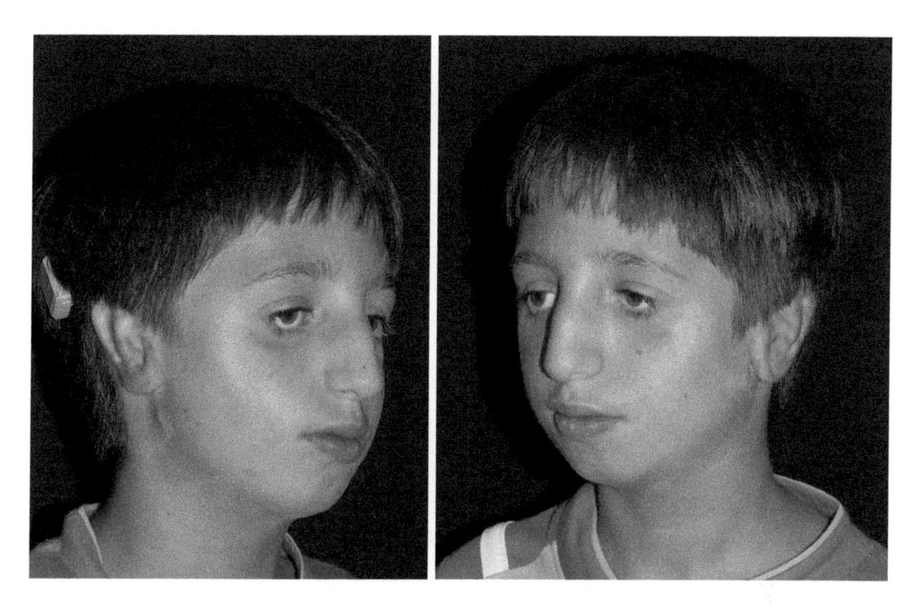

Fig. 15.15 Patient with a bilateral ear reconstruction after repositioning of the low set remnants. No malar reconstruction has been carried out

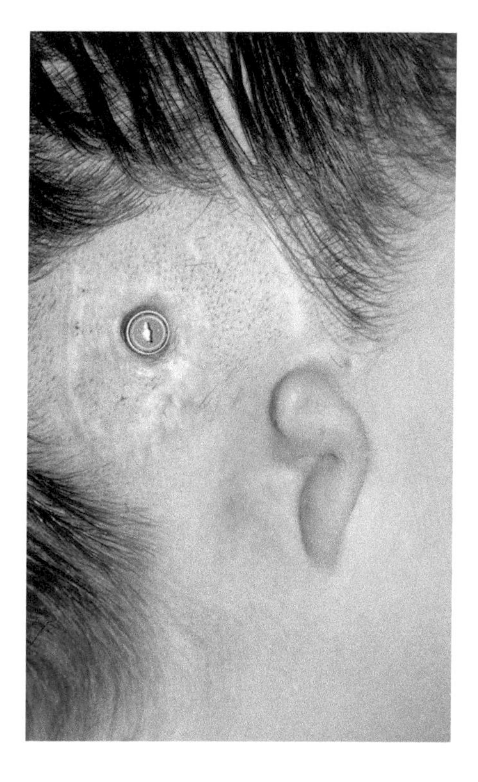

Fig. 15.16 Scars due to the previous surgical procedures, which may alter the vascular integrity of the underlying temporal and occipital fascias

Discussion

After more than 20 years of experience in treating patients affected by this complex syndrome, it is evident that the most satisfactory results that we have obtained are the adequate reconstruction of the orbito-palpebral region with long-lasting results and a progressive normalization of facial features. The same cannot be claimed for ear reconstruction with autologous cartilage. The need to wait until age 10 for an adequate cartilage harvest means that an ENT surgeon will have already placed a BAHA in the mastoid region to correct the conductive hearing loss. The possibility of reconstructing the outer ear with a porous polyethylene implant (Medpor, Styker, Kalamazoo, MI, USA) that necessitates an intact temporoparietal fascia requires planning of a different sequence. Bilateral ear reconstruction at an early age would then be the first and second procedures with the possibility of utilizing a hemicoronal incision to harvest the temporoparietal fascia. The BAHA could be positioned during this surgical stage, thus avoiding further scarring. This same incision would then allow access to the facial skeleton for the orbito-palpebral reconstruction with cranial bone grafts. In this manner, there would be a modification of the original algorithm (Fig. 15.17).

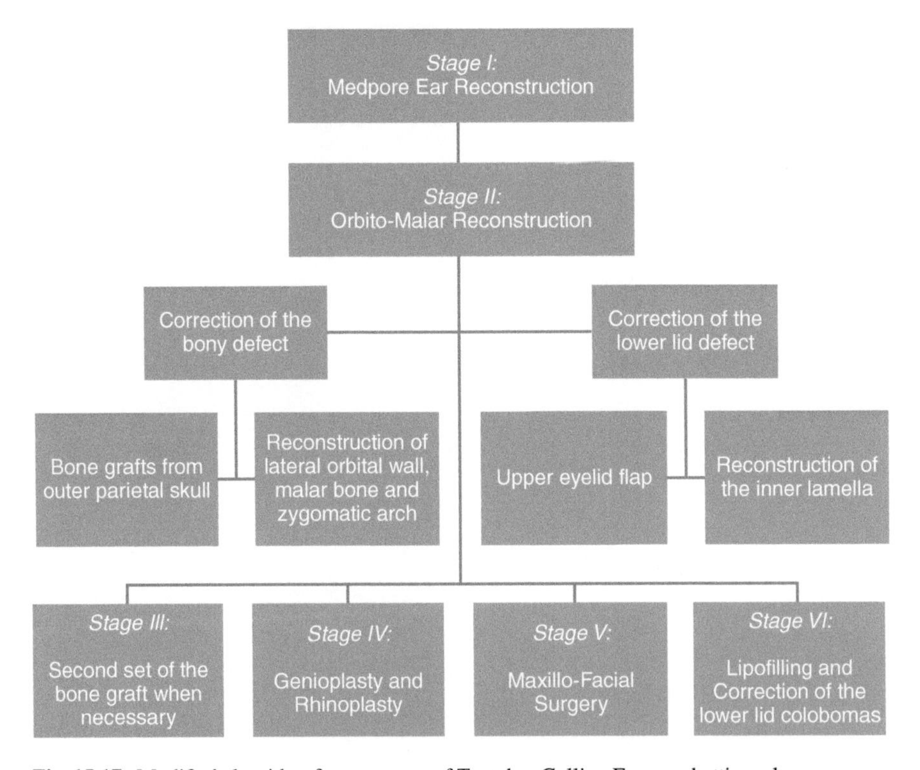

Fig. 15.17 Modified algorithm for treatment of Treacher Collins-Franceschetti syndrome

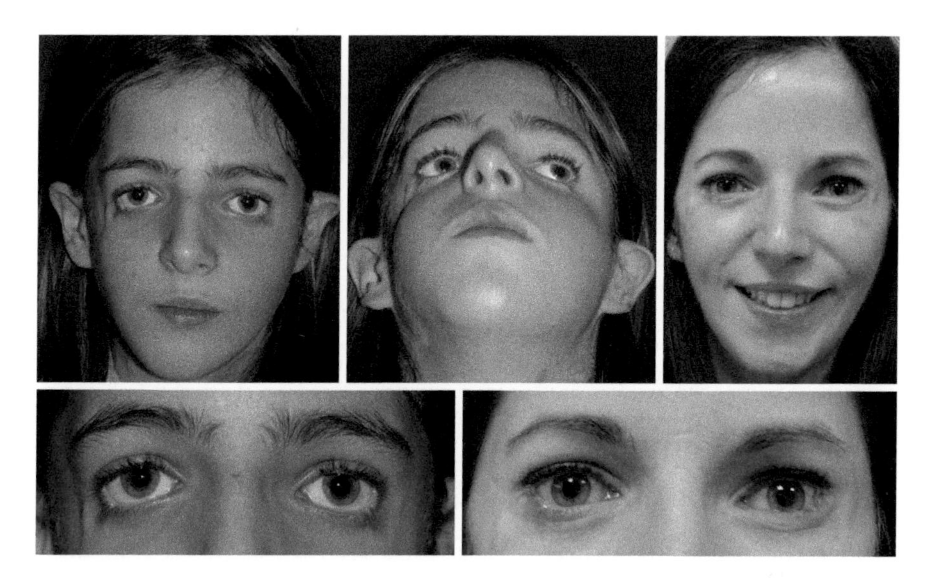

Fig. 15.18 Progressive normalization of the typical facial features

Conclusion

In TCFS like in other craniofacial anomalies, our aim is to normalize the facial structures. It is a subtle interplay in the creation of forms and volumes that may even render these faces beautiful, but our search is above all aimed at removing the typical stigmata of the syndrome (Fig. 15.18).

References

1. Schaefer E, Collet C, Genevieve D, Vincent M, Lohmann DR, Sanchez E, et al. Autosomal recessive POLR1D mutation with decrease of TCOF1 mRNA is responsible for Treacher Collins syndrome. Genet Med. 2014;16:720–4.
2. Thompson JT, Anderson PJ, David DJ. Treacher Collins syndrome: protocol management from birth to maturity. J Craniofac Surg. 2009;20:2028–35.
3. Marsella P, Scorpecci A, Pacifico C, Tieri L. Bone-anchored hearing aid (Baha) in patients with Treacher Collins syndrome: tips and pitfalls. Int J Pediatr Otorhinolaryngol. 2011;75:1308–12.
4. Fan KL, Federico C, Kawamoto HK, Bradley JP. Optimizing the timing and technique of Treacher Collins orbitalmalar reconstruction. J Craniofac Surg. 2012;23(Suppl1):2033–7.
5. Tulasne JF, Tessier PL. Results of the Tessier integral procedure for correction of Treacher Collins syndrome. Cleft Palate J. 1986;23(Suppl 1):40–9.
6. Krastinova-Lolov D. Le lifting facial sous-périosté. Ann Chir Plast Esthét. 1989;34:199–211.
7. Tessier P. Surgical correction of Treacher Collins syndrome. In: Bell WH, editor. Modern practice in orthognatic and reconstructive surgery, vol. 2. Philadelphia: Saunders; 1992.
8. Santini J, Krastinova D. Chirurgie plastique de la face, rajeunissement, embellissement, concepts et pratique. In: Rapport de la société Francaise d'ORL et de Chirurgie de la Face et du Cou. Paris: Editeur; 1999.

9. Coleman SR. Structural fat grafting: more than a permanent filler. Plast Reconstr Surg. 2006;118(suppl 3):108SY120S.
10. Miller JJ, Schendel SA. Invited discussion: surgical treatment of Treacher Collins syndrome. Ann Plast Surg. 2006;56:555–6.
11. Kobus K, Wojcicki P. Surgical treatment of Treacher Collins syndrome. Ann Plast Surg. 2006;56:549–54.
12. Posnick JC, Ruiz RL. Treacher Collins syndrome: current evaluation, treatment, and future directions. Cleft Palate Craniofac J. 2000;37:434.
13. Posnick JC, Tiwana PS, Costello BJ. Treacher Collins syndrome: comprehensive evaluation and treatment. Oral Maxillofac Surg Clin North Am. 2004;16:503–23.
14. Freihofer HP. Variations in the correction of Treacher Collins syndrome. Plast Reconstr Surg. 1997;99:647–57.
15. Plomp RG, Versnel SL, van Lieshout MJ, Poublon RM, Mathijssen IM. Long-term assessment of facial features and functions needing more attention in treatment of Treacher Collins syndrome. J Plast Reconstr Aesthet Surg. 2013;66:e217–26.
16. Firmin F. Auricular reconstruction in cases of microtia. Principles, methods and classification. Ann Chir Plast Esthet. 2001;46(5):447–66.
17. Nagata S. Total auricular reconstruction with a three-dimensional costal cartilage framework. Ann Chir Plast Esthet. 1995;40:371–99.
18. Reinisch JF, Lewin S. Ear reconstruction using a porous polyethylene framework and temporoparietal fascia flap. Facial Plast Surg. 2009;25:181–9.
19. Baluch N, Nagata S, Park C, Wilkes GH, Reinisch J, Kasrai L, et al. Auricular reconstruction for microtia: a review of available methods. Plastic Surg (Oakv). 2014;22(1):39–43.
20. Cecchi P, Bianciardi Valassina MF, Maggiulli F, Zama M. Ear reconstruction: a new flap for the retroauricular sulcus. J Plast Reconstr Aesthet Surg. 2013;66(8):1153–4.

Chapter 16
Tissue Engineering an Ear

Ananth S. Murthy

Traditional Ear Reconstruction

Surgical correction of ear anomalies continues to be a challenge for plastic and reconstructive surgeons. The ear is an intricately shaped three-dimensional structure that protrudes externally from the surface of the head. Traditional reconstruction with the use of costal cartilage remains relatively unchanged since its original description by Tanzer in 1959 [1]. The ear is an intricate framework that is not easily replicated by hand carving of costal cartilage and requires a high level of surgical skill and experience. The harvest of costal cartilage carries a significant donor site morbidity, as well as variability in age-related availability and pliability. These challenges, along with multiple-staged operations, and post-reconstruction concerns of growth, remodeling, or possible warping result in various degrees of surgical success in the constructed ear [2].

Another option is the use of a porous polyethylene framework which has been popularized by Reinisch [3]. The benefits of the polyethylene ear include a more realistic architecture with better prominence and symmetry. Surgically, it is a one-stage reconstruction removing the need for costal cartilage harvest with its complications. However, exposure and infection (although of low incidence) are a constant threat to the reconstructed ear.

A. S. Murthy (✉)
Pediatric Plastic and Reconstructive Surgery, Akron Children's Hospital, Akron, OH, USA
e-mail: amurthy@akronchildrens.org

© Springer Nature Switzerland AG 2019

J. F. Reinisch, Y. Tahiri (eds.), *Modern Microtia Reconstruction*,
https://doi.org/10.1007/978-3-030-16387-7_16

Background of Auricular Tissue Engineering

Previous Studies

Prefabrication with cartilage has been well documented in plastic surgery literature. Similarly, the use of diced cartilage grafts is also widely used in craniofacial surgery. Prefabrication with diced cartilage with the use of ear-shaped external molds was described previously by Peer in 1954 [4]. The idea of tissue engineering an ear with homologous cartilage has been a quest for several decades.

Multiple studies over 20 years have shown that auricular cartilage can be successfully engineered along predestined shapes [5–9]. Broadly, the auricular tissue has been regenerated by isolating and seeding cells (chondrocytes) onto various polymeric scaffolds and implanted in either immune-privileged rodent models or homologous animal models [10].

Despite initial success in animal models, advancement has been slow because of scaffold design flaws including poor retention of shape of the construct [8]. The success of tissue engineering depends upon an equilibrium of the biocompatible scaffold, quality and quantity of chondrocytes, growth factors, vascularization, and mechanical forces [9].

Cell and Cell Source

The chondrocyte is a 20–30 micron-sized cell (Fig. 16.1) that is easily isolated from cartilage matrix by enzymatic digestion [11, 12]. After isolation, provision of growth media and exposure to cytokines will promote cell proliferation and extracellular matrix (cartilage) production. In an animal model, after implantation, retention of the three-dimensional construct size and shape varied depending on the source of cartilage tissue (articular, auricular, costal, or nasoseptal) [13, 14]. The elastic property of auricular cartilage is unique because the large elastin extracellular matrix component is not found in other cartilage phenotypes [13] (Fig. 16.2a–c). Auricular cartilage has increased GAG content as well as elastin when compared to other chondrocyte phenotypes [15]. Histologic, gene expression analyses and mechanical properties revealed that the neocartilage generated from auricular chondrocytes was the optimal cell source for reproducing a human ear [13]. Interestingly, utilizing microtia-derived cells has yielded auricular-engineered cartilage similar to conchal harvested chondrocytes [16, 17].

One major obstacle continues to be obtaining optimal numbers of chondrocytes necessary to generate a cartilage tissue of sufficient size. Minimally 100 million cells may be required to initially seed an adult ear-shaped scaffold [18]. Insufficient cell density may lead to chondrocyte dedifferentiation and fibrous (scar) tissue ingrowth [19]. Expansion of chondrocytes in tissue culture can assure the number of

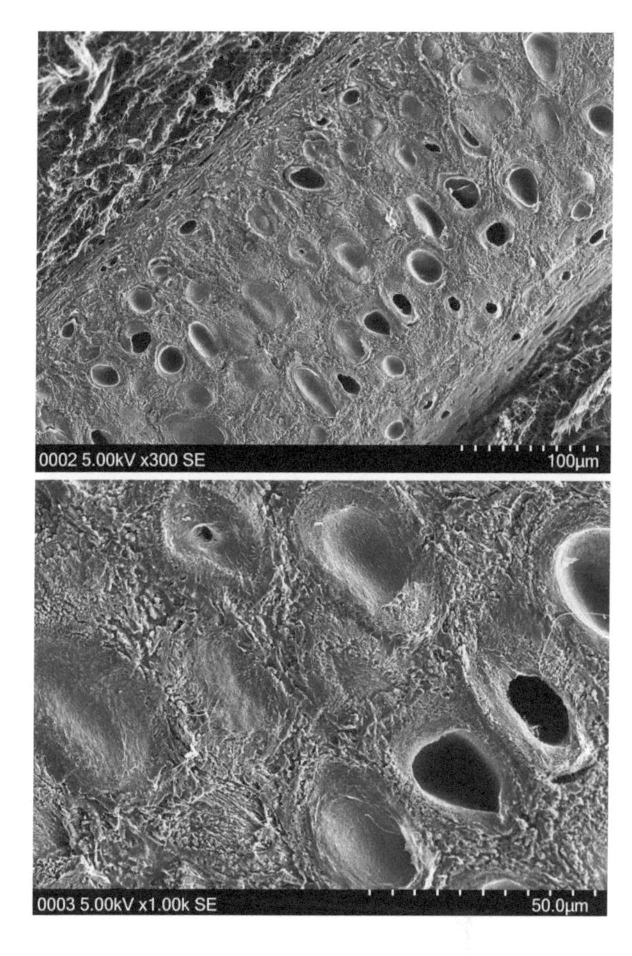

Fig. 16.1 Scanning electron microscope images of auricular chondrocytes. In electron micrographs, the matrix of ear cartilage consists of two components: chondrocytes residing in lacunae and a meshwork of extracellular molecules. (Courtesy of Dr. Noritaka Isogai, Kindai University, Osaka, Japan)

cells necessary to adequately seed a construct. Clinically, the use of cell culture has three main issues to resolve: (1) the time required to expand the cells; (2) the possible threat of contamination; and (3) dedifferentiation of chondrocytes, especially after multiple passages, into fibroblasts [18]. Surgically, the expansion of cells would require the patient initially to have a cartilage biopsy and then return to the operating room 1–2 weeks later for implantation of the expanded chondrocyte-biopolymer construct [20].

Cytokines or Growth Factors

A recent review summarizes growth factors utilized in vitro or in vivo in the field of auricular tissue engineering [9]. Expansion of chondrocytes by tissue culture (in vitro) and the use of basic fibroblast growth factor (FGF-2) have become a common

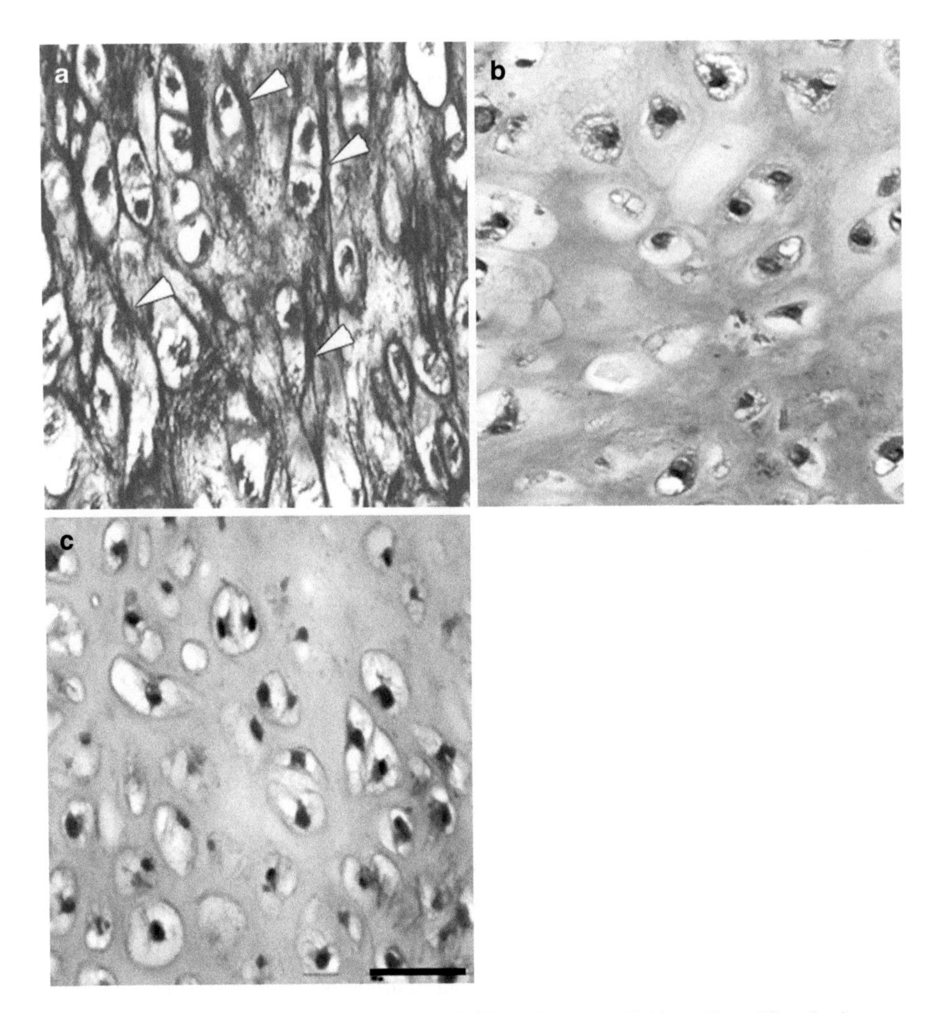

Fig. 16.2 Verhoeff stain of auricular (**a**), costal (**b**), and nasoseptal (**c**) cartilage. The elastic property of auricular cartilage is unique because the large elastin extracellular matrix component is not found in other cartilage phenotypes. The secretion of matrix molecules such as type II collagen, GAG, and elastin fibers (white arrows) in auricular cartilage provides flexibility and elasticity and is critical for deformation without failure. Bar = 50 μm

method to assure the number of cells necessary to seed an auricular-shaped scaffold [21, 22]. Scientifically, the use of FGF-2 inhibits chondrocytes from terminal differentiation allowing the rapid expansion of cells without dedifferentiation [20, 23]. This methodology can be utilized to expand auricular chondrocytes from microtia tissue or a conchal biopsy with similar outcomes [16].

Once the expanded cells are seeded onto auricular-shaped scaffolds and implanted, the chondrocytes should produce an extracellular matrix with the mechanical strength and flexibility that is maintained over time. Failures to produce cartilage after seeding and implantation have been from dedifferentiation of chondrocytes to fibroblasts or resorption of chondrocytes over time. The causes linked to chondrocyte apoptosis may be a scaffold-mediated inflammatory response, insufficient cell numbers, or weakened chondrocytes that results in fibrosis and loss of auricular shape [24]. Of the several growth factors outlined in the review, FGF-2 and osteogenic protein-1 (OP-1 or BMP-7) have been shown to improve chondrogenesis by increased cellular proliferation and extracellular matrix production in vivo. Maintaining an *auricular phenotype* certainly seems linked to a stable extracellular matrix rich in elastin fibers, GAG proteins, and type II collagen. By stimulating cell expansion in vitro and enhancing matrix production in vivo, reliable neocartilage production and shape retention can be expected.

Of note, cytokines, growth factors, and the use of stem cells (fetal, mesenchymal, and induced pluripotent) are also being studied as a means to produce chondrocyte numbers necessary for auricular tissue engineering [25]. The stability of stem cell-based expansion of human chondrocytes is unknown, and the pathways involved are complex and problematic but still may offer viable future solutions.

Matrix

The matrix provides a hospitable environment for the seeded chondrocytes and thus provides for phenotypic and genotypic stability. Several matrices for chondrocyte support have been used which broadly can be divided into alginates, pluronics, and fibrin gels. Alginate is an extraction of brown seaweed algae and has been shown to maintain chondrocytes and permit neocartilage production [26]. Alginate degradation did not promote an inflammatory response from cytokine influence [27].

Pluronic F-127 is a synthetic bioabsorbable hydrogel (70% polyethylene oxide and 30% polypropylene oxide). Similar to alginate, it supports neocartilage formation and elicits a minimal inflammatory response from the host. However, because it is a gel, the biomechanical properties will not support a 3D scaffold [28].

Fibrin gel (combination of thrombin/fibrinogen) has also been shown to support cartilage formation [29]. In fact, it was used to engineer flexible human ear-shaped constructs in nude mice [26] and in a surgically created vascularized capsule [30]. However, it offers no mechanical support and has to be maintained by either internal or external molds. Cartilage has been produced in a mouse model using fibrin gel over a polyglycolic/poly-L-lactic acid scaffold [31].

Matrices, including type I or II collagen, lack the mechanical strength to support a 3D auricular shape but have the structural properties that promote cell attachment and proliferation. In this regard, the combination of these matrices with scaffolds outlined below or reinforced with frameworks that add mechanical strength are a promising solution in the design of an auricle [22].

Scaffold

The physical microenvironment encountered by cells significantly influences attachment or adhesion, proliferation, and differentiation [32]. The consideration of the scaffold nanotopography is crucial in the support of the phenotypic maintenance of the seeded chondrocytes. Research regarding scaffolds has largely involved FDA-approved bioresorbable polymers such as polyglycolic acid (PGA), poly-L-lactic acid (PLLA), and PCL (polycaprolactone). Copolymers of different ratios of these synthetic polymers allow for different rates of bioresorption and mechanical strength [10]. Initially, the hydrophilic nature of PGA, which supports chondrocyte proliferation, was combined with the mechanical properties of PLLA, and cartilage was engineered in nude mouse models [6, 33, 34]. The more stable and longer degradation times of other resorbable polymeric scaffolds like PCL were also used but can promote an (unwanted) inflammatory reaction. This foreign body reaction may lead to compromise of the genotypic and phenotypic viability of chondrocytes as well as retention of the shape of the construct over time [7, 24, 35]. In one study, all constructs suffered from severe deformation regardless of the scaffold polymer secondary to this histologically observed inflammatory reaction [35]. Promise was seen when a PLLA/PCL copolymer maintained integrity in ear-shaped constructs, presumably secondary to the slow degradation of the PCL skeleton [33]. Unfortunately, initial success did not translate with the use of human cells in nude rodent models or large animal homologous studies.

With the advent of nanotechnology, tissue engineering was revived with the discovery that cells could easily attach to the nanofibers, rapidly proliferate which reduced cell numbers necessary for seeding. Based on the known biocompatibility of PGA, nanoscale-diameter polyglycolic acid sheets (mean fiber diameter of 1.1 μm and a fabric thickness of approximately 80 μm) have recently shown promise in long-term support of regenerated cartilage (Fig. 16.3) [16, 36]. The rapid degradation of the nanofibers does not provoke an inflammatory response, but the fabric must be used in combination with other polymers for mechanical strength [37].

Paradigm for Tissue Engineering an Ear

The success of auricular tissue engineering resides with the scaffold. Ideally, the engineered ear would be histologically, biochemically, and biomechanically similar to native cartilage. The cellular environment must be hospitable (hydrophilic) so as to improve cellular infiltration and attachment which will lead to proliferation and extracellular matrix formation. The 3D scaffold itself must have sufficient mechanical strength and flexibility to resist the skin compression (approximately 6 N/cm^2) over time [38]. Scaffold-free auricular cartilage implants have been surgically attempted by initial chondrocyte expansion abdominally with harvest and sculpting of auricular cartilage similar to current costal procedures [39]. The concern to this approach is the skin contracture over time and the need for multiple postsurgical procedures to prevent collapse of the ear.

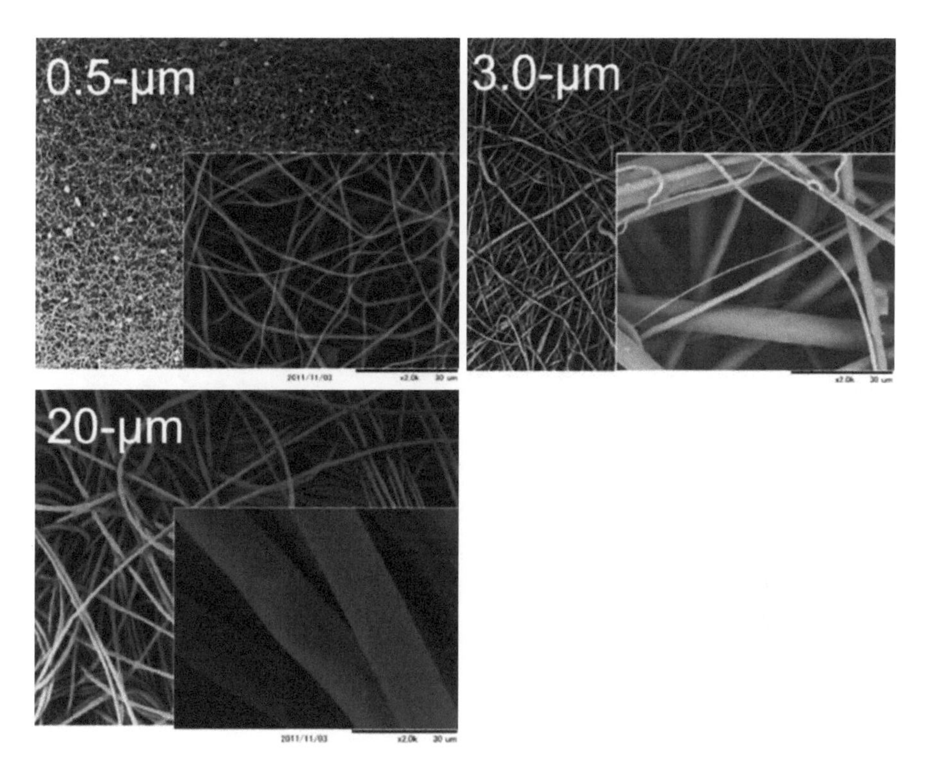

Fig. 16.3 Scanning electron microscope images of polyglycolic acid (PGA) fibers with average diameter of 0.5, 3, and 20 μm. Nano-PGA has excellent biocompatibility for chondrocytes and is a good choice for scaffolding material in cartilage regeneration studies. Nanofiber preparation of PGA (mean fiber diameter of 1.1 μm) is smaller than the seeded cell size, and resultant spacing between fibers is optimal to "trap" seeded cells which prevents cell seeping and provides high attachment efficiency. (Used with permission of Wolters Kluwer from Itani et al. [36])

Three-dimensional (3D) printing and computer-aided design (CAD) have always held the promise of creating precise copies of the unaffected ear. This patient-specific method for tissue engineering an ear scaffold would greatly improve aesthetically the reconstructed ear when compared to manual sculpting where results can be variable. The challenge for polymer engineering is to provide a substrate that is both flexible and strong enough to withstand the scar contraction forces and maintain the shape until the polymer scaffold is resorbed or replaced by cartilage [40]. Along with the appropriate scaffold, vestigial cartilage, although deformed, is usually present in the majority of microtia cases. These remnants can be used and avoid harvest of additional cartilage and associated donor site morbidity. The secretion of matrix proteins such as type II collagen from this source, with flexibility and elasticity provided by elastin fibers, is the key to success as it allows for deformation without failure. Combining an optimal chondrocyte source with a supportive scaffold will allow for a replacement tissue (like with like) that restores normal structure and appearance. This paradigm may require in vitro and in vivo phases to obtain adequate number of chondrocytes for seeding the scaffold (Fig. 16.4). In fact, Zhao et al. recently pub-

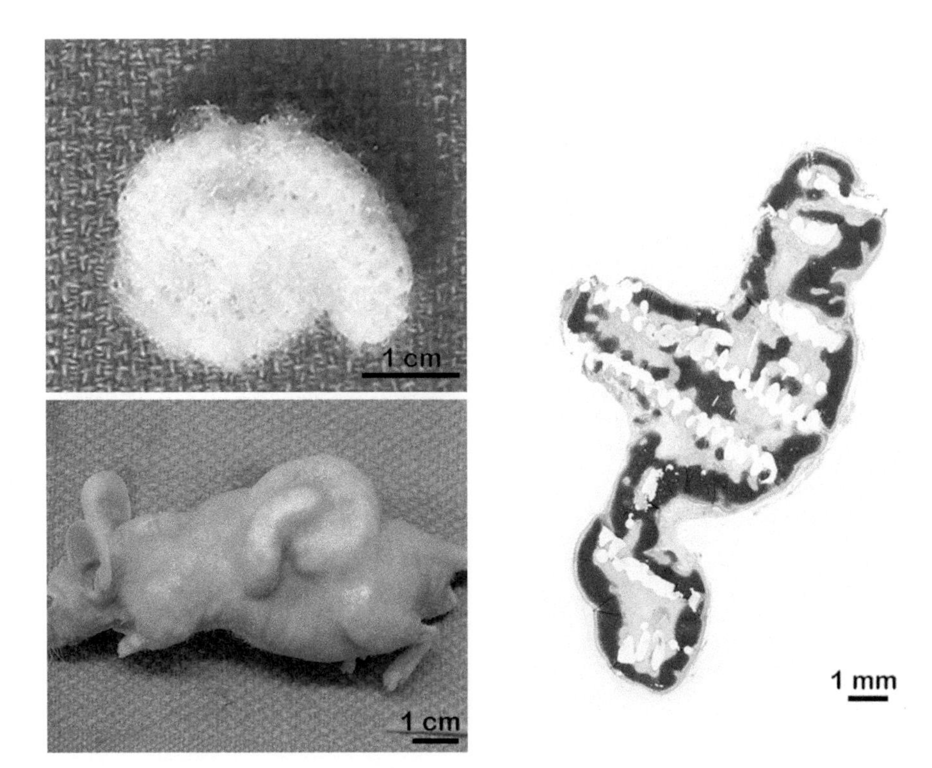

Fig. 16.4 Current state of tissue engineering in an animal model. A copolymer ear scaffold (KLS-Martin, Tuttlingen, Germany; and Gunze LTD, Kyoto, Japan) is seeded with passaged human microtia chondrocytes. A nude mouse behaves like a bioreactor, and cartilage is produced along the scaffold. After explantation, Safranin-O staining demonstrates cartilage production along the three-dimensional surface of the scaffold. (Courtesy of Robin DiFeo Childs, MS, Akron Children's Hospital, Akron, OH, USA)

lished the first clinical translation for this technique with histologic and radiologic evidence of cartilage matrix formation and scaffold resorbtion at 2.5 years after implantation [41]. However, after all the research with cell expansion, recently the FDA issued a statement that allows only for "minimal manipulation" of grafted tissue [42]. Until this statement is reversed or modified, expansion in vitro and its use in tissue engineering are in limbo.

Intermediate Steps and Future Directions

Nondegradable constructs are an attractive solution for ear reconstruction because they would definitely maintain the original dimensions over time. The concept of developing a cartilage bioshell over a nondegradable scaffold may prevent issues such as extrusion and skin erosion and has been previously described [43]. A collagen matrix with an embedded titanium wire framework has been shown to preserve auricular shape and size as well as allow for flexibility [44].

The successful use of this scaffold in a large animal model has now proceeded to a preclinical trial [45]. The nondegradable components of the scaffolds allow for an intermediate solution to the skin contracture and enhances the success of the ear reconstruction, but ultimately there is always the possibility of migration of the nondegradable portion.

Another possible intermediate step would be the use of diced cartilage which has long been used in plastic surgery. Auricular vestigial cartilage subjected to limited digestion and then suspended in a commercially available fibrin gel matrix could be used to cover the scaffold. Contralateral conchal cartilage graft may provide additional number of cells as well and obviate the need for a costal donor site. Customized constructs as a result of CAD and 3D printing can be made from resorbable polymers [44, 45]. A scaffold made from emerging copolymers would be a formulation of nanofibers which supports chondrocyte proliferation along with a strong long-lasting bioresorbable inner core which would provide stability and flexibility, as an example. Placing this hybrid cartilage-polymer construct under a temporoparietal fascial flap to promote construct-tissue integration would be optimal for coverage [21]. The adjunct use of FDA-approved growth factors may further stabilize the genotype and phenotype of the seeded diced cartilage.

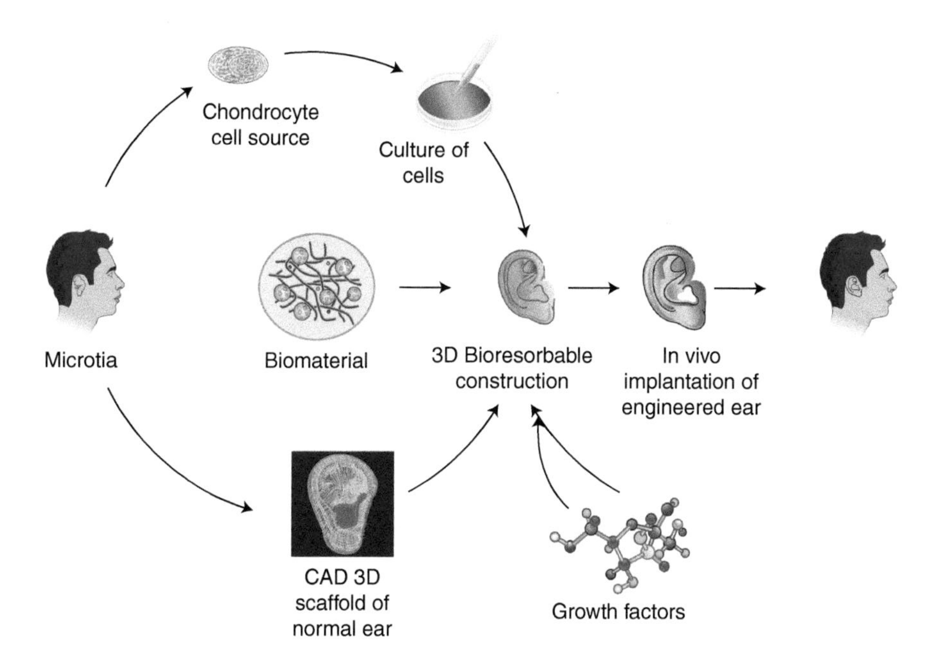

Fig. 16.5 A proposed schema for tissue engineering a human ear. Vestigial auricular cartilage is subjected to digestion and expanded to provide the optimal quality and quantity of cells. Customized constructs as a result of CAD and 3D printing can be made from resorbable polymers. A scaffold made from emerging copolymers supports chondrocyte proliferation along with providing stability and flexibility. The adjunct use of cytokines and growth factors may further stabilize the genotype and phenotype of the seeded cartilage. Placing this hybrid cartilage-polymer construct under a temporoparietal fascial flap to promote construct-tissue integration would be optimal for coverage

However, auricular tissue engineering currently would be most successful with the use of a resorbable scaffold and expanded auricular cell source. Future studies will need to delineate optimal biocompatible scaffolds, cytokines, or growth factors to maintain the cartilage and prevent dedifferentiation and biomimetic engineering to allow for normal appearance, contour, thickness, and flexibility of the construct [46] (Fig. 16.5).

Future clinical applicability will emphasize personalized bedside products. Research is already in progress with an instrument that would combine patient cells in the 3D printing of their CAD-generated ear-shaped construct [47]. Following proper expansion of homologous chondrocytes in an FDA-approved, in-house tissue processing center, the cell-construct hybrid would be delivered to the surgery suite.

Acknowledgments The author thanks Robin Childs, our lab manager, for reviewing, editing, and teaching me the intricacies of auricular tissue engineering; Dr. Noritaka Isogai, for encouraging my research and being an inspiration in tissue engineering; Dr. William Landis, for always being the voice that demands good evidence and science behind our research studies; and KLS-Martin and Gunze LTD companies, for allowing me to use their proprietary scaffold both for our ongoing study and for this publication.

References

1. Tanzer RC. Total reconstruction of the external ear. Plast Reconstr Surg Transplant Bull. 1959;23(1):1–15.
2. Bauer BS. Reconstruction of microtia. Plast Reconstr Surg. 2009;124(1 Suppl):14e–26e.
3. Reinisch J. Ear reconstruction in young children. Facial Plast Surg. 2015;31(6):600–3.
4. Peer LA. Extended use of diced cartilage grafts. Plast Reconstr Surg. 1954;14(3):178–85.
5. Kim WS, Vacanti JP, Cima L, Mooney D, Upton J, Puelacher WC, Vacanti CA. Cartilage engineered in predetermined shapes employing cell transplantation on synthetic biodegradable polymers. Plast Reconstr Surg. 1994;94(2):233–7.
6. Cao Y, Vacanti JP, Paige KT, Upton J, Vacanti CA. Transplantation of chondrocytes utilizing a polymer-cell construct to produce tissue-engineered cartilage in the shape of a human ear. Plast Reconstr Surg. 1997;100(2):297–302.
7. Shieh SJ, Terada S, Vacanti JP. Tissue engineering auricular reconstruction: in vitro and in vivo studies. Biomaterials. 2004;25(9):1545–57.
8. Xu JW, Johnson TS, Motarjem PM, Peretti GM, Randolph MA, Yaremchuk MJ. Tissue-engineered flexible ear-shaped cartilage. Plast Reconstr Surg. 2005;115(6):1633–41.
9. Nayyer L, Patel KH, Esmaeili A, Rippel RA, Birchall M, O'toole G, Butler PE, Seifalian AM. Tissue engineering: revolution and challenge in auricular cartilage reconstruction. Plast Reconstr Surg. 2012;129(5):1123–37.
10. Bichara DA, O'Sullivan NA, Pomerantseva I, Zhao X, Sundback CA, Vacanti JP, Randolph MA. The tissue-engineered auricle: past, present, and future. Tissue Eng Part B Rev. 2012;18(1):51–61.
11. Kawiak J, Moskalewski S, Darzynkiewicz Z. Isolation of chondrocytes from calf cartilage. Exp Cell Res. 1965;39(1):59–68.
12. Klagsburn M. Large scale preparation of chondrocytes. Methods Enzymol. 1979;58:560–4.
13. Kusuhara H, Isogai N, Enjo M, Otani H, Ikada Y, Jacquet R, Lowder E, Landis WJ. Tissue engineering a model for the human ear: assessment of size, shape, morphology, and gene expression following seeding of different chondrocytes. Wound Repair Regen. 2009;17(1):136–46.
14. Haisch A. Ear reconstruction through tissue engineering. Adv Otorhinolaryngol. 2010;68:108–19.

15. Park SS, Jin HR, Chi DH, Taylor RS. Characteristics of tissue-engineered cartilage from human auricular chondrocytes. Biomaterials. 2004;25(12):2363–9.
16. Nakao H, Jacquet RD, Shasti M, Isogai N, Murthy AS, Landis WJ. Long-term comparison between human normal Conchal and microtia chondrocytes regenerated by tissue engineering on nanofiber polyglycolic acid scaffolds. Plast Reconstr Surg. 2017;139(4):911e–21e.
17. Kamil SH, Vacanti MP, Vacanti CA, Eavey RD. Microtia chondrocytes as a donor source for tissue-engineered cartilage. Laryngoscope. 2004;114(12):2187–90.
18. Saadeh PB, Brent B, Mehrara BJ, Steinbrech DS, Ting V, Gittes GK, Longaker MT. Human cartilage engineering: chondrocyte extraction, proliferation, and characterization for construct development. Ann Plast Surg. 1999;42(5):509–13.
19. Puelacher WC, Kim SW, Vacanti JP, Schloo B, Mooney D, Vacanti CA. Tissue-engineered growth of cartilage: the effect of varying the concentration of chondrocytes seeded onto synthetic polymer matrices. Int J Oral Maxillofac Surg. 1994;23(1):49–53.
20. Shasti M, Jacquet R, McClellan P, Yang J, Matsushima S, Isogai N, Murthy A, Landis WJ. Effects of FGF-2 and OP-1 in vitro on donor source cartilage for auricular reconstruction tissue engineering. Int J Pediatr Otorhinolaryngol. 2014;78(3):416–22.
21. Isogai N, Nakagawa Y, Suzuki K, Yamada R, Asamura S, Hayakawa S, Munakata H. Cytokine-rich autologous serum system for cartilaginous tissue engineering. Ann Plast Surg. 2008;60(6):703–9.
22. Pomerantseva I, Bichara DA, Tseng A, Cronce MJ, Cervantes TM, Kimura AM, Neville CM, Roscioli N, Vacanti JP, Randolph MA, Sundback CA. Ear-shaped stable auricular cartilage engineered from extensively expanded chondrocytes in an immunocompetent experimental animal model. Tissue Eng Part A. 2016;22(3–4):197–207.
23. Wroblewski J, Edwall-Arvidsson C. Inhibitory effects of basic fibroblast growth factor on chondrocyte differentiation. J Bone Miner Res. 1995;10(5):735–42.
24. Santavirta S, Konttinen YT, Saito T, Grönblad M, Partio E, Kemppinen P, Rokkanen P. Immune response to polyglycolic acid implants. J Bone Joint Surg Br. 1990;72(4):597–600.
25. Zhao X, Hwang NS, Bichara DA, Saris DB, Malda J, Vacanti JP, Pomerantseva I, Sundback CA, Langer R, Anderson DG, Randolph MA. Chondrogenesis by bone marrow-derived mesenchymal stem cells grown in chondrocyte-conditioned medium for auricular reconstruction. J Tissue Eng Regen Med. 2017;11(10):2763–73.
26. Xu JW, Zaporojan V, Peretti GM, Roses RE, Morse KB, Roy AK, Mesa JM, Randolph MA, Bonassar LJ, Yaremchuk MJ. Injectable tissue-engineered cartilage with different chondrocyte sources. Plast Reconstr Surg. 2004;113(5):1361–71.
27. Chang SC, Tobias G, Roy AK, Vacanti CA, Bonassar LJ. Tissue engineering of autologous cartilage for craniofacial reconstruction by injection molding. Plast Reconstr Surg. 2003;112(3):793–9. 20.
28. Cao Y, Rodriguez A, Vacanti M, Ibarra C, Arevalo C, Vacanti CA. Comparative study of the use of poly (glycolic acid), calcium alginate and pluronics in the engineering of autologous porcine cartilage. J Biomater Sci Polym Ed. 1998;9:475.
29. Silverman RP, Passaretti D, Huang W, Randolph MA, Yaremchuk MJ. Injectable tissue-engineered cartilage using a fibrin glue polymer. Plast Reconstr Surg. 1999;103(7):1809–18.
30. Neumeister MW, Wu T, Chambers C. Vascularized tissue-engineered ears. Plast Reconstr Surg. 2006;117(1):116–22.
31. Haisch A, Duda GN, Schroeder D, Gröger A, Gebert C, Leder K, Sittinger M. The morphology and biomechanical characteristics of subcutaneously implanted tissue-engineered human septal cartilage. Eur Arch Otorhinolaryngol. 2005;262(12):993–7.
32. Marszalek JE, Simon CG Jr, Thodeti C, Adapala RK, Murthy A, Karim A. 2.5D constructs for characterizing phase separated polymer blend surface morphology in tissue engineering scaffolds. J Biomed Mater Res A. 2013;101(5):1502–10.
33. Isogai N, Asamura S, Higashi T, Ikada Y, Morita S, Hillyer J, Jacquet R, Landis WJ. Tissue engineering of an auricular cartilage model utilizing cultured chondrocyte-poly(L-lactide-epsilon-caprolactone) scaffolds. Tissue Eng. 2004;10(5–6):673–87.
34. Liu Y, Zhang L, Zhou G, Li Q, Liu W, Yu Z, Luo X, Jiang T, Zhang W, Cao Y. In vitro engineering of human ear-shaped cartilage assisted with CAD/CAM technology. Biomaterials. 2010;31(8):2176–83.

35. Britt JC, Park SS. Autogenous tissue-engineered cartilage: evaluation as an implant material. Arch Otolaryngol Head Neck Surg. 1998;124(6):671–7.
36. Itani Y, Asamura S, Matsui M, Tabata Y, Isogai N. Evaluation of nanofiber-based polyglycolic acid scaffolds for improved chondrocyte retention and in vivo bioengineered cartilage regeneration. Plast Reconstr Surg. 2014;133:805e–13e.
37. Lee SJ, Yoo JJ, Lim GJ, Atala A, Stitzel J. In vitro evaluation of electrospun nanofiber scaffolds for vascular graft application. J Biomed Mater Res A. 2007;83(4):999–1008.
38. Edwards C, Marks R. Evaluation of biomechanical properties of human skin. Clin Dermatol. 1995;13:375–80.
39. Yanaga H, Imai K, Fujimoto T, Yanaga K. Generating ears from cultured autologous auricular chondrocytes by using two-stage implantation in treatment of microtia. Plast Reconstr Surg. 2009;124(3):817–25.
40. Cohen BP, Hooper RC, Puetzer JL, Nordberg R, Asanbe O, Hernandez KA, Spector JA, Bonassar LJ. Long-term morphological and microarchitectural stability of tissue-engineered, patient-specific auricles in vivo. Tissue Eng Part A. 2016;22(5–6):461–8.
41. Zhou G, Jiang H, Yin Z, Liu Y, Zhang Q, Zhang C, Pan B, Zhou J, Zhou X, Sun H, Li D, He A, Zhang Z, Zhang W, Liu W, Cao Y. In vitro regeneration of patient-specific ear-shaped cartilage and its first clinical application for auricular reconstruction. EBioMedicine. 2018;28:287–302.
42. https://www.fda.gov/downloads/BiologicsBloodVaccines/GuidanceComplianceRegulatoryInformation/Guidances/Tissue/UCM469751.pdf
43. Lee SJ, Broda C, Atala A, Yoo JJ. Engineered cartilage covered ear implants for auricular cartilage reconstruction. Biomacromolecules. 2011;12(2):306–13.
44. Zhou L, Pomerantseva I, Bassett EK, Bowley CM, Zhao X, Bichara DA, Kulig KM, Vacanti JP, Randolph MA, Sundback CA. Engineering ear constructs with a composite scaffold to maintain dimensions. Tissue Eng Part A. 2011;17(11–12):1573–81.
45. Wiggenhauser PS, Schantz JT, Rotter N. Cartilage engineering in reconstructive surgery: auricular, nasal and tracheal engineering from a surgical perspective. Regen Med. 2017;12(3):303–14.
46. Sterodimas A, de Faria J, Correa WE, Pitanguy I. Tissue engineering and auricular reconstruction: a review. J Plast Reconstr Aesthet Surg. 2009;62(4):447–52.
47. Kang HW, Lee SJ, Ko IK, Kengla C, Yoo JJ, Atala A. A 3D bioprinting system to produce human-scale tissue constructs with structural integrity. Nat Biotechnol. 2016;34(3):312–9.

Chapter 17
Anesthesia Considerations in Ear Reconstruction

Richard J. Novak

Introduction

Ear reconstruction surgery for patients with microtia is primarily a pediatric practice, and these surgeries are most often performed in an ambulatory setting. Providing safe pediatric anesthesia care in a surgery center or office-based operating room is a vital aspect of the success of these procedures on outpatients. The anesthetic management presents preoperative, intraoperative, and postoperative challenges.

Preoperative Evaluation

Ambulatory surgery on pediatric patients is common in the United States. At least 60% of pediatric surgical procedures are now performed in an outpatient setting [1]. Because the prevalence of microtia is low, at only 2–3 patients per 100,000 population [2], a busy surgical and anesthetic team specializing in microtia reconstruction must accept patients from a wide geographical area. Our team routinely operates on patients from throughout the United States as well as Asia, Central and South America, Australia, and Europe. Families make long and expensive journeys to California for their surgery. It is imperative that preoperative screening for appropriate candidates is done prior to arrival. Screening requirements for pediatric ambulatory surgery in a freestanding surgery center or an office-based operating room include:

R. J. Novak (✉)
Adjunct Clinical Professor of Anesthesiology, Perioperative and Pain Medicine,
Stanford University, Stanford, CA, USA

© Springer Nature Switzerland AG 2019

J. F. Reinisch, Y. Tahiri (eds.), *Modern Microtia Reconstruction*,
https://doi.org/10.1007/978-3-030-16387-7_17

1. A history and physical from the primary care physician.
2. A medical workup of all cardiac, respiratory, or congenital abnormalities prior to travel to the surgical site city.
3. Absence of any active cardiac or pulmonary symptoms.
4. No preoperative laboratories or tests are ordered unless indicated by the history and physical.

The surgical office gathers the initial history and physical data. Blood tests and laboratory workup are not required unless indicated by the patient's history or physical exam. Microtia patients with associated congenital cardiac, respiratory, gastroenterologic, or airway abnormalities may require additional consultation by appropriate specialists nearer to the patient's geographical home. Accepted surgical patients should have no active cardiac or pulmonary disease and must not have dyspnea, productive cough, or fever. Patients with active or compensated cardiac or pulmonary disease may mandate their microtia surgery be performed in a hospital setting.

Healthy patients are booked for surgery without anesthesia consultation.

If a patient has a significant health abnormality, an anesthesiologist associated with the surgical team will review the chart and approve the case prior to the surgical date. If the anesthesiologist recommends further consultation or testing and the patient resides a great distance from the operating room location, these recommendations are carried out before the patient makes the journey to the surgical site.

Freestanding ambulatory centers are ideal locations for ear reconstruction surgeries because these procedures involve limited surgical trauma, blood loss, perioperative fluid shifts, or need for complex postoperative care. The lack of inpatient or emergency cases at an ambulatory surgery center enables surgical and anesthetic teams to work efficiently on stable, healthier patients. Freestanding surgery centers lack laboratory or blood bank services, radiology services, or intensive care units. If a patient becomes acutely ill, a freestanding surgery center must have a transfer arrangement with a local hospital.

Office-based operating rooms are becoming more commonplace in the United States and offer the surgeon the advantage of being able to manage their outpatient clinic practice and their surgical procedures in close proximity. Additional advantages include increased convenience for the patient's family as well as decreased costs for the surgery when compared to a hospital or a surgery center. Because most office facilities have only one operating room, the anesthesiologist staffing the facility each day must be highly qualified and experienced and must usually work alone without any backup from other anesthesia colleagues. State laws regulate office-based operating rooms, and oversight by regulatory organizations in many states is less rigorous than it is for surgery centers. Anesthesia care in an office-based operating room must comply with the same standards of care as anesthesia in hospitals and freestanding surgery centers. A supply of dantrolene for the treatment of malignant hyperthermia is required, as well as drugs to treat an acute cardiac emergency or cardiac arrest. Equipment requirements for office-based pediatric anesthesia care include:

1. An anesthesia machine equipped to deliver a sevoflurane/N2O/O2 anesthetic
2. Oxygen and nitrous oxide supply
3. All pediatric airway equipment described in the ASA difficult airway algorithm, including a video laryngoscope
4. A drug cart containing all the necessary anesthetic drugs
5. Suction
6. Drugs to treat acute cardiac emergencies or cardiac arrest, per Pediatric Advanced Life Support guidelines
7. Dantrolene for the treatment of malignant hyperthermia

Anesthesiologists must be certain that all necessary routine equipment, emergency equipment, and drugs are available in an office-based operating room prior to undertaking any anesthesia care. If a patient becomes acutely ill, an office-based operating room must have policies and procedures to facilitate emergency transfer to a local hospital.

We limit the number of anesthesiologists who staff our office-based ear reconstruction anesthesia practice, so that each individual sees an adequate volume of pediatric microtia/atresia patients to keep their skills honed. Not all of these anesthesiologists are fellowship-trained pediatric anesthesiologists, but all have long careers of anesthetizing children without complications.

For freestanding ambulatory centers, the University of Pennsylvania lists patient disqualifiers as age under 6 months of age, any cardiac disease, asthma with a recent emergency room visit or hospitalization, postoperative pain which is not easily controlled, known susceptibility to malignant hyperthermia, and any procedure over 4 hours in duration [3]. Our anesthetic team adheres to these recommendations, with the exception that we are comfortable with procedures longer than 4 hours providing that none of the other above factors are present.

A Canadian study showed a low incidence of unanticipated admission in ambulatory pediatric surgery, with only 0.97% of patients admitted to a hospital postoperatively [4]. Age <2 years, ASA physical status III, duration of surgery >1 hour, dental, ear-nose-and-throat or orthopedic procedures, and obstructive sleep apnea were all risk factors for unexpected admission. A study from Cincinnati, Ohio, showed that adverse respiratory events occurred in 2.8% of pediatric ambulatory surgeries and were the most common reason for unanticipated admission. Risk factors for adverse respiratory events were age less than or equal to 3 years of age, ASA physical status II and III (versus ASA I), morbid obesity, or a preexisting pulmonary disorder [5]. Our ear reconstruction anesthetic team respects these limits, with the exception that our surgeries routinely exceed 1 hour.

The child with a preoperative upper respiratory infection (URI) is of concern. A recent URI carries an increased risk for laryngospasm, bronchospasm, postintubation croup, and/or episodes of oxygen desaturization. The risk of these complications can continue for up to 6 weeks following a viral infection, so cancellation of surgery for less than 6 weeks does not ensure safety. If a child has a fever >38 degrees centigrade, chest symptoms of an approaching viral illness, wheezing, productive cough, or dyspnea, they are not a candidate for elective ear reconstruction, and the surgery is postponed until symptoms resolve [6]. If a child appears stable and only has symptoms of nasal discharge, we discuss the risks with the parents and routinely decide to proceed with the surgery. Because many patients travel long distances for their microtia surgery, cancelling surgery at the last moment is disruptive and disappointing to the family.

A preoperative anesthesia evaluation clinic is not essential for these patients. Arriving patients visit the surgeon's clinic 1 day prior to surgery. Any change in their physical or functional status at that time is reported to the anesthesia service. The scheduled anesthesiologist telephones the patient's parent(s) the night prior to surgery to discuss the anesthetic. Instruction to the family includes reminders that the child may not have solid food or milk after midnight and that clear liquids such as water or apple juice are safe until 2 hours prior to anesthetic induction [7]. The anesthesiologist typically meets the family for the first time immediately prior to the surgery the following day.

Preparation for Anesthetic Induction

On the day of surgery, a registered nurse performs the intake functions of documenting the patient's vital signs, weight, allergies, and medications history. The anesthesiologist reviews the medical chart and obtains an up-to-date history from the parents, utilizing an interpreter if the patient is non-English speaking. The anesthesiologist performs a physical exam with particular attention to the airway, lungs, and heart and explains the anesthetic plan and options to the parents. Efforts are made to decrease the anxiety of the parent(s) and the child. The anesthesiologist explains that the medications ensure that the child has no awareness or pain and that the child will reawaken when the anesthesia medications are discontinued. The anesthesiologist explains that the child will be as comfortable as possible on awakening. Reassurance is given that the child will not receive any shots or needles prior to going to sleep. The anesthesiologist explains to the parents the common minor risks of anesthesia (postoperative sleepiness, nausea, sore throat from the endotracheal tube, possible nausea, and possible postoperative agitation) as well as the remote chance of life-threatening complications, and parental consent is obtained.

Premedication with oral midazolam (0.5–0.7 mg/kg) is offered 20–40 minutes prior to induction as indicated. Midazolam is most useful in children 3–8 years old, ages when anxiety at the time of separating from the parent(s) is most common. Video games or video movies are an effective alternative and provide excellent non-pharmacologic cognitive distraction to relax a child prior to anesthetic induction [8].

Induction of Anesthesia

We ask parents to say goodbye to their child at the door of the operating room suite. The anesthesiologist and circulating nurse then bring the child to the operating table. Monitors are applied to the patient prior to inhalation induction. The child is allowed to continue playing a handheld video game or to continue watching a handheld iPad movie. The circulating nurse may hold the electronic device in front of the child's eyes as the child falls asleep. We do not permit or recommend parental presence inside the operating room at induction. Although one study showed a child's anxiety was significantly lower in a parental-presence group when compared to a parental-absence group at the time point when the child is separated from their parents, no significant difference occurred at any other time point and no outcome difference exists [9]. In our practice, we value inhalation induction as a critical medical procedure involving airway management and believe that the presence of an emotional layperson/parent in the operating room adds an unpredictable element should any complication occur during induction.

Inhalation induction by mask is initiated with 8% sevoflurane with or without 67% nitrous oxide. The anesthesiologist calms the patient with verbal reassurances such as stating how the child is "flying a plane and wearing a jet pilot mask" or asking the child to "blow up the balloon" of the anesthesia ventilation bag.

In an office-based operating room, there are usually no other anesthesia providers for miles around. The anesthesiologist must work alone with only the assistance of the circulating nurse and the surgeon. Prior to beginning inhalation induction, the anesthesiologist must be prepared for any or all airway emergencies, as described in the ASA difficult airway algorithm [10]. A well-stocked pediatric anesthesia cart is essential. Immediately available equipment must include an oral airway, a properly sized laryngeal mask airway, and a syringe loaded with succinylcholine/atropine in case of unresolved laryngospasm. Should upper airway obstruction or stridor occur, the anesthesiologist can apply 5–10 cm water of positive airway pressure via the ventilation bag and the pressure relief valve on the anesthesia machine to assist effective respiration during spontaneous ventilation.

Once the child has lost consciousness and their gaze is conjugate [11], an intravenous line is placed. Three methods are recommended if the anesthesiologist is working alone:

1. If the airway is easily maintained, the surgeon or circulating nurse can hold the mask while the anesthesiologist moves to the patient's upper extremity and starts the IV.
2. If the airway is easily maintained, the anesthesiologist can strap the anesthesia mask over the patient's airway while the anesthesiologist moves to the patient's upper extremity and starts the IV.
3. The anesthesiologist can continue to hold the mask over the patient's face with his or her non-dominant hand while the circulating nurse tourniquets and flexes one of the patient's hands back toward the anesthesiologist, who then inserts the IV into the back of the patient's hand with his or her dominant hand.

Once the intravenous line is in place, this author prefers to inject rocuronium (0.5 mg/kg) to facilitate endotracheal intubation. Although otologic surgery may require a seventh cranial nerve monitor to be used during the surgery, the rocuronium dose will have dissipated during the 30–50 minutes of surgical preparation before the actual surgery begins. Succinylcholine should never be used for non-emergency muscle relaxation in children, because of its FDA black box warning regarding cardiac arrest in children with undetected muscular dystrophies [12]. If the anesthesiologist chooses to avoid a muscle relaxant altogether, the child may be intubated with an intravenous bolus of 2–3 mg/kg of propofol administered after sevoflurane induction.

Uncuffed endotracheal tube size selection follows the formula (age + 16)/4 = endotracheal tube size. Thus a 4-year-old child would require a size 5 uncuffed endotracheal tube. If the anesthesiologist prefers a cuffed endotracheal tube, a tube one half-sized smaller, i.e., a 4.5 cuffed endotracheal tube for the same patient, is used.

A variety of pediatric laryngoscopes should be available, as well as a pediatric video laryngoscope (VL). A straight blade such as a Miller 1 is recommended for toddlers. Either a straight or a curved blade may be used for older children. If visualization of the larynx proves difficult, the anesthesiologist should consider early use of the VL. Microtia patients may have facial congenital anomalies which make endotracheal intubation difficult. The incidence of difficult laryngoscopy in school-aged children with bilateral microtia is 42%, and the incidence in patients with unilateral microtia is 2% [13].

Maintenance of adequate mask ventilation between laryngoscopic attempts is critical. Patients with known difficult airways may require VL as the initial laryngoscopic technique. If a congenital airway anomaly is of extreme concern, that patient may require scheduling in a pediatric hospital setting with the planned presence of a second anesthesiologist at anesthesia induction.

For the 8–9-hour anesthetic duration of CAM surgeries, our surgeons routinely suture the endotracheal tube to the maxillary periodontal tissue to assure the tube cannot become dislodged during surgery. Inadvertent intraoperative extubation of the trachea must be avoided.

Intraoperative Management

Pediatric ambulatory surgery requires the same level of monitoring as utilized in a pediatric hospital, including end-tidal gas monitoring and temperature monitoring. All pressure points are well padded prior to the beginning of surgery. The surgical team may request an age-appropriate dose of antibiotic prophylaxis. Because microtia reconstruction can include implantation of a plastic prosthesis, vancomycin is frequently requested for antibiotic prophylaxis. The vancomycin dose must be initiated prior to surgical incision and infused over 1 hour via a piggyback intravenous infusion set.

General anesthesia is typically maintained with a combination of sevoflurane, nitrous oxide, and propofol, with incremental bolus doses of fentanyl as needed. The end-tidal sevoflurane concentration is varied from 1% to 2%, the nitrous oxide concentration is varied from 0% to 50%, and the propofol infusion rate is varied from 50 to 100 mcg/kg/min. Ventilation is typically controlled. If the surgeons utilize a facial nerve monitor, no muscle relaxants are administered after the intubation dose. Ondansetron, dexamethasone, and metoclopramide are usually given as intravenous antiemetics to decrease the incidence of postoperative nausea and vomiting.

Combined atresia-microtia (CAM) reconstruction surgeries require 8–9 hours of anesthesia time. This long duration poses unique challenges. In the office setting, a solo anesthesiologist must remain in attendance the entire time. A vigilant anesthesiologist must contend with the issues of his or her own food, water, and bathroom breaks. During an 8–9-hour anesthetic, our surgery-anesthesia team manages with these issues by allowing the solo anesthesiologist brief food, water, and bathroom breaks as necessary during stable moments of the anesthetic, while the surgeon and the circulating nurse remain with the patient.

The surgical team contributes to the anesthetic management by infiltrating the surgical fields with local anesthesia throughout the procedure. Injected doses of lidocaine and bupivacaine provide the primary intraoperative and postoperative analgesia. The chief purpose of the general anesthetic is to blunt the stimulus from the endotracheal tube, as well as to keep the patient free of awareness, pain, and movement.

A forced-air warming blanket is draped over the patient to prevent hypothermia. Core temperature is monitored by a rectal or esophageal temperature probe. Because a forced-air warming blanket covers much of the patient's torso, the potential exists for overheating the patient. Care must be taken to discontinue forced-air heating as the body temperature approaches 37 degrees centigrade.

Emergence from Anesthesia and Post-anesthesia Recovery Room Care

The final hour of the anesthetic is planned to render an awake, comfortable patient at the time of extubation. The anesthesiologist will initiate gradual tapering of the sevoflurane and propofol doses while maintaining sufficient anesthetic so that the patient will not cough or buck on the stimulus of the tracheal tube. A final IV dose of fentanyl 0.5 mcg/kg may be administered approximately 45–60 minutes prior to extubation. General anesthetics should be continued during the application of the surgical dressings, which is an exacting procedure that may take 10–20 minutes to complete.

When the head dressing is finished, all anesthetics are discontinued, and the operating table is rotated once again so that the head of the patient is near the anesthesia machine. If a suture was used to secure the endotracheal tube, this suture is cut. If the patient's spontaneous respiratory rate exceeds 20 breaths/minute, small incremental intravenous doses of fentanyl may be titrated into the IV. When the patient's spontaneous respiratory rate reaches 10–20 breaths/minute, the level of narcotic analgesia is likely to be adequate for postoperative comfort. At the time of awakening and eye opening, the pharynx is quickly suctioned and the trachea is extubated [14]. This author recommends remaining in the operating room where all emergency airway equipment and drugs are at easy access, until the patient's airway, breathing, and analgesic level are stable before transporting the patient to the recovery room.

On arrival at the recovery room, monitors are reapplied to the patient and supplemental oxygen is administered as needed to maintain oxygen saturation at or above 95%. After the initial vital signs are documented to be stable, the anesthesiologist proceeds to the waiting room to inform the parent(s) that their child is safe and awake, and the parents then return to the recovery room to reunite with their child.

With appropriate infiltration injections of local anesthesia during surgery and carefully titrated narcotics at the conclusion of surgery, the patient should have minimal recovery room pain. Utilizing local anesthetic infiltration to block postoperative pain is known to result in decreased need for hospitalization following pediatric surgery [15]. It is rare for a child to require additional intravenous narcotics in the recovery room. For this reason, the post-anesthesia stay rarely lasts more than 1 hour. Once the patient's Aldrete score returns to baseline in terms of activity, respiration, consciousness, blood circulation, and color, the child may be discharged. Because many families travel long distances to seek microtia reconstruction, at times patients are discharged to a hotel rather than to their home. The parent is given detailed written instructions regarding vigilance for complications following discharge.

Post-anesthesia Complications

In the past decade, our team has anesthetized hundreds of patients in our office-based and freestanding surgery center practice of pediatric ambulatory surgery for ear reconstruction, with no patient requiring hospitalization. We attribute this statistic to strict preoperative patient selection as well as excellent surgical and anesthetic care. Our statistics also include a total of over 300 CAM reconstruction procedures. Even though these CAM procedures require an average of 8–9 hours of general anesthesia, and each patient was discharged to a hotel or home environment directly from the post-anesthesia recovery room, we have had no adverse respiratory events.

Our results compare favorably to the published complication rates for pediatric ambulatory surgery. In a series of over 13,000 pediatric day surgery patients in Scotland, 1.8% of patients required unplanned admissions to a hospital. The cause of admission was nausea and vomiting (23%), postoperative bleeding (13.9%), and unexpected extent or difficulty of the procedure (11.8%) [16]. A second study of 21,957 pediatric ambulatory surgery patients from Canada showed an unanticipated admission rate for pediatric ambulatory surgery of 0.97% [4].

Anesthesia Care for Adult Ear Reconstruction

Anesthesia care for adult ear reconstruction is ideally suited for office-based or freestanding surgery center ambulatory anesthesia. Preoperative patient selection and preoperative assessment are done per the guidelines discussed for pediatric patients above. Adult anesthetics are induced by intravenous propofol and are followed by a similar endotracheal anesthetic plan as discussed for children above. Adult patients are extubated awake and discharged to their home or hotel after a 60–90-minute recovery room stay.

Summary

1. Ear reconstruction surgery in children can be safely done in office-based or freestanding surgery centers.
2. Proper patient selection is critical to minimize anesthetic risk. Preoperative screening and clearance is often done at a distant geographic location. We do not utilize or require an anesthesia preoperative clinic.
3. In an office setting, anesthesiologists must be highly qualified, highly experienced, and comfortable working alone without the backup of additional anesthesia colleagues.
4. General anesthesia with endotracheal intubation is used. The level of general anesthesia can be light because of the intraoperative analgesia supplied by the surgeon's infiltration of local anesthetics at the surgical site(s).
5. Postoperative pain is minimized by local anesthetic infiltration by the surgeons.
6. Postoperative nausea and vomiting are minimized by limiting the quantity of narcotic given and by administering prophylactic antiemetics during surgery.
7. Postoperative bleeding and surgical complications are minimized by careful surgical technique.
8. Cases of up to 9 hours of anesthesia time can be done safely, and these patients can be discharged to their home or hotel after a 60–90-minute stay in the postoperative recovery room.

References

1. Emhardt JD, Saysana C, Sirichotvithyakom P. Anesthetic considerations for pediatric outpatient surgery. Semin Pediatr Surg. 2004;13(3):210–21.
2. Luquetti DV, Leoncini E, Mastroiacovo P. Microtia-anotia: a global review of prevalence rates. Birth Defects Res A Clin Mol Teratol. 2011;91(9):813–22.
3. Fishkin S, Litman RS. Current issues in pediatric ambulatory anesthesia. Anesthesiol Clin North Am. 2003;21(2):305–11, ix.
4. Whippey A, Kostandoff G, Ma HK, Cheng J, Thabane L, Paul J. Predictors of unanticipated admission following ambulatory surgery in the pediatric population: a retrospective case-control study. Paediatr Anaesth. 2016;26(8):831–7.
5. Subramanyan R, Yeramaneni S, Hossain MM, Anneken AM, Varughese AM. Perioperative respiratory adverse events in pediatric ambulatory anesthesia: development and validation of a risk prediction tool. Anesth Analg. 2016;122(5):1578–85.
6. Cote CJ. Pediatric anesthesia. Chap. 93. In: Miller R, editor. Miller's anesthesia. 8th ed. Philadelphia: Elsevier; 2015. p. 2757–98.

7. ASA practice guidelines for preoperative fasting and the use of pharmacologic agents to reduce the risk of pulmonary aspiration: application to healthy patients undergoing elective procedures: and updated report by the American Society of Anesthesiologists Committee on Standards and Practice Parameters. Anesthesiology. 2011;114:495–511.
8. Patel A, Schieble T, Davidson M, Tran MC, Schoenberg C, Delphin E, Bennett H. Distraction with a hand-held video game reduces pediatric preoperative anxiety. Paediatr Anaesth. 2006;16(10):1019–27.
9. Wright KD, Stewart SH, Finley GA. When are parents helpful? A randomized clinical trial of the efficacy of parental presence for pediatric anesthesia. Can J Anaesth. 2010;57(8):751–8.
10. Apfelbaum JL, Hagberg CA, Caplan RA, Blitt CD, Connis RT, Nickinovich DG, et al. Practice guidelines of the difficult airway: an updated report by the American Society of Anesthesiologists task force on management of the difficult airway. Anesthesiology. 2013;118:251–70.
11. Lee SY, Cheng SL, Ng SB, Lim SL. Single-breath vital capacity high concentration sevoflurane induction in children: with or without nitrous oxide? Br J Anaesth. 2013;110(1):81–6.
12. PharmGKB, U. S. Food and Drug Administration (FDA) label information for succinylcholine. Available at https://www.pharmgkb.org/view/drug-label.do?id=PA166122970.
13. Uezono S, Holzman RS, Goto T, Nakata Y, Nagata S, Morita S. Prediction of difficult airway in school-aged patients with microtia. Paediatr Anaesth. 2001;11(4):409–13.
14. Tsui BC, Wagner A, Cave D, Elliott C, El-Hakim H, Malherbe S. The incidence of laryngospasm with a "no touch" extubation technique after tonsillectomy and adenoidectomy. Anesth Analg. 2004;98(2):327–9.
15. Lonnqvist PA, Morton NS. Paediatric day-case anaesthesia and pain control. Curr Opin Anaesthesiol. 2006;19(6):617–21.
16. Blacoe DA, Cunning E, Bell G. Paediatric day-case surgery: an audit of unplanned hospital admission Royal Hospital for Sick Children, Glasgow. Anaesthesia. 2008;63(6):610–5.

Chapter 18
Medical Photography

Christopher A. Derderian

Introduction

Today, digital cameras provide excellent resolution with many automatic functions to improve the image quality captured under varying conditions. A variety of proprietary computer programs are also available to improve image quality after the photo is taken, such as allowing for adjustments of suboptimal lighting effects. These tools make it easier today to obtain quality photos. However, a controlled and systematic setup is still needed to provide consistency and accuracy to the documentation process. This chapter will highlight the important considerations for taking patient photos in the clinic and in the operating room. These considerations include organizing a dedicated photo suite, lighting and camera body, and lens properties.

The Basics of Cameras and Lenses

A camera is made up of several key elements. The lens captures light from the subject that is directed though an adjustable diaphragm that controls the amount of light allowed through the aperture per unit time. The shutter has variable durations of opening "shutter speeds" that allow more or less light to reach the digital sensor (or film) in the body of the camera per exposure.

Point-and-shoot cameras have many features and are commonly used. They have the advantage of being smaller and more portable. Typically, point-and-shoot cameras will have a zoom lens, autofocus, and built-in flash. This makes them an attractive option to keep in one's bag for intraoperative photos. In the office setting, where

C. A. Derderian (✉)
Department of Plastic Surgery, University of Texas Southwestern Medical Center, Dallas, TX, USA
e-mail: Christopher.derderian@utsouthwestern.edu

© Springer Nature Switzerland AG 2019

J. F. Reinisch, Y. Tahiri (eds.), *Modern Microtia Reconstruction*,
https://doi.org/10.1007/978-3-030-16387-7_18

portability is less important, a digital SLR camera is better suited to interface with appropriate lighting systems to achieve the reproducibility and fine details wanted for medical documentation, operative planning, and publication quality photos we desire.

Today, a standard digital SLR camera will have more than enough pixels to achieve the resolution and publication quality one could desire. Standard publication resolution is 300 pixels per square inch. For a single-page printed photograph of 8 × 10 inches, you would need (8 × 300 pixels) 2400 × (10 × 300 pixels) 3000, which equals 7.2 million pixels. Today, most digital SLR cameras have resolution that is many times this number of pixels.

The aperture is the diameter of the opening in the diaphragm. This is frequently referred to as the F-stop (f/1.2, f/2, f/4, etc.). The F-stop and aperture values have an inverse relationship. The larger the F-stop is, the smaller the aperture is.

The depth of field is how wide or narrow a distance that objects in front of or beyond the main subject appear sharply in focus. The larger the F-stop (smaller the aperture) is, the greater the depth of field will be: images at different distances will both be in focus. Higher F-stops are frequently used for landscapes to have the entire image in focus. The smaller the F-stop (the larger the aperture) is, the narrower the depth of field will be: slight changes in distance from the primary subject will cause images to be blurred. This is often desirable for portraits. A sufficient aperture setting should be maintained to keep the entire subject in focus.

Appropriate lighting conditions and studio setup facilitate keeping the aperture settings ideal.

Short/fast shutter speeds are used for moving subjects such as athletes, animals, or children in motion to prevent blurring. When a camera is being held in hand versus on a tripod, a faster shutter speed can reduce or eliminate the blur created by shaking or movement of the photographer's hands. Having a tripod will also eliminate this blur, particularly in low light. In an office photo studio, the distance from where the patient stands/sits to the camera and the lens properties will be relatively fixed. Therefore, adjusting the aperture of the lens changes the depth of field – how much of the scene is in focus.

The focal length of the lens is the distance of the lens to the film or sensor. A "standard" lens has a fixed focal length and does not distort the image. The photographer must move closer or farther away from the subject to change the portion of the image (field of view) that the subject takes up. A "standard zoom" lens has an adjustable focal length that allows the photographer to remain in the same position and change the portion of the field of view that the subject occupies by adjusting the lens.

The "standard lens" is the lens that causes minimal image distortion in focus. Traditionally, this is determined by the diagonal dimension of the negative size that is 43 mm for 35 mm film. The 50 mm lens was closest to this dimension. This property at 50 mm is why many "standard zoom" lenses center their focal range on 50 mm, such as a 24–70 mm lens.

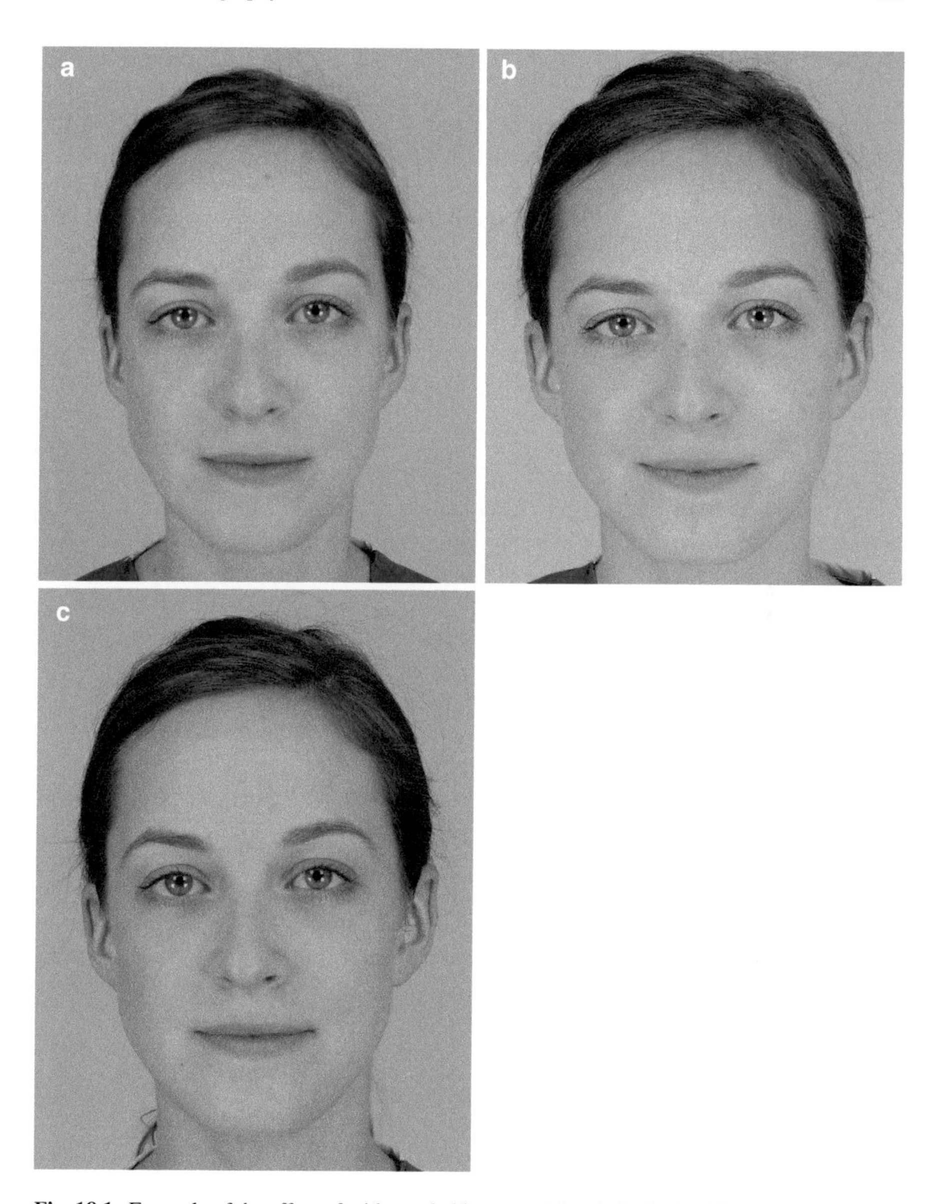

Fig. 18.1 Example of the effect of wide-angled lenses: subject is "spherized." In the AP view, the central facial features will appear full (exaggerated projection) (**a**), Example of the effect of telephoto lenses: central portion of the image is centrally pinched (features closer together) (**b**), Example of AP view (**c**)

Lenses with a focal length less than the diagonal of the film/sensor are considered wide-angled lenses. For 35 mm film, focal length less than 50 mm is a wide-angled lens. Telephoto lenses are those with a focal length longer than the diagonal dimension of the film/sensor.

Barrel distortion is a lens effect that occurs with wide-angled lenses, particularly at the wide end of a zoom lens focal length. The subject is "spherized." In the AP view, the central facial features will appear full (exaggerated projection) (Fig. 18.1). Pincushion distortion is a lens effect that occurs with telephoto lenses or the telephoto end of zoom lenses. The central portion of the image is centrally pinched (features closer together). Therefore it is critical that if a zoom lens is being used for patient photos, the middle range of the zoom lens should be used and should be an approximation of the standard lens to avoid image distortion.

Digital cameras often have sensors of smaller dimensions than traditional 35 mm film. The change in the dimensions of the sensor can cause the image obtained from a particular focal length to differ from what would be obtained with 35 mm film. This difference is in the field of view of the image the lens captures which is referred to as a crop factor.

The focal length is a property of the lens that does not change, but the field of view will appear as though a longer focal length was used because the image captured by the lens is larger than the sensor. The image captured will be a percentage of the center of the image that 35 mm film or a sensor with the dimensions of 35 mm film would capture. Imagine a projector image that is 1.6× larger than the projection screen that it is projected on. This effect is compensated for by using a crop factor or "focal length multiplier (FLM)." The FLM is typically 1.5–1.6. Using 1.6 as the crop factor to compensate for a smaller sensor area, a 50 mm lens will provide a field of view that an 80 mm lens would capture on 35 mm film.

In general, portrait lenses should be used for medical studio photography. I recommend a 50 mm or an 85 mm prime lens or a zoom lens that centers on this focal length.

Lighting and Studio Setup

The flash greatly impacts the settings and lens choice. In patient photographs, the primary role of the flash is to appropriately light the patient to appreciate fine features and coloring and eliminate shadows behind the patient. Reliability of the flash and how much light is emitted will impact the consistency of the photos. Built-in flash or flashes mounted on the body of the camera frequently produce harsh and uneven lighting with shadows behind the subject. These suboptimal light levels are also not sufficient to allow a larger F-stop to be used to provide a greater depth of field. One superior aspect of using a digital SLR in the operating room is the ability to use a ring flash that provides uniform flat lighting of the subject. In the office, ideally a studio setup should be used that allows symmetric lighting of the patient's face with strobe lights with a soft box and back lighting positioned at a 45-degree angle to minimize visible shadows behind the patient (Fig. 18.2a, b). When this degree of space cannot be dedicated to a photo studio, smaller strobes or a remotely mounted external flash should be used to provide even lighting and avoid shadows. A consistent, nonreflective background behind the patient is important. Light blue provides adequate contrast to all skin tones and hair color. Appropriate white balancing of the camera will help achieve consistency in color temperature.

Patient Positioning

Surgery of the ears requires adequate views to illustrate the projection of the ears, the position and axis of the ear in relation to other facial features, and the detailed anatomy of the affected and normal ears (when present). The relationship of the brow, lateral canthus, and nose to the axis and vertical position of the ear is captured in the AP, three-quarter, and lateral views (Fig. 18.3a–d). Projection and vertical positioning are key determinants of perceived symmetry. The views that aid in assessing the projection are AP upward and downward gazes and a direct posterior view (Fig. 18.4a–c).

Consent for Use of Images

When there is any possibility that patient photos may be used in a presentation or publication, it is imperative to have the patient's permission to use their photos. In general, institutions will have guidelines for the wording to be used on a photo consent. For surgeons in private practice, it is best to have an "all-or-none" approach to photo consents to avoid any confusion. Be explicit in the consent form that the photos may be used in any online, digital, or print media that may include protected health information. The American Society of Plastic Surgery offers resources for HIPPA compliant photo consent on the ASPS website.

Conclusion

In summary, a basic understanding of photography and a standardized approach allows plastic surgeons to reproducibly obtain high-quality standardized preoperative, intraoperative, and postoperative photos.

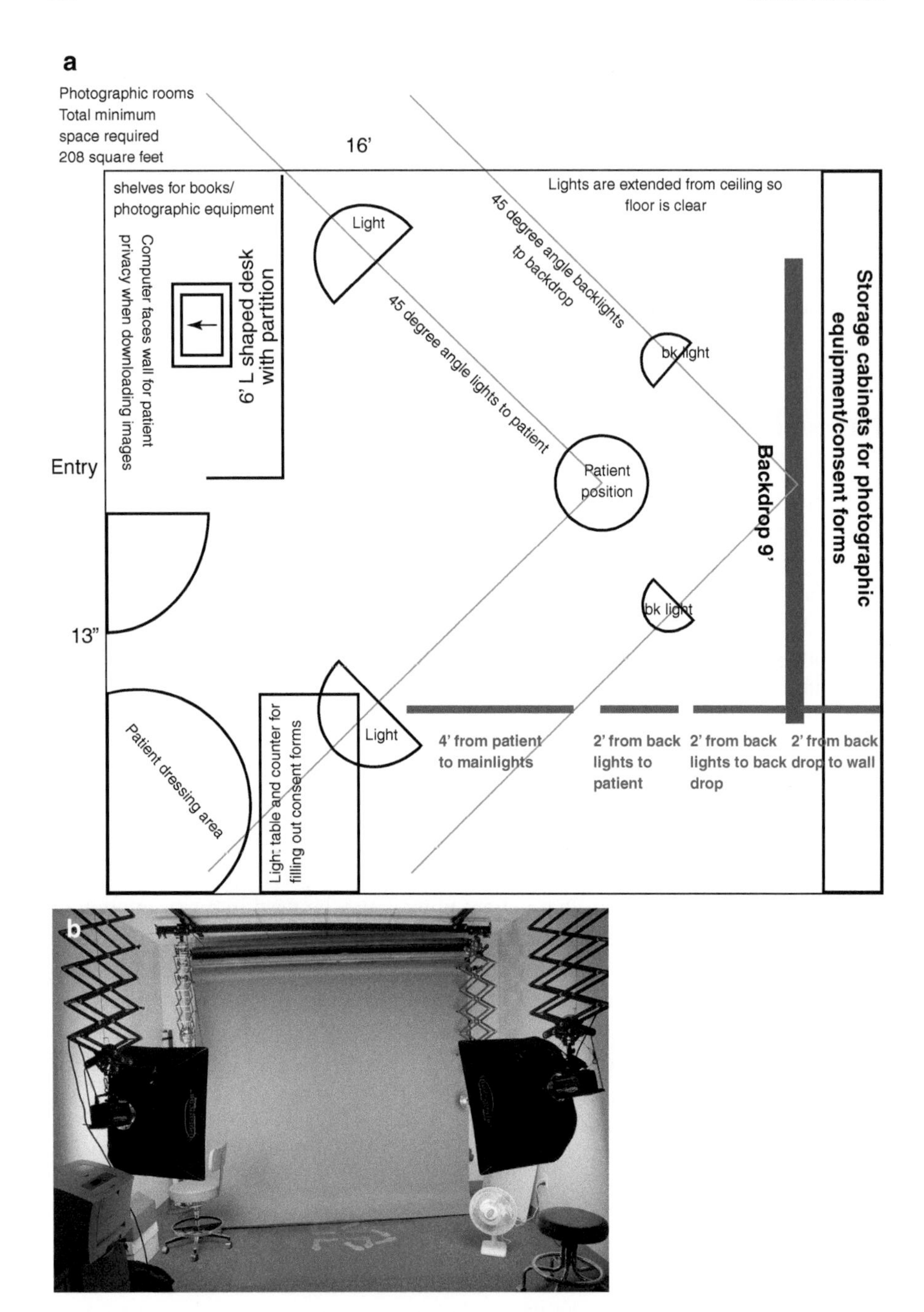

Fig. 18.2 (**a**) Diagram showing setup for photographic room. (**b**) Example of lighting setup

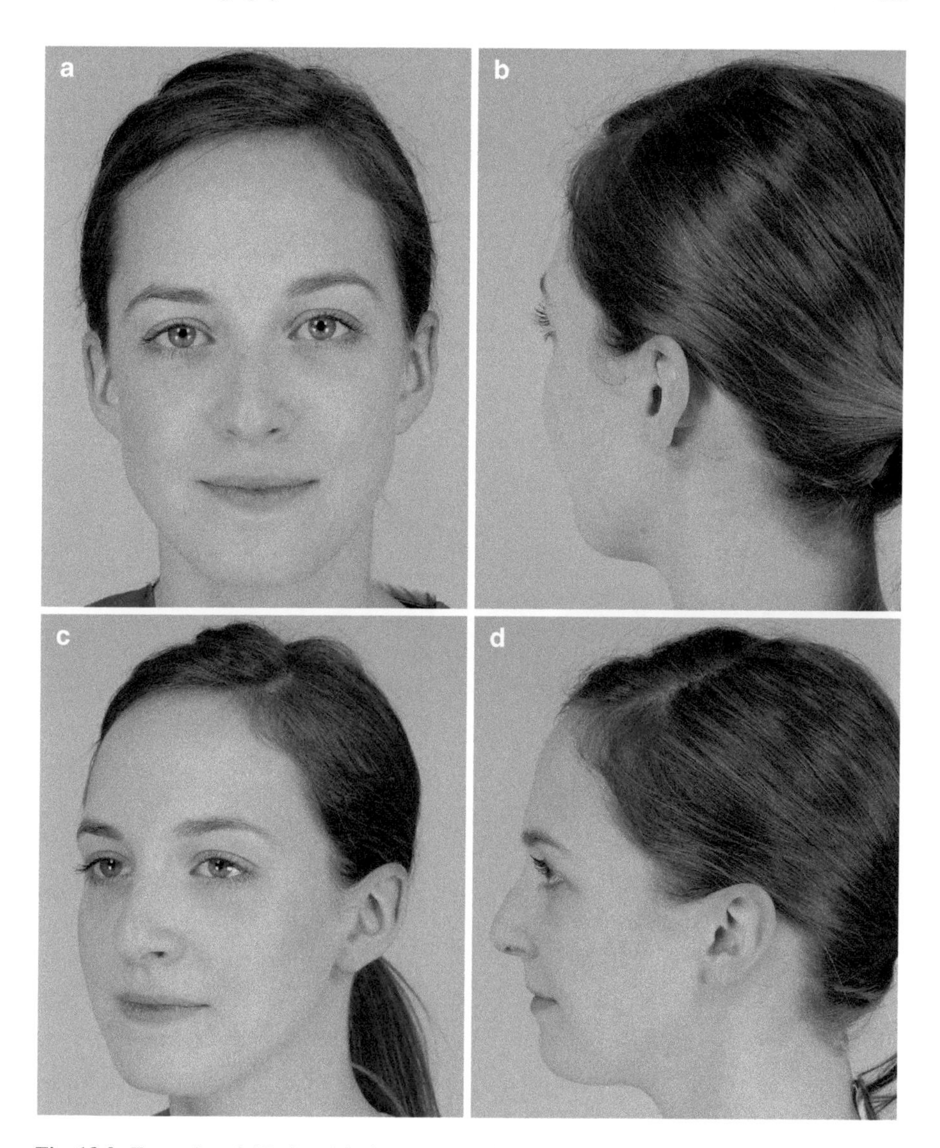

Fig. 18.3 Examples of AP view (**a**), three-quarter views (**b**, **c**), and lateral view (**d**)

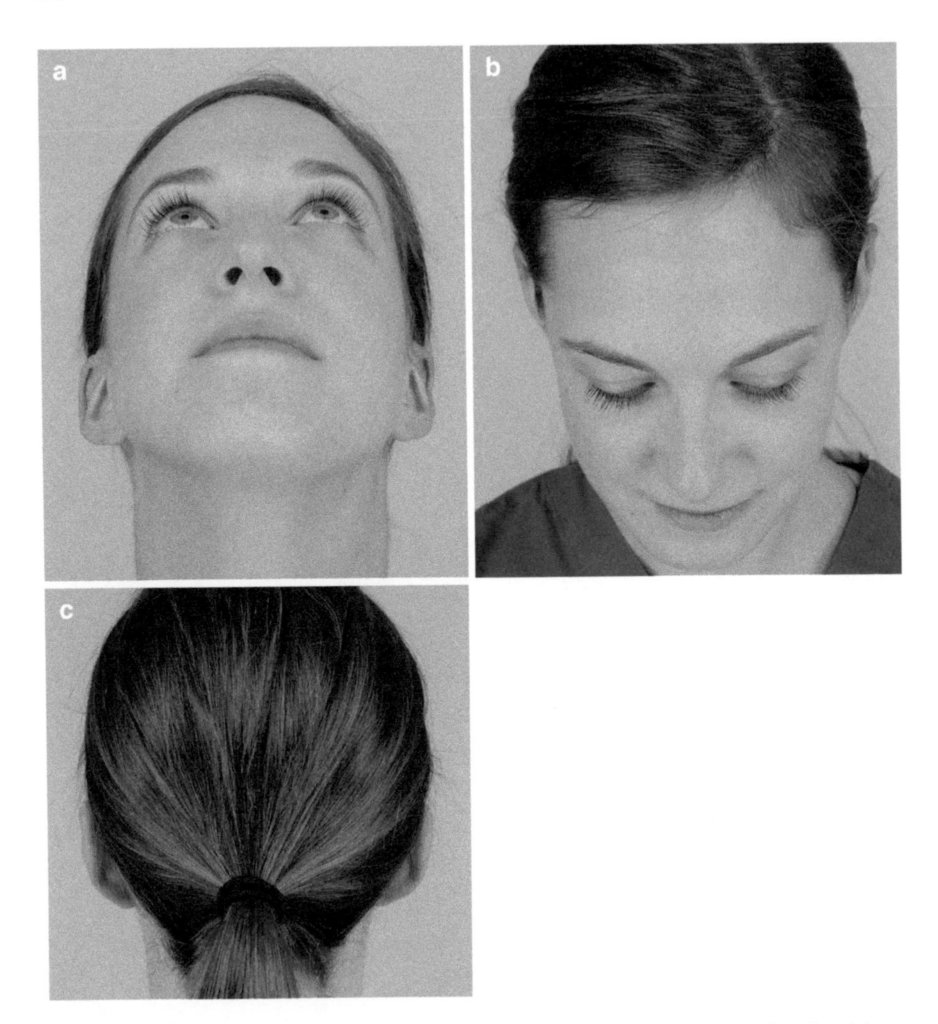

Fig. 18.4 Examples of AP upward and downward gazes (**a**, **b**) and a direct posterior view (**c**)

Bibliography

1. Afrooz PM, Amirlak B. Digital imaging and standardized photography in rhinoplasty. In: Rohrich RJ, Adams WP, Ahmad J, Gunter J, editors. Dallas rhinoplasty: nasal surgery by the masters. 3rd ed. Boca Raton: CRC Press; 2014.
2. Behr AY, Smith HP. Photography for the plastic surgeon. In: Janis JE, editor. Essentials of plastic surgery. 2nd ed. New York: Thieme; 2017.
3. Hoffman WF. Photography in plastic surgery. In: Mathes SJ, editor. Plastic surgery. Philadelphia: WB Saunders Elsevier; 2006.
4. Nahai F, Hoffman WY. Photographic essentials in aesthetic surgery. In: Nahai F, editor. The art of aesthetic surgery: principles and techniques. 2nd ed. Boca Raton: CRC Press; 2011.

Chapter 19
Evolution of Porous Polyethylene Ear Reconstruction

John F. Reinisch

Introduction

The technique of PPE ear reconstruction has evolved over the past three decades to reduce complications, improve the appearance of the reconstructed ear, and minimize the trauma of microtia reconstruction for the patient and their family. Over this time, all aspects of the reconstruction including the implant, soft tissue coverage, instrumentation, postoperative care, anesthesia, and hearing loss have been modified. A review of these changes is helpful because it explains the rationale for the currently used technique and hopefully will shorten a surgeon's learning curve.

Implant

Tad Wellisz, MD, a resident in our USC program, introduced me to PPE made by Porex Surgical, a small division of Porex Corporation (Fairburn, GA, USA), a manufacturer of porous plastics and filters for industry and healthcare. Porex Surgical was acquired by Stryker (Kalamazoo, MI, USA) in 2010. Alexander Berghaus first reported the use of PPE for ear reconstruction in 1983 [1]. Porex Surgical did not make an ear implant but did make a chin implant. To form the base component of the two-piece implant, we divided one end of a chin implant to replicate the two crus. The company made a straight, rain gutter-shaped implant which we heated in hot water and bent into the curved helical component of the implant. Tad eventually joined the USC faculty and worked at Rancho Los Amigos Hospital, which had a large population of burn reconstruction patients. Tad used the PPE implant for ear

J. F. Reinisch (✉)
Keck School of Medicine, University of Souther California, Los Angeles, CA, USA

Craniofacial and Pediatric Plastic Surgery, Cedars Sinai Medical Center, Los Angeles, CA, USA

© Springer Nature Switzerland AG 2019

J. F. Reinisch, Y. Tahiri (eds.), *Modern Microtia Reconstruction*,
https://doi.org/10.1007/978-3-030-16387-7_19

reconstruction in burn patients. He designed a dedicated ear base, which he patented, receiving royalties from Porex.

The helical rim tended to crack, and we persuaded Porex to make a curved rim. The initial iteration looked like a large corkscrew. It was an improvement over the straight rim, but still cracked. In 1995, I designed the currently used helical rim. It maintains a thin outer edge but has a thicker medial edge to increase its strength. To eliminate a conflict of interest when recommending alloplastic ear reconstruction, I never patented the rim design or ever had any financial arrangement related to the sale or design of the PPE ear implant.

Tad and I disagreed about the assembly of the ear implant. He felt that the helical rim should not be attached to the implant base so that the helical rim would be mobile and theoretically would pivot like a bucket handle. He published a series of ear reconstructions in burn patients with the unattached helical rims in 1993 [2]. This was a preliminary report of 24 reconstructions in 18 patients with the longest follow-up being 2 years. Shortly after this publication, Tad left clinical medicine to start Bioplate® (Los Angeles, CA, USA), a cranial plate and screw fixation company.

I felt that the contraction of the overlying soft tissue would pull an unattached rim medially. I started doing polyethylene ear reconstruction in pediatric patients in 1991 and rigidly attaching the rim to the base to produce rim projection. Because many of the burn patients Dr. Wellisz reported in his paper developed exposures and had subsequent removal of their alloplastic ear frameworks (Libby Wilson MD, Rancho Los Amigos Medical Center, personal communication), I waited until 1999 to present our initial results [3].

Ralf Seigert, MD, an otolaryngologist from Recklinghausen, Germany, had a large ear reconstruction practice. Because his cases were limited by the number of in-patient beds his hospital allocated to his service, he became interested in outpatient alloplastic ear reconstruction and visited Los Angeles to watch our method of reconstruction. He later designed a single-piece polyethylene framework for Porex Surgical. Because of the inability to precisely match the size of the opposite ear and the need to stock multiple sizes of both right and left implants, the single piece was never popular.

In 2004, I met Dr. Joseph Roberson, a neurotologist from Palo Alto, California. From him, I learned that the brain is the organ that actually hears. The ear simply converts sound waves to electrical impulses that go to the brain. Dr. Roberson feels that early hearing is important for brain development. Hearing restorations beyond an early critical window is less effective [4]. Although he shared an office and many patients with Dr. Burt Brent, Dr. Roberson became interested in the PPE method of ear reconstruction because, unlike the traditional cartilage method of reconstruction, it was compatible with an early atresia repair, prior to outer ear reconstruction. In 2005 Dr. Roberson started referring me patients that had prior, early atresia repairs.

In order to make room for a canal, I moved the attachment of the helical root superiorly by making the notch in the base higher. The presence of the helical root in the conchal bowl reduced the size of the concha and occasionally would erode into the superior portion of the canal. Eventually, I removed the helical root from below its attachment to the inferior curs (Fig. 19.1a–h).

Dr. Roberson and I began to *c*ombine the aural *a*tresia repair and *m*icrotia (CAM) reconstruction in a single procedure in early 2009. As the number of ear reconstruction patients with either a prior or simultaneous canal repair increased, I began to notice

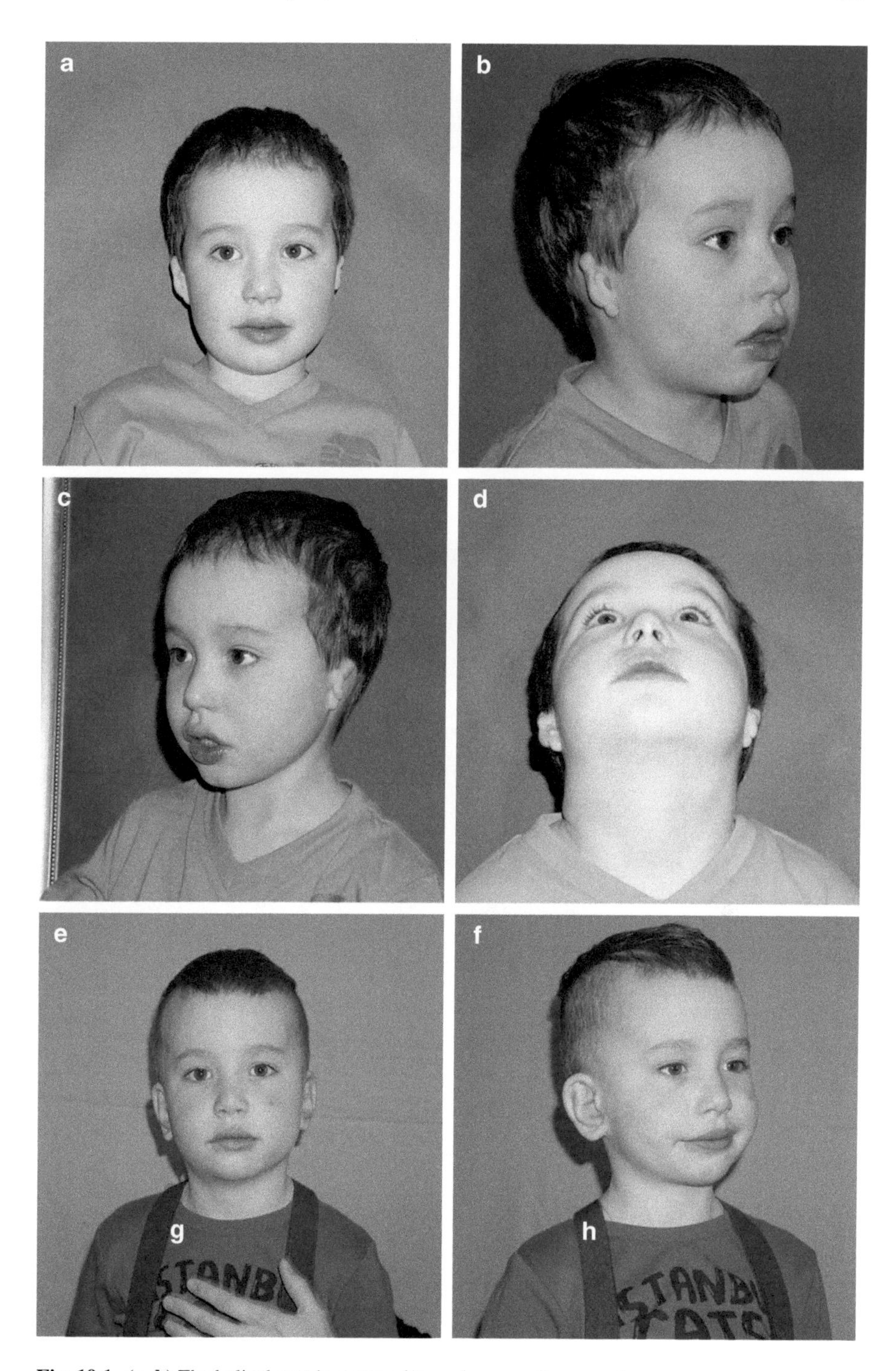

Fig. 19.1 (**a–h**) The helical root is removed to make room for a canal

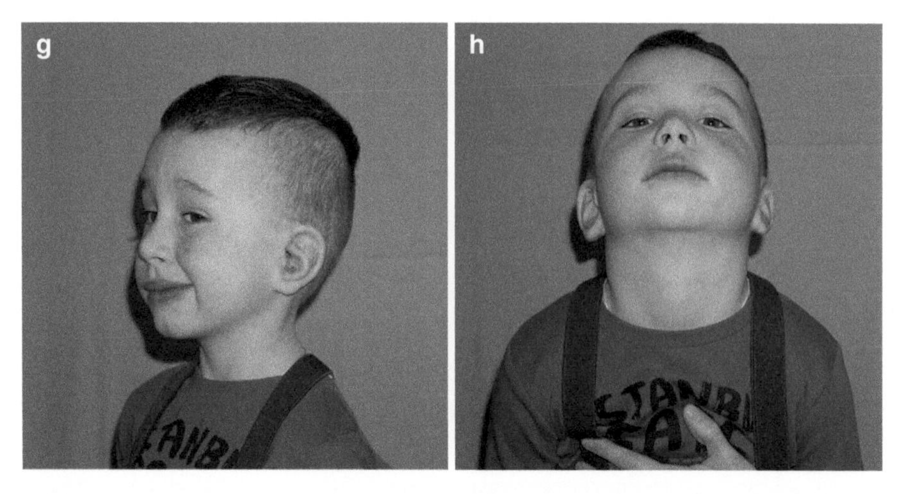

Fig. 19.1 (continued)

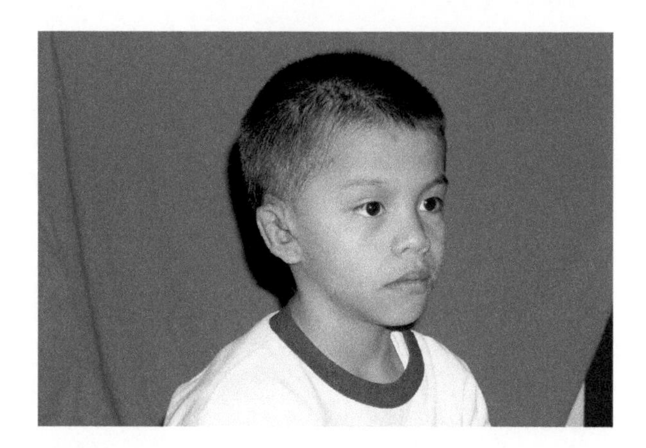

Fig. 19.2 Medial subluxation of the rim: the rim is no longer projected lateral to the superior crus of the base implant

implant fractures with increasing frequency. There were two distinct types of fractures. The first type was the medial subluxation of the rim so that the rim is no longer projected lateral to the superior crus of the base implant (Fig. 19.2). The second type of fracture seen was a disruption of the smooth arch of the helical rim (Fig. 19.3). The fractures were often subtle and only noticed on late follow-up exam. These fractures did not result in collapse of the framework or implant exposures, but they did cause a loss of ear definition or shape.

In late 2011, I calculated the 5-year postoperative implant fracture rate. Implant fractures occurred in 15% of our CAM patients, 9% of patients with a prior atresia repair, and 3% of patients without a canal reconstruction. I attributed the greater fracture rate in canal patients to the reduced mobility of the implant when an atresia repair was present, causing the implant to absorb more of an impact if struck.

To minimize the implant fractures, I incorporated two modifications when assembling the implant. I stopped thinning the thickness of the superior crus and began to add a strut between the superior crus and lateral helical rim (Fig. 19.4). These changes dramatically reduced the implant fractures rate with only three fractures seen in the last 700 cases.

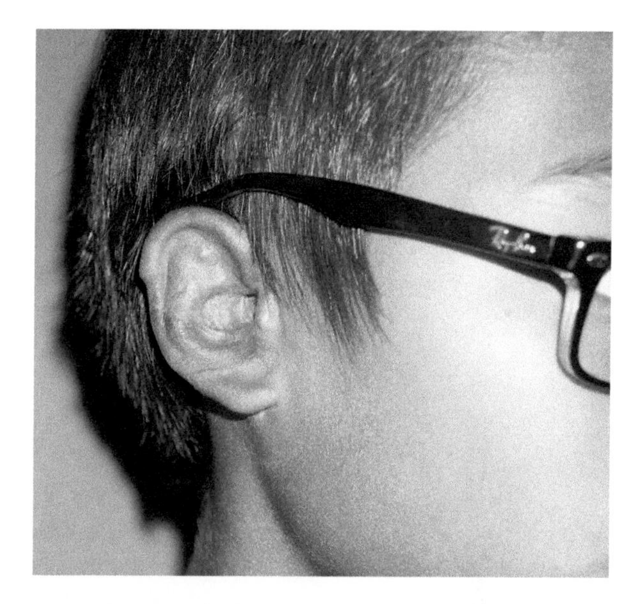

Fig. 19.3 Helical rim fracture causing disruption of the smooth arch of the helical rim

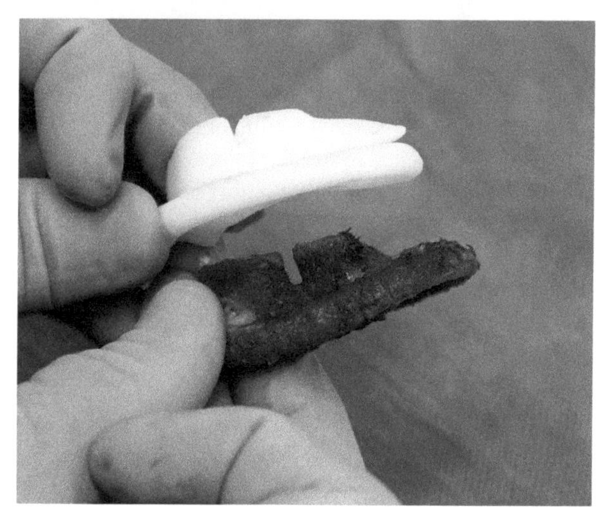

Fig. 19.4 Modification done to the implant to decrease the risk of fracture

Soft Tissue Coverage

At the beginning of our experience with alloplastic ear reconstructions, we placed the majority of the PPE implant framework under the existing mastoid skin. The upper, protruding portion of the implant was covered by transposing a relatively small, inferiorly based, superficial temporal parietal fascia (STPF) flap. These flaps were randomly based and were covered with a full-thickness skin graft. The lobule was transposed and inset at a subsequent stage. Looking at our first 25 ear reconstructions, we found that there were 11 implant exposures within the first 3 years of reconstruction. The exposures occurred over the lower part of the implant, not over the portion of the implant covered by the STPF and skin graft. When we began to

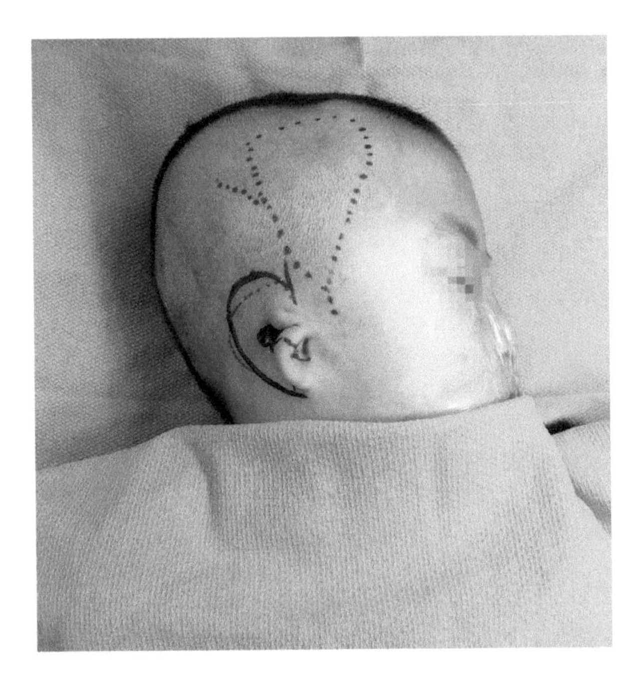

Fig. 19.5 The distal anterior branch of the STA arches in a posterior direction and runs transversely to form a distal arcade. The transverse portion of the branch is found about 12.0 cm superior to the canal or where the canal should be

cover the entire ear implant with a much larger fascia flap in 1995, we saw a dramatic reduction in the rate of implant exposures.

The larger fascia flap needed to cover the entire implant required the incorporation of the superficial temporal artery (STA) to provide sufficient distal circulation. The inferior portion of the implant was covered by the most distal part of the STPF. The occasional exposure in this area was completely eliminated when we realized that the distal anterior branch of the STA arches in a posterior direction and runs transversely to form a distal arcade. The transverse portion of the branch is found about 12.0 cm superior to the canal or where the canal should be (Fig. 19.5). The upper extent of our scalp elevation must be at least a centimeter more cephalic to this important landmark. By harvesting a flap of sufficient length to incorporate the distal transverse portion of the anterior branch of the STA, one can eliminate the occasional distal ischemia, which can lead to an inferior exposure.

Scalp Incisions

The scalp incision used to harvest the STPF flap has evolved with time. The original vertically oriented "Y" incision left noticeable alopecia in the long vertical component of the scar because the adjacent scalp hair grew parallel to the scar, not across it. We converted our access incision to a large zigzag to better conceal the scar as the vertically growing hair could better cross the oblique incisions. We noted that the scalp incisions reduced the blood supply to the temporal parietal scalp so that the pressure from a protective Glasscock® cup dressing (Grace Medical, Memphis,

TN, USA) or from a bone conduction hearing aid would occasionally cause a small area of alopecia. As we became more comfortable with elevation of the STPF from beneath the scalp, we converted our approach to a single transverse scalp incision. The incision was placed approximately 10 cm above the position of where the ear canal should be. The scalp was then elevated from the surface of the STPF with a Colorado tip using a blended cautery setting. Care was taken to avoid injury to the STA and its more distal anterior and main branches. The transverse incision was placed where the scalp hair would run perpendicular to the incision to minimize its visibility. Through the transverse incision, the scalp could be dissected caudally to connect with the dissection from below. Through the incision one could then extend the scalp elevation 3.0–4.0 cm in a more cephalic direction to make the division of the distal STPF easier. With experience, the length of the transverse incision could be reduced. Peter Wang, one of our craniofacial fellows, published a series of STPF elevations made through a small distal incision using an endoscope [5]. Tae Ho Kim, another former fellow, was able to divide the distal flap without a cephalic transverse incision by extending transverse scalp incisions anterior and posterior to the ear more inferiorly to make the distal exposure easier. In 2007, both my former associate, Dr. Sheryl Lewin, and I started to raise the STPF flap through an incision limited to the outline of the ear without addition scalp incisions.

Skin Grafts

Because the PPE implant projects when covered with a large STPF flap, one must cover both the lateral and medial surfaces of the reconstructed ear. The lateral skin must match the color of the lobe and adjacent cheek.

In the usual unilateral microtia patients, the skin of both the microtia ear and adjacent non-hair-bearing mastoid has a good color match. Since there will not be a sufficient amount of color-matched skin to provide a uniform color to the lateral surface of the reconstructed ear, one will need additional skin for the lateral and medial aspect of the reconstructed ear.

Initially, we harvested a large amount of skin from behind the opposite ear, since the skin from the posterior surface of the opposite ear has a similar thickness and color as the anterior aspect of the ear. We then used a lower abdominal skin graft to cover the posterior surface of the reconstructed ear and replace the donor skin from the opposite ear. While the lower abdominal skin healed with a very nice scar, the post-auricular skin on both the reconstructed and donor ear often would grow hair after puberty. Additionally, the opposite donor ear would occasionally become deformed from the contracted post-auricular skin graft.

Now, we routinely use the skin from both the microtia ear and adjacent non-hair-bearing mastoid as well as a FTSG from the posterior aspect of the contralateral ear (because of this similar thickness and color) to cover the anterior and lateral aspect of the reconstructed ear. The medial or posterior surface of the reconstructed ear is covered with the thicker, less matched skin of the abdomen or groin if its junction is hidden behind the helical rim.

In bilateral microtia, there is no available opposite post-auricular skin. We tried using the ipsilateral post-auricular non-hair-bearing skin along with the adjacent hair-bearing scalp skin. We aggressively defatted the scalp to remove the hair follicles. Occasionally, this was successful, but usually the scalp skin still grew hair and left a visible, abnormal post-auricular hairline.

Split thickness grafts (STSG) harvested from the scalp were used for several years. The donor site was hidden beneath the scalp hair, and reasonable results were often obtained especially after using steroid ointment postoperatively to minimize contracture of the fascia beneath the STSGs. Unfortunately the color match of the STSGs was not ideal and not infrequently the epithelium lining the hair shafts would form inclusion cysts in the skin grafts.

Now for bilateral microtia patients, where there is no available opposite ear skin, we prefer to use of FTSG from the medial upper arm to cover the lateral aspect of the reconstructed ear. The donor site requires careful closure and prolonged postoperative taping to minimize postoperative scar widening. If parents object to having a medial arm scar, we will use a scalp STSG. I have not used neck or supraclavicular skin in children.

Because of the risk of hair growth after puberty, we have abandoned the use of the lower midline abdominal skin as a source of full-thickness skin for the posterior aspect of the ear. We currently use a FTSG from the groin, taking the ellipse more laterally in non-Asian children, who are more likely to have a larger escutcheon.

Concha and Faux Canal

The features that define an excellent reconstructed ear are a thin, defined helical rim, good projection that matches the normal ear, and a deep concha bowl to give the appearance of a canal. The helical rim and ear projection can be achieved with the PPE ear implant. The appearance of a large concha bowl, ear canal, and tragus is not easily achieved.

The base component of the ear implant comes with a tragus extension. I almost never use it because it requires coverage with fascia like the rest of the implant. Draping the STPF flap over the implant, concha, and tragus requires a very wide flap. The additional tissue in the bowl and the contraction of the overlying skin minimize the chance for a deep bowl when healed. Therefore, our early ear reconstructions were done in two stages. The implant was placed and covered with the fascia and skin grafts in the first stage. The second stage addressed the bowl and tragus. The loss of ear projection often seen in our early ears could also be improved at the second stage with the release of the sulcus and addition of more skin.

At the second stage, the tragus was constructed using a “whale’s tail” design. Two vertically oriented pre-auricular flaps were elevated and used for the medial tragus lining. The cheek was advanced posteriorly to close the pre-auricular donor sites and provide lateral tragal lining. Tragal support was provided by a thin, curved PPE lower eyelid implant. These implants would occasionally become infected and had to be removed. The creation a tragus at the first stage involves the use of the microtic cartilage remnant as a cartilage graft for tragal support.

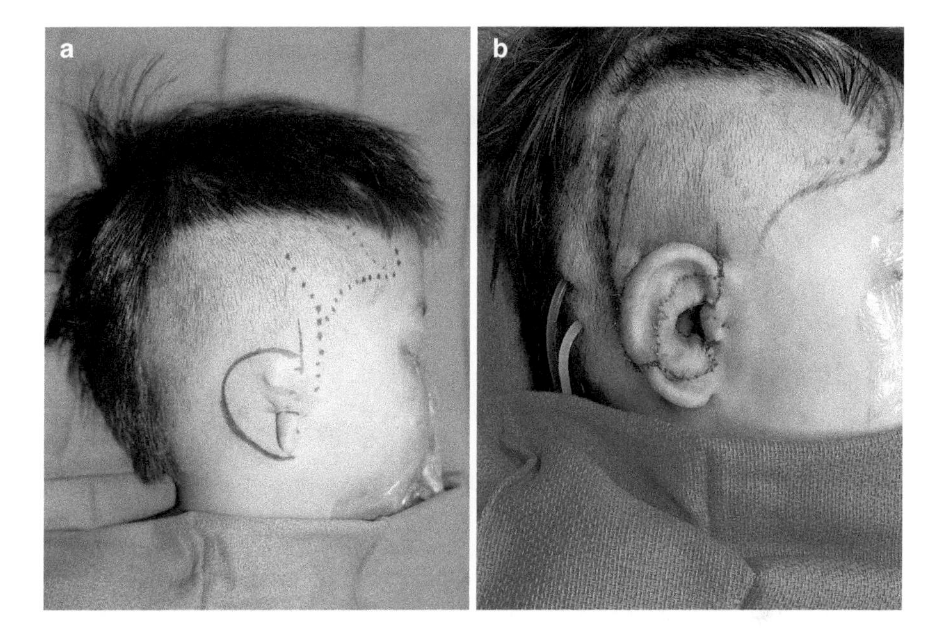

Fig. 19.6 (**a**, **b**) The size and depth of the bowl are improved by removal all of the cartilage remnant and the soft tissue. The tragus is created by placing a piece of the previously harvested microtic cartilage under an anterior base skin flap and sutured in place with a mattress 6-0 chromic catgut suture

To improve the size and definition of the concha and allow room for the increasingly frequent ear canal, the attachment of the helical root was repositioned superiorly from the notch provided in the implant base. With the increasing number of atresia repairs in our patients, we eventually amputated the helical rim completely. This provided more room for the atresia repair and allowed a large concha.

In the patient without a prior atresia repair, tragal reconstruction is now done at the initial surgery by folding a horizontally oriented, anteriorly based mastoid skin flap medially. A portion of the resected cartilage remnant is placed as a graft between the tragal flaps and secured with temporary 6-0 mattress suture for support (Fig. 19.6a, b).

Equipment

In most children the course of the STA can be either visualized or palpated through their relatively thin scalp. The use of a Doppler to outline the position of the STA is only helpful in adults and the rare child with weak pulsations. Early in the evolution of the technique, when the STPF fascia was harvested through an open scalp incision, no special equipment or instrumentation was needed.

Elevation of the scalp from the surface of the STPF fascia is facilitated by dissection with electrocautery which is set to a low blend of cutting and coagulation currents. Different lengths and shapes of Colorado needle tips are helpful. Once I

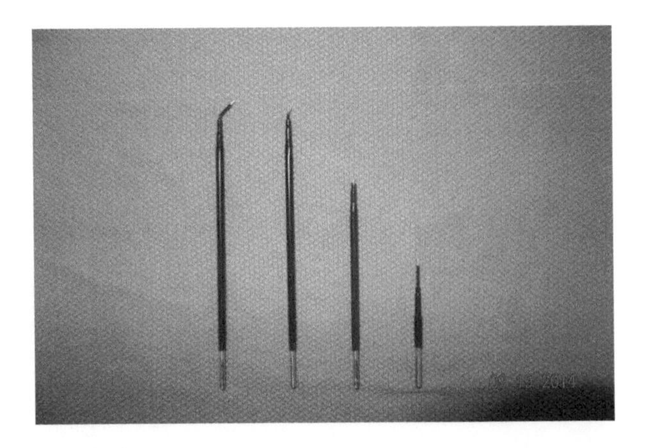

Fig. 19.7 Various lengths of Colorado needle tips are needed

began to limit the scalp access incision, first to an upper transverse and later to only the lower ear incision, a better lighting source became important. I used several lighted retractors but found a light battery powered headlight to be best. Using it with a black Tessier, soft tissue retractor eliminated the need for an extra fiber-optic cord and an external light source. To dissect the scalp, I now use a short straight electrocautery needle (Colorado® N1038, Stryker, Kalmazoo, MI, USA) and then switch to a longer needle with a short-angled tip (Colorado® E1134, Stryker, Kalamazoo, MI, USA) once the pocket is more developed (Fig. 19.7). A McAndrews suction tip helps to remove smoke and can act as a retractor to provide tension when cutting tissue. A bulb saline irrigation of the scalp and fascia helps to counteract the drying effect of the increased airflow caused by the suction.

The distal end of the STPF flap is more robust if one includes the transverse portion of the distal anterior branch of the STA. It is found around 12.0 cm above the external auditory canal or where the canal should be. The realization that the distal anterior branch runs in a posterior direction to form a distal vascular arcade was important in eliminating exposures of the inferior portion of the implant. The division of a sufficiently long flap to incorporate the distal arcade is facilitated by using a #22 urethral sound (Jarit® 475/557, Integra Life Sciences, Plainsboro, NJ, USA) to strip the upper scalp from the periosteum. One can then divide the sub-galeal fascia and galea from inside out beyond the area of scalp elevation and connect the incision to the more proximal scalp dissection to increase the length of the flap. A long right-angled clamp is helpful to dissect the STPF flap from the deep temporal fascia.

Finally, in order to see at the correct angle, it is helpful to use a hydraulic sitting stool which allows fine up and down movements.

Anesthesia

Our anesthesia protocol also has evolved along with our surgery technique. Ear reconstruction was initially done as an inpatient procedure with discharge 1–2 days following surgery. The lack of rib cartilage harvest and the infiltration of bupivacaine into the scalp drain and the FTSG donor sites at the end of the procedure reduced postoperative discomfort to the point that hospitalization was unnecessary. With the exception of a handful of cases, all reconstructions have been done as an outpatient procedure since May 1996.

With the proper selection and timing of anesthetic agents, anesthesiologists familiar with the procedure (see Chap. 17) allow a shorter recovery room stay despite the long operative time. A smooth, comfortable recovery reassures anxious patients and minimized postoperative oozing and swelling for better postoperative healing.

The length of the procedure makes careful positioning and padding critical to prevent pressure points and postoperative neck stiffness. With teenagers and adults, prolonged elbow extension during surgery results in a surprising degree of postoperative elbow discomfort. This joint discomfort is completely eliminated when the elbows are kept in slight flexion during surgery. It is interesting that children and adolescents do not experience elbow pain when the joint is kept in extension.

Draping of the patient has evolved. Initially, we used a head drape, but it was difficult to keep the drape in place during a long procedure, especially when the head was rotated back and forth. Stapling of the drapes helped, but prepping the entire undraped head made surgery easier. Sealing the eyes, nose, and mouth with an adherent transparent film dressing before prepping protects the eyes, provides better sterility, and stabilizes the endotracheal tube. It is important to make sure that the tube does not put pressure on the lower lip (Fig. 19.8a, b).

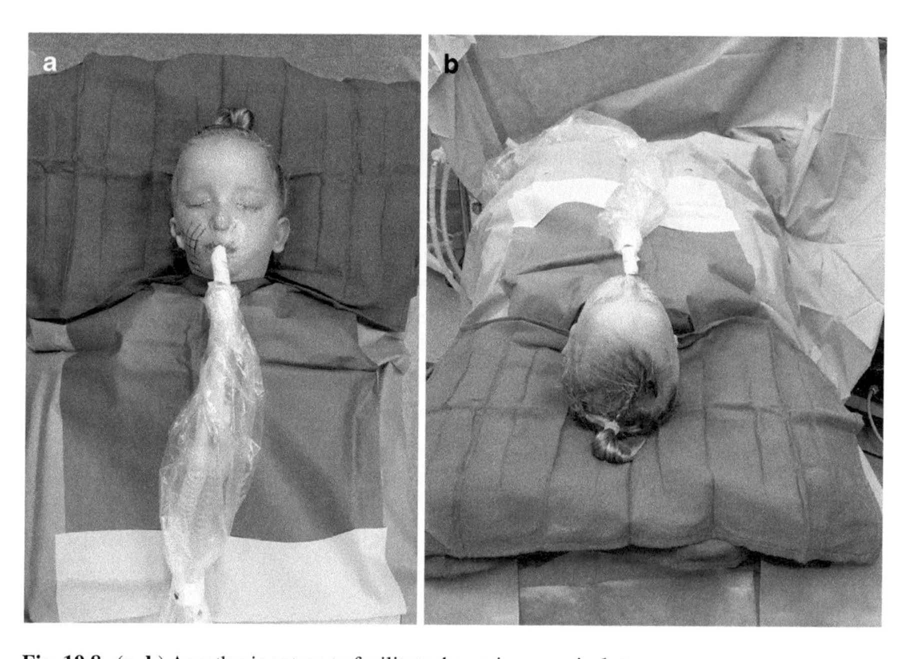

Fig. 19.8 (**a**, **b**) Anesthesia set up to facilitate the various surgical steps

The need to harvest post-auricular skin from the opposite ear requires head turning during surgery. With the endotracheal tube under the drape, occasional inadvertent extubation from traction on the endotracheal tube occurred. Since we began suturing the endotracheal tube to the upper central gingiva and placing the tubing in a sterile camera sleeve above the drapes, we have not had any extubations. The sterile tubing also gives us more flexible access to the umbilicus for harvesting abdominal fat for correction of soft tissue cheek hypoplasia.

Hearing Restoration

Since the great majority of microtia patients usually have a normal contralateral ear with adequate hearing for speech and language acquisition, it is common for both surgeons and parents to ignore the functional issues of the conductive hearing loss that accompanies unilateral microtia. Like most plastic surgeons, I only focused on the external ear early in my career. My only experience with early atresia repairs were in older bilateral microtia patients who had prior atresia repairs for hearing. Because of the local scarring from their prior surgery, they were denied the standard cartilage ear reconstruction. They were candidates for reconstruction using TPF coverage as it was unaffected by the prior surgery. I reconstructed a number of these patients with alloplastic frameworks. Some of my ear reconstructed patients decided to have atresia repairs years after alloplastic ear reconstruction. The otologists performing the canalplasty surgery were unfamiliar with alloplastic frameworks. Many of these patients returned to me with implant fractures when the implant was drilled to make room for the canal or became exposed because of inadequate soft tissue coverage lining the canal.

In 2005, I started collaborating with Dr. Joseph Roberson, an otologist in Palo Alto, California. He was interested in our methods of ear reconstruction because it permitted an early atresia repair before the ear reconstruction. As a plastic surgeon with only a superficial understanding of hearing, our association gave me a better understanding of the importance of binaural hearing. I learned that the ear does not actually hear. It is a converter of sound waves to electrical impulses which are then interpreted by the brain as sound. The brain not only hears sound but does the auditory processing necessary for sound localization, better hearing in noisy environments, and hearing low volumes by binaural summation. Most surgeons are aware of the importance of early visual stimulation for the development of the visual cortex and the avoidance of amblyopia. Amblyaudia is a term used to describe persistent hearing difficulty experienced by individuals with a history of asymmetric hearing loss during a critical early window of brain development. The concept of amblyaudia is not well known, but clearly exists as late restoration of hearing beyond an early period of brain plasticity is less able to provide the brain with auditory processing abilities [6].

Parents see little difference between their unilateral microtia children and their normal siblings in terms of early development and speech and language acquisition. As children become older and experience more complex social, educational, and language situations, the effect of unilateral conductive hearing loss becomes more evident.

Initially, our collaboration consisted of ear reconstruction after a prior aural atresia repair in patients who had good middle ear anatomy as determined by CT scan and whose parents wanted to improve their conductive hearing loss. In January 2008, we started to combine the atresia repair and ear reconstruction in a single surgery: the CAM procedure or combined atresia microtia. This procedure is especially popular with families whose children have bilateral microtia because two combined procedures can restore both their hearing and cosmetic appearance before starting school.

Dressing and Postoperative Care

Initially we covered the reconstructed ear with a cup dressing for postoperative protection. We have never used a bolster dressing on the skin grafts for fear of compromising the blood flow of the underlying fascia flap. We placed an unfolded gauze dressing between the ear and cup to apply minimal pressure and absorb drainage. We used two bulb suction drains, one beneath the scalp and the second beneath the ear framework. The drains were removed at 1 week, and the cup dressing was removed and replaced. The ear was very swollen, and the grafts were dark when observed at 1 week. It could look as if there was a hematoma under the fascia. The swelling slowly resolved and the color improved in the ensuing months.

In 2006, I started to cover the reconstructed ear with silicone putty used for making hearing aid molds (A-Zoft by Oticon, Kongebakken, Denmark). The protective ear cup was placed over the silicone splint. The silicone mold reduced the postoperative swelling. When the ear cup and mold were removed at 1 week, it was difficult to determine the viability of the underlying skin and fascia because of the normal early discoloration of the skin grafts. We would see some further swelling of the reconstructed ear after the mold was removed.

In 2011, I stopped using the plastic ear cup and simply sutured the silicone mold to the scalp with 2-0 Prolene® (Ethicon, Somerville, NJ, USA) mattress sutures tied over cottonoid pledgets to prevent suture marks (see Chap. 6). Once the mold was sutured in place, I placed plain bupivacaine in the scalp drain and removed the drains in the operating room at the end of the procedure. Leaving the mold on for 2 weeks allowed the grafts to take and minimize the postoperative swelling once the mold was removed.

The initial projection of the ear at the end of the procedure often was not maintained in the months following surgery. I attributed the loss of projection to both the contracture of the post-auricular skin grafts and pressure on the ear while sleeping. To compensate we either had to increase the initial projection or add a second surgery to add skin to the contracted sulcus. For the last 8 years, I have used a silicone mold at night and found that the loss of projection could be eliminated when the mold was used for the first 4 months after surgery. Parents need to make a new splint several times during the 4 months as swelling diminished over time.

Current Technique

The current technique of alloplastic ear reconstruction has evolved over time to reduce complications, improve outcomes, and minimize the trauma of having reconstructive surgery for the patient and family. Reconstruction of the external ear is a cosmetic procedure. Patients and their families have the expectation that the new ear will closely match the opposite ear in size, shape, and projection. For the surgeon beginning alloplastic reconstruction, the hope is for survival of the ear without complications. With more experience and confidence, the surgeon's efforts are directed to subtle refinements to give their patients more of what they are expecting. A surgeon's critical assessment of his or her results and the continuous striving for improvement lead to more satisfactory outcomes. I hope that understanding the evolution of our technique will shorten one's journey and help improve ear reconstruction for both the patient and surgeon.

References

1. Berghaus A, Axhausen M, Handrock M. Porous synthetic materials in external ear reconstruction. Laryngol Rhinol Otol. 1983;62:320–7.
2. Wellisz T. Reconstruction of the burned external ear using a medpor porous polyethylene pivoting helix framework. Plast Reconstr Surg. 1993;91:811.
3. Reinisch J. AAPS 1999, Colorado Springs, CO.
4. Jensen D, Grames L, Lieu J. Effects of aural atresia on speech development and learning: retrospective analysis from a multidisciplinary craniofacial clinic. JAMA Otolaryngol Head Neck Surg. 2013;139(8):797–802.
5. Helling E, Okoro S, Kim G, Wang P. Endoscope-assisted temporoparietal fascia harvest for auricular reconstruction. Plast Reconstr Surg. 2008;121(5):1598–605.
6. Kaplan AB, Kozin ED, Remenschneider A, Eftekhari K, Jung DH, Polley DB, et al. Amblyaudia. Review of pathophysiology, clinical presentation, and treatment of a new diagnosis. Otolaryngol Head Neck Surg. 2016;154(2):247–55.

Index

© Springer Nature Switzerland AG 2019
J. F. Reinisch, Y. Tahiri (eds.), *Modern Microtia Reconstruction*,
https://doi.org/10.1007/978-3-030-16387-7

B

R

S

T

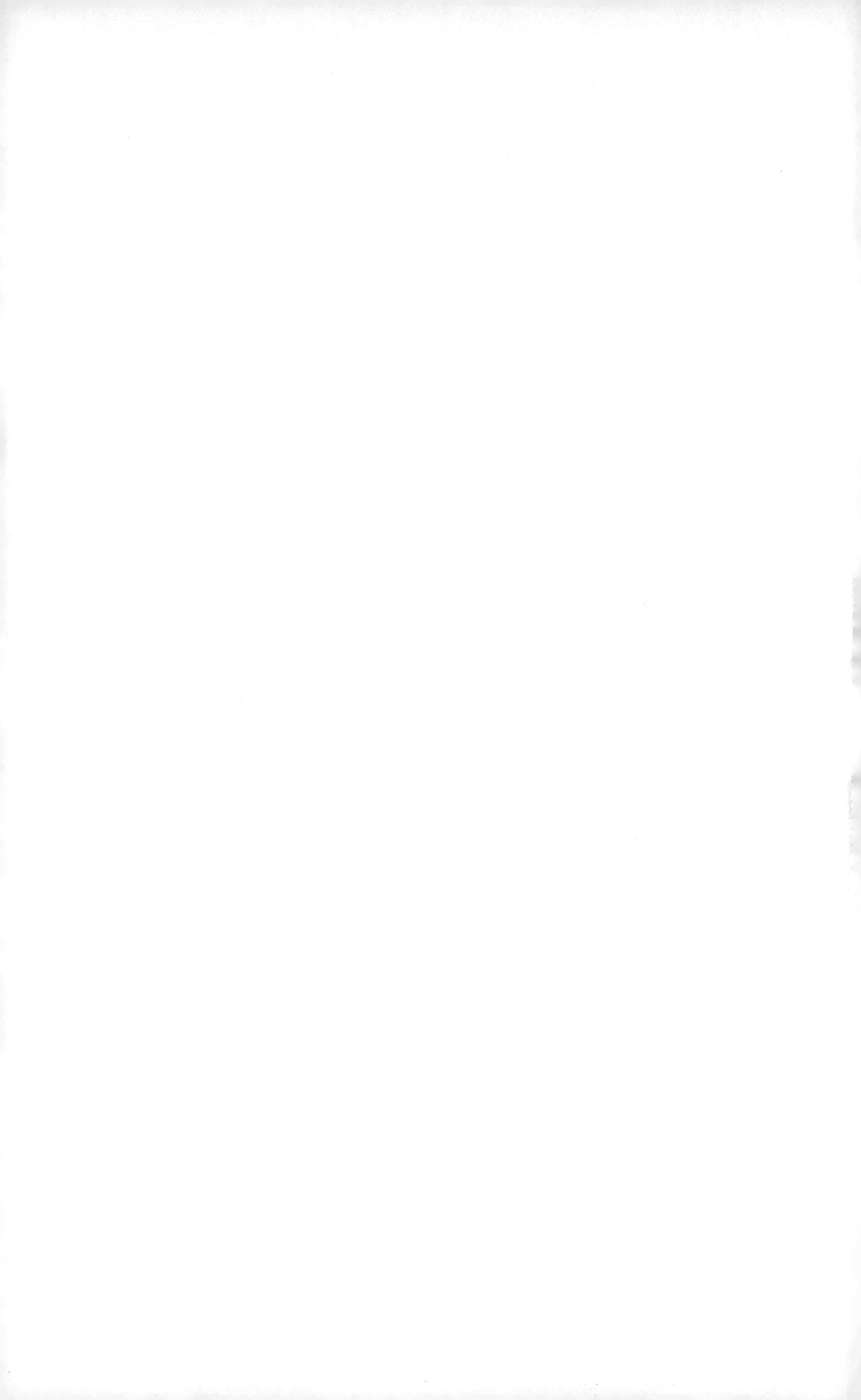

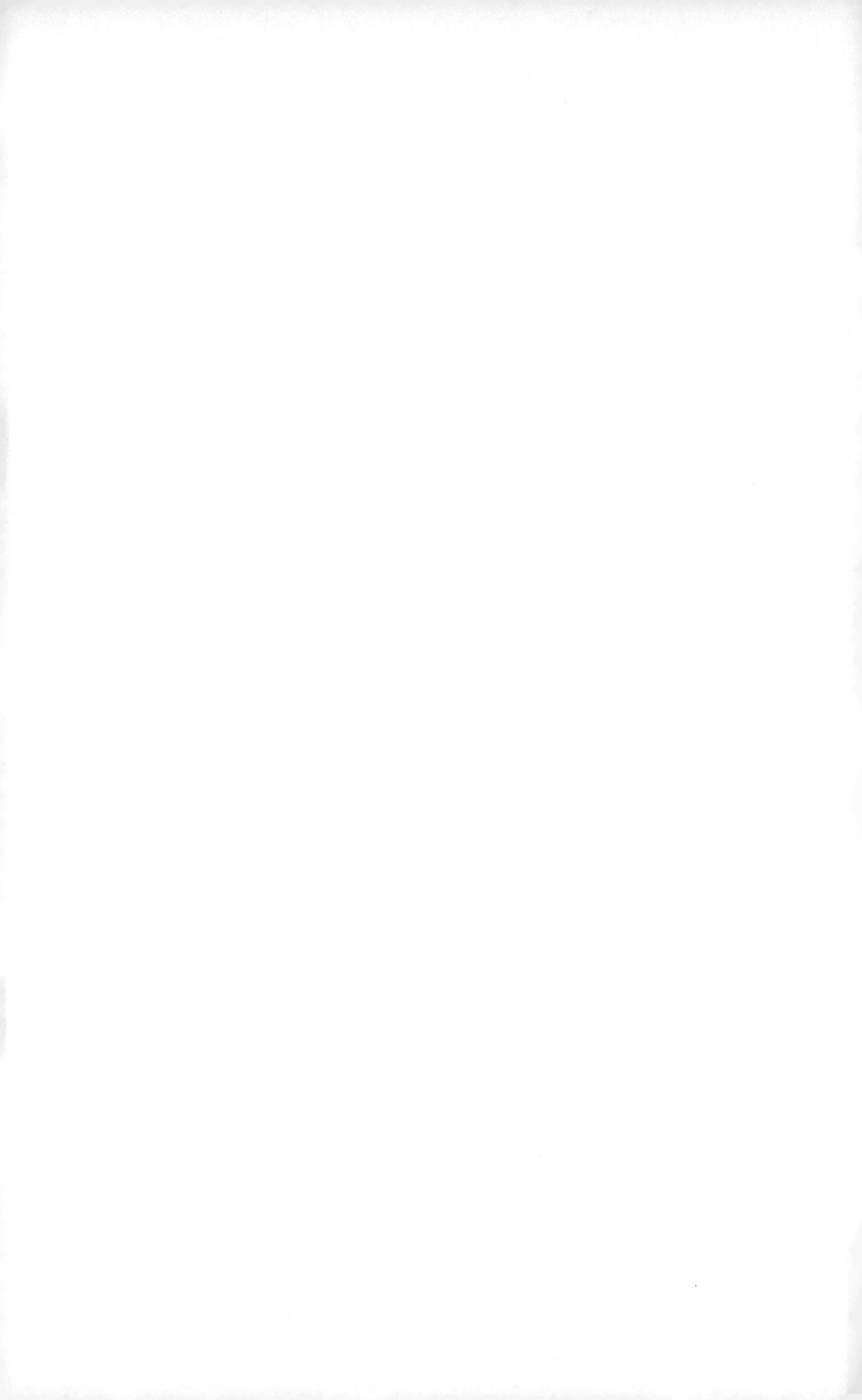